MW01485502

For Paula,

May you & your
family always be safe!

Lots of love!

SECURITY FOR WOMEN

The Evolution of Empowerment

Laura Clark
William E. Algaier

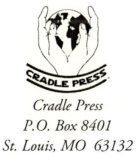

Cradle Press
P.O. Box 8401
St. Louis, MO 63132

SECURITY FOR WOMEN
The Evolution of Empowerment
Copyright © Laura Clark and William E. Algaier, 2006
All rights reserved.

No part of this book may be reproduced, stored in a retrieval system, or transmitted by any means without written permission of the authors and publisher.

ISBN: 978-0-9789499-0-7

Library of Congress Control Number: 2006908150

Cover Design by Jim Mosley and book layout by Scott Eagle at Outflow Media
www.outflowmedia.us

This book is printed on acid-free paper.

Disclaimer

This book and all information contained herein is intended for educational and entertainment purposes only, therefore the authors, editors, and publishers of this work are not responsible for the use or misuse of any information contained herein or any consequence (whether foreseen or reasonably foreseeable) of said use or misuse. This book is not to be used as a manual or substitute for relevant training and the authors, editors, and publishers expressly state that this book is not intended or otherwise considered to be a substitute for applicable training in self-defense, martial arts, evasive driving, or personal protection. The authors, editors, and publishers hereby disclaim all responsibility and liability for any loss or harm suffered or caused by the use of any technique, content, or information contained herein (whether applied correctly or incorrectly) and expressly reiterates that any such risk, responsibility, and liability for the use or misuse of any content within this book is expressly assumed and consented to by the reader or user of said content.

This book contains both true and fictitious characters and stories. All names of individuals and characters within this book have been altered in order to protect the privacy and identity of the individuals involved.

ABOUT THE COVER

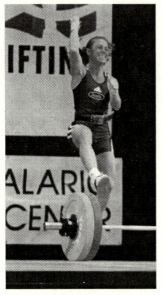

Bruce Klemens Photo

The inspiration for our cover design began with this photograph of Tara Nott. Tara won the gold medal in the 2000 Olympics in Sydney, Australia for women's weightlifting. This photo was taken when Tara made the Olympics, an exhilarating moment after years of training, trials, and injuries. What we love about the photo is Tara's triumphant expression. She embodies the feeling of empowerment and achievement we hope to convey to our readers regarding their ability to participate in strengthening their personal security practices and preventing violence.

When we spoke with Tara about using the photo, she was eager to contribute to helping women learn to be safe. We spoke of the irony that even though at one time, pound for pound, she was one of the strongest women in the world, she would have been hard pressed to defend herself against a male attacker. Tara immediately registered how important it is for women to learn about prevention against violence, as physical strength will only take us so far. For Tara, physical strength is where she found her power and triumph. We hope all women will feel that same triumphant jump in their lives once they learn to protect themselves.

For my parents,
who kept me safe and taught me
that I am worth protecting.

(Laura Clark)

I dedicate this book to all women.
I pray the ideas and techniques bring you
happiness, peace, and security.

(William E. Algaier)

CONTENTS

PART ONE
PREVENTION TECHNIQUES

PART TWO
INTEGRATION: PREVENTING,
DEFENDING, AND SURVIVING

FORWARD

A REALLY BIG IDEA

Hidden inside me
this woman I see
self-contained and idealized
her own hybrid
twenty-first century species
love and power welded
using her hands for grace

Centuries of women have lived and died before you, the currents of their lives swiftly carrying you forward. Yet the steady undercurrent of their fear continues into your present day reality. Were they alive today, they would wonder as you might: "*Should I carry mace? Will I be stalked? Should I own a gun? Could I defend myself against a rapist? Am I safe at home alone? Will my husband beat me? Will my child go missing? Will a woman I know be murdered?*"

It is time we transform our approach to the violence against us and pass on a safer way of living to the generations of women to come. This book is that big idea set in motion. If you have arrived to read this sentence, you are ready to transform your personal security practice. Trust in that and that alone. You are meant to receive this information. Welcome to your own evolution. Now you have more.

What you will learn and assimilate just by virtue of the act of reading this entire book is a life changing approach to personal security and a safer way of living. We are offering you the promise of becoming empowered with prevention methods which will exponentially improve your odds of avoiding being victimized by predators. Because this book is a comprehensive guide, it is admittedly over the top, meaning we intentionally provide you with an excess of information. We do so in an attempt to correct the disparity between the gross amount of violence against women and their lack of ability to protect themselves. It is not our desire to make you paranoid every second of your life. It *is* our desire to make you empowered with prevention.

Your opportunity to transform your personal security practice is dependent upon your commitment to reading all of the information provided, as we take you through a progressive approach that builds with each chapter. Do not doubt in your ability to grasp the information in this book. Survival is instinctive. Instinct is instant. The real question boils down to this: Would you prefer to remain a potential victim or are you willing to take responsibility for your own security? Stated another way: Are you willing to learn to rescue yourself or would you rather continue to entrust your personal security to others? It should be evident to you by now that our criminal justice system and law enforcement are unable to protect many women from becoming victims of violent crimes. The reasons for this are varied and complex, but the hard truth you must accept is that you are largely on your own against predators. This truth combined with the preponderance of stories in the news about women whose lives have been shattered or have ended prematurely at the hands of predators should be enough for you to say: *"Enough! I need to take charge of my own security."*

We can relate to how over-burdened your life may be, for that is the twenty-first century malaise from which we all suffer. This is why we created a *prevention oriented* book that takes into account your need for legal, affordable, easy methods of staying safe that will benefit you for the rest of your life without taking up too much of your valuable time or requiring you to become an expert in self-defense. Although we discuss crime deterrence and attack survival, our primary objective is to teach you how to *avoid becoming a victim* in the first place. We will accomplish this by exposing you to crime prevention methods about which you have very likely never been informed. We call our unique methodology "getting SASD™" (rhymes with jazzed). SA stands for Situational Awareness. SD stands for Surveillance Detection.

The first part of our methodology, situational awareness, involves learning an easy, daily practice for enhancing your awareness that will impact your ability to detect danger early on and take action to avoid it. When you combine situational awareness with the second half of our methodology, surveillance detection, you will exponentially increase your ability to identify threats, detect early warning signals, avoid danger, and outsmart predators.

Surveillance detection is a technique that has been kept quietly under wraps and has been used rather selectively for preventing terrorist and criminal attacks against heads of state, government facilities, diplomats, politicians, and wealthy corporate executives. Now you can use surveillance detection (SD) to undermine any predator intent on targeting you. In a nutshell, the premise behind surveillance detection is that few attacks are impulsive; most criminals plan their deviant acts and part of their planning phase involves conducting surveillance on their targets. If you are a woman who is being targeted by a predator, that predator will study you. He (or she) must collect information on you in order to attack you successfully. Surveillance detection is a method by which you can discreetly see your predator as he is out there collecting information on you and then use the information you collect against him in order to prevent being attacked by him. This book teaches you where, when, and how to detect him early on in his plot against you so that you can avoid coming into contact with him and involve the appropriate authorities *before* becoming his victim.

We spent years training surveillance detection teams around the world (for our government and other governments) as part of the efforts to fight global terrorism. We have also used surveillance detection operationally on a variety of government and privately contracted jobs. We know it is a proven, highly effective prevention method. We feel so strongly about its value that our goal is to introduce it into the mainstream and make SD a household word. SD works and anyone can learn to integrate it into his/her personal security practice.

In addition to learning how to get SASD, you will also learn how to become empowered, even if you are in a high threat situation. In order for women to become truly empowered around the issue of their personal security they need to take two actions: concentrate more on prevention and reshape their evolutionary process. The big idea behind "The Evolution of Empowerment" is that women are capable of and entitled to becoming fully endowed with the power of their innate survival instincts. We believe women can participate in their own evolutionary process by becoming proactive about their security and by *refusing to be victimized.* Prevention is the vehicle to this refusal. What fascinates us about the victimization of women is that, no matter how progressive our societies become, women remain grossly victimized by men, sometimes even by educated and sophisticated men. We find it ironic that women, the people who know best what it is like to have to be prepared on a daily basis for violence against them from the opposite sex, are the very same people who deflect the majority of the responsibility for their safety *to* the opposite sex. Our vision is a world in which all women get SASD so that whenever predators target women they will hit roadblock after roadblock. The more we spread this methodology throughout the world, the less able predators will be to target women. It is that simple.

We are using the word evolution as an equal opportunity concept that women of all faiths or beliefs can apply to their lives. You can be propelled forward by our concept of evolutionary momentum while remaining true to your God. In fact, it will bring you closer to your God in that you will reconnect with parts of yourself that God bestowed upon you that you have simply forgotten. If you do not believe in any God, you will perceive this reconnection as the innate female asset you have always possessed but have never explored to this extent. We want each reader to know that you are included in the big idea and you can improve your life by reading about it.

As collaborators we are excited about fusing both a female and male perspective on the violence against women, defenses against it, and solutions for prevention and empowerment. Our vision for women's security comes out of our years of working in the field and from our unique perspectives on what it means to be a warrior rather than just a survivor. Our hope is to advance your mindset as well as your skill set. We are excited and honored to have you as a reader.

By presenting a holistic approach to security, our intention is to teach you how to integrate security solutions into your life so that you can transform your fears about being attacked into confidence about avoiding attacks. Getting SASD is easy, legal, possible, doable, and fun. With little effort on your part, it will change your life. We believe that the empowerment of women will propel the gender into the next phase of its evolution and the consequences will add depth and vision to the theory of "Survival of the Fittest." It is a big idea and a vision worth aspiring towards if we want this world to be a better place.

HOW TO USE THIS BOOK

NOW YOU HAVE MORE

As a Comprehensive Guidebook...

This book is partially designed to be used as a guidebook. We provide you with a unique and comprehensive approach to personal security which will allow you to keep yourself safe without having to live in constant fear and paranoia. We do this by providing you with exercises, diagrams, and map studies so that you can learn to apply the techniques to your life in order to address your specific security needs. By conducting our simple exercises and following our instructions for creating your own map studies and charts, you will be given the opportunity to teach yourself state of the art prevention techniques. We have done our best to provide you with samples of the charts and diagrams we ask you to make for yourself. It is our hope that you find the process of studying yourself as a target to be one of the most eye opening and profoundly valuable experiences you have had in a long time.

As a Reference Book...

This book is also designed as a reference book that serves as your Bible for personal security and crime prevention. This means that, after you have read the book in its entirety, it will remain a source of protection for you. A chapter you read now may not apply to your current situation but may apply to your future. Or, perhaps a friend will need guidance on a particular subject in the book and you can read up on it and help her or direct her to the book.

The point is, keep this book handy so that when you need instruction, information, or inspiration, it will be accessible.

As an Inspirational and Philosophical Guide...

Finally, this book was designed as an inspirational and philosophical approach to the subject of women's empowerment as it applies to personal security. This is not a feminist treatise or a self-help book. This is a book about empowerment, self-protection, and the evolution of women. We do not fault women for being victimized because we know a void exists in terms of the accessibility of information regarding violence prevention. Women have been doing their best to protect themselves with what they have. *Now you have more.*

How to Get the Best Read...

First, we want to clarify that we intentionally opted for me (Laura) to write the book because it is a book about and for women. As a result, the pronoun "we" is used for speaking about women collectively (for example: "As women, we need to take a stand against the violence"). However, since Bill and I are equal collaborators on this book we consider ourselves to be co-authors in the respect that we are offering a fused perspective, methodology, and philosophy. Therefore, we often refer to ourselves in the book by using the pronoun "we" (for example: "We believe women can become empowered by getting SASD").

Because we present a progression of techniques, your best bet is to start at the beginning and read through to the end. We encourage you to take your time with the material. This is not an easy read like a novel that sweeps away your imagination and gives you momentary escape from life's responsibilities. However, if you commit to reading the entire book, by the time you get to the end you will feel proud of yourself for having invested time and energy in *yourself.* You will be well ahead of any predator out there who targets you.

Most of all, you will have rebooted yourself with so many new and exciting ideas and techniques that you will walk away from this book a changed woman.

In order to provide you with a variety of approaches to the material, we have created three fictional characters who appear throughout the book. These characters represent women who face varied levels of threat. As we introduce each new prevention technique, we will draw on one or more of these characters (or other stories from real women) to exemplify how to apply the technique according to the level of threat you face (low, medium, or high).

1. **Tammy** is a sixteen year old high school student. She is our *low threat* character, meaning she has not identified any potential threats or any credible threats in her life at this time. With Tammy, we give you a simplified version of the techniques we are presenting so that you can get the overall concept (before you learn how to delve deeper into prevention if your threat escalates).

2. **Victoria** is a fifty-one year old mother. She is divorced and lives with her twelve year old son, Jake. She is our *medium threat* character, meaning she has identified a potential threat in her life at this time (she recently encountered a man whom she believes may be a threat). Victoria is our character who, early on, applies preventative measures. She will teach you how to use the techniques we provide to your greatest advantage.

3. **Kate** is our *high threat* character, meaning she currently has a credible threat in her life. Kate has a stalker but by the time she confirms this, she is well on her way to being attacked. With Kate we will show you how to catch up to a threat and apply preventative measures late in the game.

You will notice that we do not include a *no threat* character. The reason for this is that there is no such thing as "no threat." No matter who you are or where you live or what you do, you are always part of the constant flux between danger and security. Your life can totally change in a moment if you are in the wrong place at the wrong time or if someone turns his propensity for violence against you.

In this book we concentrate mainly on defending oneself against male predators, though certainly women are capable of violence and female predators are a viable threat. Although we refer to predators using masculine pronouns (he/him/his), this is not a male-bashing book. The majority of men in our world respect, love, and care about grandmothers, mothers, sisters, wives, daughters, girlfriends, female co-workers, and women in general. The truth, however, is that the majority of crimes against women are committed by men, thus our reason for describing predators using masculine pronouns.

As one half of the species, we are responsible for educating and preserving the women who will inherit this world when we are gone. Perhaps through our guidance they will evolve and dispel the myth that women are the "weaker sex." Perhaps they will invent a new definition of strength, one that we cannot yet see. We advise mothers, sisters, and teachers to take the responsibility to read the information and impart it to the younger girls (and boys) in your lives. Some of what you read in here will be too complex for children, but much of it can be made applicable to their ride on the school bus, their interactions with strangers, and their encounters with people they know who might be predators. In addition, if any of the grown women in your life are developmentally disabled or suffer from some illness that inhibits their mental abilities, please use your communication skills to impart as much of this information as possible. Women who have challenges that are based on an illness or mental condition are often victimized simply because they are soft (easy) targets.

We invite you to take this opportunity to learn something new; even if you do not need it today, you may in the future. So relax, enjoy the read, and trust that you are capable of becoming an evolved, empowered, woman who refuses to be victimized.

PART ONE

PREVENTION TECHNIQUES

CHAPTER ONE

SITUATIONAL AWARENESS: THE FORGOTTEN INSTINCT

"…keep your attention focused on the work, be alert and ready to handle ably and intelligently any situation which may arise—this is mindfulness."

--Thich Nhat Hanh

Women seek a happy ending. It is our nature to appease, apologize, and provide a solution. Women nurture the child, mend the torn shirt, offset the argument with a smile, and dilute conflict with compassion. It seems to be an innate trait for us to want to work together towards positive solutions. Perhaps this part of our nature is estrogen driven. Perhaps it is the result of our conditioning and upbringing. What really matters is that, by some design, we generally tend to *avoid* conflict rather than perpetuate it. In this chapter we take a fresh look at what women can do to bolster this innate quality and utilize it for their own protection. We begin by introducing what we consider to be the most powerful and effective skill any woman can use to prevent being attacked. Oddly enough, this skill is closely tied to our nurturing, conflict avoiding nature, yet we have become separated from it. It is called situational awareness and it has become our forgotten instinct.

Situational awareness is an extremely broad topic that we will funnel into the specific channel of women's security. Everyone from pilots to soldiers to business people to health care professionals uses situational awareness for his/her own purposes. There is no reason why women cannot be trained to integrate this practice into their lives to protect themselves.

Defined, situational awareness (SA) is the practice of remaining alert in the present moment and aware of the reality of the present situation. Having situational awareness means developing a habitual awareness of your surroundings in order to be able to discern if any indicators of suspicious or potentially dangerous activity are present in your midst and then acting accordingly to offset the danger. By rebooting your forgotten instinct and implementing situational awareness, you buy yourself more time to react to potential danger and avoid it altogether. If you are unable to escape the danger, your SA is what will give you the best chance of surviving the threat because you will have identified the exits and nearest safe locations where you can find help. You have to be aware of what is going on around you, what could go on that would change the situation into something dangerous, and what options you have to avoid and survive that danger. You must be aware of the present situation, while at the same time be thinking ahead to the future problem and solution.

Below are examples of three levels of situational awareness: poor, moderate, and excellent:

Poor SA

Margot is standing at the back of her SUV loading groceries into the car. It is night time and she is wearing a pair of headphones, rocking out to the music blaring in her ears from her MP3 player. Her purse is wide open on the seat of her grocery cart, where a child normally rides. Her back is turned to the parking lot as she makes space for the groceries and loads them into the vehicle. She is singing away and cannot even hear the cell phone ringing inside her purse.

Margot gets an "F" because she is completely unaware of her surroundings and, depending on the area, she may be seriously tempting any prospective purse snatcher or pickpocket. She is basically broadcasting herself as a target by her obvious lack of awareness. She can neither hear nor see danger approaching.

Moderate SA

Stella is riding on the subway in New York. She is on her way to meet a friend in Soho for drinks. A young man sitting next to her strikes up a conversation with her and introduces himself as 'Zach.' It turns out he goes to NYU also and they have one professor in common. As they continue to ride along, it becomes apparent to Stella that Zach is interested in her. She notices that he is asking more and more personal questions and is closing in on her physical space, making her feel uncomfortable. Stella casually mentions that she is on her way to meet her boyfriend and continues on with friendly banter. Because Zach has already indicated where he will disembark, Stella decides to get off two stops before his stop and get back on the subway to go meet her friend.

Stella gets a "C+" because she gave Zach, a total stranger, too much personal information. However, she did recover well by using her analytical skills to assess the potential threat and by mentioning the boyfriend and getting off the train early.

Excellent SA

Alison is getting ready for her first date with Peter. They met at a bar a week ago and he has called her every night since then. Although flattered by the attention, she is also the slightest bit uneasy. Still, she agreed on a date, not wanting to think the worst of him or make assumptions. She arranged to meet Peter at the restaurant so that she could drive herself in case he turned out to be a heavy drinker. As Alison is getting ready to leave she grabs her purse and puts in the right shade of pink lipstick, eye pencil, and her compact. Of course her cell phone, keys, and "mad money" (her credit card, cash, and some coins) are musts. Alison adds her mini flashlight (hard enough to use as a weapon) and programs her speed dial so her friend Sam's number is one button away. Almost out the door, she has a sudden urge to call her friend Melissa. She listens to the urge and tells Melissa where she is meeting Peter. Melissa says she'll give her a 'check in' call on her cell in a couple of hours. Alison looks in the mirror, confident, excited, and ready to go out and have a good time.

Alison gets an "A" for several reasons. First, she refuses to give Peter, a basic stranger, control over her by allowing him to drive. She also does not allow Peter to pick her up at home on the first date (that way, if Peter turns out to be a threat, he does not know where she lives). Next, she is well prepared to take care of herself, financially and physically. Her car and monetary options give her the choice to break contact with Peter if necessary. Alison has a 'what if' plan (a back up plan, including the check in call from Melissa and Sam's phone number) in case she gets into any kind of trouble. If the flashlight part sounds extreme to you, consider that Peter is a total stranger and he has exhibited signs of possibly being smothering and coming on too strong. Light is a key element to survival and the flashlight can double as a defensive weapon. Alison is realistic about her date, yet she is also excited and willing to give Peter a chance. However, she will not compromise her own safety. Because she is so well prepared and has arranged for outside support, Alison can feel much more at ease on her date and can enjoy herself.

Your situational awareness is constantly in flux. Sometimes the situation warrants that your alertness level be elevated. Other times, it is obvious that you can relax. Think of a mother with her toddler: she is not constantly on high alert, but she is ever watchful and ready to immediately respond to any danger. The point is, if you accept this constant state of flux as a given, then you will be able to remain calm and on a baseline until, even at a moment's notice, the situation changes and you are forced to elevate your awareness and alertness level. You could be in the most relaxed state and suddenly something causes that to shift (such as: an unfamiliar noise in your home in the night; a strange man approaching you on the street; or a car driving erratically) and you must immediately jump on board and raise your SA level so that it matches the new level of danger. It would be too exhausting to walk around all the time in a constantly heightened state of alertness. Likewise, it is foolish to remain in a perpetually relaxed state. Having good situational awareness means having the ability to shift in and out of a heightened state of alertness whenever necessary and retaining your composure all the while.

Now that you have the basic concept of SA, we will break it down into its components and teach you how to integrate it into your life. In order to help you reconnect to your forgotten instinct, we will look at ways you can strengthen your practice of situational awareness. We will also give you simple exercises for each SA component so that you can practice and train yourself. The best way to improve your SA is to, over time, practice integrating the following skills into your daily life:

- Respecting Your Intuition
- Developing Sensory Awareness
- Maintaining Solid Stature and Balance
- Identifying Early Warning Signals
- Creating 'What If' Plans

Respecting Your Intuition

In order to respect your intuition you must learn to listen to, trust in, and act on it. Listening to your intuition in any given situation or environment is a critical part of allowing your awareness to remain focused on the present moment. Intuition is visceral; that is why we say "I could feel it in my gut" or "my gut tells me not to go there." We all experience our intuition in a unique way. Sometimes it may feel like a subtle nudge from our higher selves. Other times it takes the shape of a little voice that deeply sighs "ah ha!" or curiously wonders "hmm…" No matter how you experience the voice of your intuition, it is the launching pad of your early warning system. Sometimes you know, in your gut, not to go into an area of a shopping mall or parking lot. Sometimes you intuit that it would be better to stay home instead of going out to the party. Other times your intuition kicks you in your center and cries out "stay away from that person."

Once you have heard the cry of your intuition, you must then place your trust in it. It is paradoxical how often women ignore their intuition regarding their personal security. The reasons they ignore it are varied. Perhaps they are in denial or feel embarrassed about being wrong. Perhaps they feel they may be overreacting and will cause trouble. At other times they may rationalize away their intuitive nudges by concocting reasons to ignore them. Ignoring your intuition where your security is concerned, more often than not, is a critical mistake. Women who do so often have a difficult time recovering from an attack because they know they ignored their built-in early warning system. In order to trust your intuition, you must remain alert to it. As previously mentioned, each of us experiences intuition in our own, unique way. For some, the heart begins to race. For others, a little voice speaks the warning. Regardless if your specific intuitive signals manifest themselves physically, visually, emotionally, or mentally, remain alert to these signals and practice trusting them. Trusting your intuition will help you to discern why you feel apprehension and to spot danger. Rather than wasting time second-guessing your intuition, you will be better able to respond immediately and appropriately to potential threats.

After you practice listening to and trusting in your intuition, you must then take the next step and act on it. Acting on your intuition is sometimes a conscious decision and at other times happens automatically. However, in order to act on your intuition you need support from the rest of your being, including your senses, your physical being, and your analytical mindset. Again, we have noticed a missing link in women when it comes to acting on their intuitive nudges pertaining to their personal security. Often women will hear the voice of their intuition but they do not take that necessary step of acting on what it is telling them to do or not do. It is curious that mothers normally have no problem acting on their intuition when it comes to protecting their children, yet their instinct to protect themselves is not equally honed. Our intention is to assist you in rebooting your instinct to protect *yourself*.

Remember that intuition alone does not provide you with overall situational awareness. Intuition evokes emotion; it is a visceral response. Situational awareness separates emotion from the equation and allows you to assess the situation *as it is*, not how you would like it to be. Your intuition will alert you to the reality that danger is in your midst, but fully developed SA is what will enable you to respond successfully to the situation at hand without allowing your emotions to place you in even greater danger.

Exercise 1: Intuition

Enter any public location (a hotel lobby; a restaurant; a bar; a waiting room; a subway; a shopping mall, etc.) and find a place to either sit or stand still. Take a moment to focus on your breathing and tune in to your overall sense of the place. Do not close your eyes. Listen to your intuition. Is it telling you that everything is okay here? Are you at all uncomfortable in this location? Perhaps you may feel a twinge of nervousness that someone might be watching you and wondering what you are doing. Let it go and tune in again to your intuition. Find a word or phrase that describes what it is telling you. Maybe the words "I'm fine here" will arise. Maybe you will find yourself saying "I feel happy here today" or "Something feels off about this place." Perhaps you will utter something that makes no sense to you such as "I wish I had chosen another location." Whatever it is, do not judge it. Just listen. Give your intuition its voice.

Spend some time in your location and move around. Tune in to that intuitive voice every few minutes and see if you notice any changes in what it is telling you. Are any people present in the location causing you to feel uncomfortable? Put your feeling into words or phrases. You might hear your intuitive voice saying: "Don't make eye contact with that man."

Do you notice any physical sensations that arise, such as nervousness or nausea or a racing heartbeat? Does your body feel relaxed? Be present with yourself in the location and see what happens. Perhaps nothing out of the ordinary will grab your attention. What is important is that you are taking time to mindfully focus on your intuition while out in public. This is the first part of activating situational awareness.

Developing Sensory Awareness

Once you have responded to the visceral, emotional cry of your intuition, you must shift gears and begin to utilize all of your tools for action. Your first tool is sensory awareness. In order to develop your sensory awareness you simply must pay attention to it. You must make it a habit to take in your surroundings by using all of your senses:

- **Sight:** Get eyes on the situation. Scan the area and re-scan every fifteen seconds if you sense potential danger. Establish ground truth; what is really happening around you? Where are the avenues of approach into the area and who is entering? How many people are in the area? Are there any people whose behavior is suspicious? Where are the exits? What escape routes exist?

- **Sound:** Listen for trouble. Are any aggressive, angry voices in your midst? Are there any alarming sounds or unfamiliar noises that seem out of place?

- **Smell:** Breathe in through your nose and smell the environment. Are there any uncomfortable or incongruent odors?

- **Taste:** Do you notice any odd taste in your mouth (sometimes odors will also cause us to experience a peculiar taste)?

- **Touch:** Assess the energy or overall feeling of the area (for example, an overcrowded subway station has a very different feel than a lazy Sunday afternoon in a park). Notice the temperature. Does the chill of a sudden draft indicate that someone has just entered the room? Be aware of any tactile threats, such as broken glass, sharp edges or corners, or any obstacles that could cause you to trip and fall.

Developing sensory awareness requires you to simply be alert to any indicators that something you perceive through one or more of your senses is out of sync. Rarely would you notice a strange taste, but you might if some chemical odor or the stench of a dead animal were released into the air. In many cases your senses will alert you without you consciously instructing them to do so. But, like intuition, we sometimes ignore our sensory warning signals. Pay attention and respect your body's ability to keep you safe.

The benefits of improving your sensory awareness are profound. Stated simply, you will become more alive. Our senses help us tremendously in avoiding danger of all kinds. We see the brake lights of cars stopped ahead of us on the highway. We hear the panic in the voice of a child crying for help. We smell the smoke of a fire. We taste the rotten food. We touch the sharp edge of the broken glass beneath our feet. We already automatically rely on our senses to protect us everyday, thus it is not too great a leap for women to further cultivate their sensory awareness for the purpose of averting danger from an attacker. By conducting the exercise below you can train yourself to detect danger just like a security professional would.

Exercise 2: Sensory Awareness

Enter any public location and begin visually scanning the area. Take a look behind you, above and below you, and scan the horizon of the location from one end to another. This should take you all of twenty to thirty seconds. Activate your peripheral vision and take in an overall visual snapshot of the place. Identify all of the entrances and exits in the location. Look for 'dead spaces' such as corners or underneath staircases (or any spaces that are normally not occupied by or within line of sight to people). Notice any movement around you. Pay attention to the men in the area: what are they doing? Do any of them alarm you or cause you to feel wary?

Now focus on the sounds around you. Is the sound affecting you in any positive or negative way? What about any particular smells? Perhaps, if you are at a grocery store, you might notice that the smell of the bakery makes you feel warm and safe. If you are in a restaurant and someone lights a cigarette, do you become agitated? Do you notice that any of the smells affects the taste in your mouth? Is the temperature affecting you in any positive or negative way? Again, try not to judge yourself but listen to your reactions and give yourself an accurate assessment.

Notice any emotional reactions you may be having. Does your sensory awareness prompt any intuitive reaction?

Notice the level of presence you attain when you take just a few moments to focus on your sensory awareness. We are so accustomed to ignoring our sensory awareness or taking it for granted. When we become mindful of it, we enhance our ability to allow it to send us early warnings about potential danger.

Maintaining Solid Stature and Balance

Your physical stature and balance are as important as your intuition and sensory awareness. You can train yourself to maintain your bearing and physical integrity (see Chapter Twelve). If you have ever studied dance or yoga or any type of movement, you know what it feels like at the end of class when you emerge physically revitalized and energized in your body. You project a physical self-confidence that is apparent to the onlooker. The same idea applies to maintaining solid stature when you are out in public. The idea is to reduce your chances of becoming a target of opportunity by emanating a physical presence that keeps predators at a distance. Why would a predator choose a woman who emits a capable physical demeanor? Normally, if you physically cower when danger lurks, you undermine your ability to survive it. In some situations, however, cowering may be part of your ploy to stay safe. For example, if you were abducted you might at some point physically cower to send your abductors the message that you will not be causing them trouble by trying to escape. Your cowering might buy you time to craft a more effective response and ensure your escape when the opportunity arises. Every attack is different; you must use your judgment and respond the best way you see fit.

When you are in prevention mode, your stature is an important element, both physically and psychologically. Stand tall when you sense danger. Lift your chest (this does not mean stick out your breasts; it means raise your chest from the inside). Take a moment to feel your connection to the ground below you. Check your balance. Are you weighed down by grocery bags? Are you standing close to the edge of the curb or a set of stairs? Where is your body in time and space? Adjust your stance so that you feel a solid connection to the ground below and you are ready to move in any direction at any moment. Even if you are sitting inside a car, you can still raise your physical posture and connect your body to the space around you.

Breathe. Lift your body tall and connect your body down. If all you do is lift and stand tall, you will be empty and off balance in the lower half of your body. Likewise, if all you do is ground yourself by sinking your body to connect below, you will be too heavily weighted and will not have the ability to move quickly. Maintain this solid but flexible stature throughout the situation. It will embolden you and prepare you physically to move out of harm's way.

Use your peripheral vision to help you expand your awareness of what and who is in front of you, at your sides, behind you, above you, and below you. If you are riding up an escalator in a shopping mall your awareness of above and below is different than if you are standing in an elevator. Heighten your body's ability to feel the presence of others. Our skin is one of the most valuable organs we have. You can sense the heat and energy of another's body standing behind you if you are paying attention. Do your best to keep physical distance from hazardous areas and potentially dangerous people. In addition, pay attention to others' personal space and notice if they are invading yours. In some cultures it is normal to close in on another when standing in lines. Consider what is appropriate for your given location.

Occupying your body in the present moment and solidifying your stature will immediately boost your self-confidence and allow you to experience much greater control over your environment. The attacker's most important weapon is the element of surprise. If you have listened to, trusted in, and acted on your intuition, have heightened your sensory awareness, and have adjusted your physical stature so that you are strong, balanced, and present, you are seriously compromising any attacker's ability to surprise you. Predators generally avoid strength of presence in their victims because they want to attack successfully, without getting caught. A physically strong presence may deter them and send them looking for 'weaker' victims, ones they feel confident they can overpower.

Exercise 3: Maintaining Solid Stature and Balance

Take a short stroll on your street, in a park, in a shopping mall or some other public place. Move slowly so that you can focus, but not so slowly that you draw attention from others. Pay attention to your body and your stature. Are you at once rooted and raised up in your posture? What is your balance like? Are you stable or could you easily be physically compromised and thrown off balance? Use your peripheral vision as you negotiate the people and objects around you. Are you aware of the people behind you? Are you mindful of the ground beneath you? Use one word or short phrase to describe how you feel moving in this space. If the word "awkward" comes to mind, ask yourself if you are just experiencing the natural nervousness of wondering if others think you are crazy because you are conducting this exercise. If that is the case, ignore it and find a word that truly reflects how your body feels moving around in this space. Perhaps the words "safe, confident, lonely, or vulnerable" will come to mind. Whatever it is, just listen and do not judge yourself.

Identify your escape routes. If you had to move quickly, in which direction would you travel? Is there any safe location nearby? To whom would you turn for help? If in one moment your reality in this place changed and you were suddenly in serious danger, how would you respond physically? Would your body be ready to move?

Again, this is simply an exercise in being mindful and present in your body in a particular environment. Our bodies move around all day from place to place. Do we adjust our attention and stay present in our bodies in each of these places? Normally we are so distracted that we ignore our bodies unless we feel uncomfortable because we are tired, hungry, cold, or have a headache. The more often you practice this exercise in different environments, the easier it becomes to develop the habit of maintaining solid stature and balance.

Identify Early Warning Signals

Now that your intuition, your senses, and your body are activated, it is time to bring your intellect into the situation. With your alertness heightened, you will be able to access and sharpen your analytical skills so that you can effectively inform your brain and reshape your mindset to match the level of danger. Analyze that fearful, apprehensive or nagging feeling you have. What is occurring around you that may be the cause of it? What early warning signals are present that give you reason to be stirred?

Your mind's ability to distinguish correlating activities or suspicious behaviors now comes into play. Correlating activities are any activities that relate to your movements or actions. For example, if you get off the bus and a man gets off at the same stop, his movement has correlated with yours. It may be completely coincidental and innocuous, but you are wise to pick up on this correlation and remain alert to his actions. Does he walk in your direction? Does he strike up a conversation with you? In addition to (or rather than) correlating to your movements, someone might correlate with your location and/or actions. For example, imagine you meet a friend every Friday at a particular lunch spot. Each Friday when you arrive at your regular time the same man is sitting parked in a car in a location that gives him line of sight to the restaurant entrance. When you arrive you notice he writes down something on a small pad of paper. His location and activity correlate with your location and actions.

Predators have a variety of techniques they use to ready themselves to first choose and then pursue victims. If you start to think like the bad guy you will be able to spot early warning signals of danger. In order to help you to do this, you must first educate yourself on typical tactics used by predators. First, when choosing a target the predator will be particularly interested in detecting any signs of the following from his potential victim:

- Weakness (either physical or emotional)
- Distraction

- Any compromised emotional state (such as crying or anguish)
- Any vulnerability he can exploit (if a woman's car is broken down or she is lost)
- Isolation
- Lack of awareness
- Overt friendliness or approachability

Next, the predator will approach his potential victim to either assess if he will have an opportunity to put her under surveillance in the future, attack her in the present, or to set the stage for the attack. His objective is to somehow close the distance between himself and the potential victim, (this could be either a literal physical distance or a psychological one). His approach is sometimes called the "interview phase" and it is chock-full of early warning signals. Be on the lookout for any of the following:

- **Mr. Intruder:** He will initiate physical proximity by devising an approach or finding a plausible entry into your physical space (for example: "Excuse me, did you drop this pen?"; "Let me help you with the door"; "Here, this flower is for you"). Once he closes the physical distance between you he may make an inappropriate advance (by touching you) or he may use the physical proximity to imply that an intimacy is forming between the two of you (for example: "You smell wonderful; what is your perfume?" or "That is a very beautiful necklace you are wearing.").
- **Mr. Charming:** He will use compliments and flattery to make you drop your guard and give you a false sense of security. His intention is to make you feel at ease in his presence, thereby creating an opening for him to initiate further contact with you. He might begin by complimenting you on your work or some ability you have (for example: "I noticed the way you handled that rude customer. How do you put up with people like that? You seem to have the patience of a saint!"). Once he establishes rapport and a false sense of trust, he may then progress by trying to secure a date with you or some type of future contact.

- **Mr. Politician:** He will try to win rapport with you in order to maintain contact, even after you have made it clear that you are not interested in conversing. Perhaps he will point out a common plight you share, such as a late bus you are both waiting for, or he may talk about the weather or a recent event in the news. He is constantly trying to sell himself as a man you can trust and should get to know better.

- **Mr. Persister:** He will not take your "No" for an answer or he will try to continue the conversation by circumventing or downplaying your "No" (regardless if your "No" is stated assertively or tentatively). His tactics are similar to those of an aggressive car salesman and he will manipulate the conversation until you agree to his terms. Unless you break contact from him, he will persist until he gets what he wants.

- **Mr. Generosity:** He will attempt to give you something for nothing and will try to barter for a response by reassuring you (for example, he may insist you take his seat on the train and then begin telling you a story, to which you now feel obligated to listen because he has just been so polite in offering his seat).

- **Mr. Trickster:** He will create a ruse or con to draw you into his sphere, like opening his briefcase and allowing papers to spill to the ground. Be on the lookout for any partner (male or female) with whom he may be working. Once he has engaged your help, he will use the opportunity to con you further and obtain information from you that he can potentially exploit (such as where you work, live, etc.).

- **Mr. Distracter:** He will fabricate smoke and mirrors to occupy your mind with extraneous information so that he can distract you. He might point to something happening in the distance and ask you about it while he pulls your wallet out of your opened purse.

- **Mr. Nosy:** He will attempt to elicit information about you, such as your name, address, phone number, where you work, any details about your schedule or habits, and information about your family. He will normally create a conversation and plug in key questions so that you do not even realize how much information you gave him until later. Sometimes he will give you information about himself first so that you feel obligated to reciprocate (for example: "I live in an apartment over on 5th Street. How about you?).

• **Mr. New Best Friend:** He will try to convince you that he is just like you by pointing out that the two of you have some type of bond or connection. Perhaps he will see a bumper sticker on your car for a sports team and he will use that as his entry (for example: "Another Cubs fan. Aren't they the greatest team ever?").

• **Mr. Master and Commander:** He is the guy you meet on the street who tells you to "smile" as you walk past him. He will attempt to take charge and to control your mood, appearance, and reaction to him. He wants to evoke a reaction from you so that he can be gratified if you follow his commands. He will try to use his commands and your response to them as a means of leading you into a conversation, one that he intends to control in order to elicit information from you.

• **Mr. Out of Sorts:** This guy needs some kind of help from you. Perhaps he is lost, has dropped something, or needs a recommendation for a good restaurant in the area. He will use his feigned disorientation to manipulate you into helping him somehow. He might even resort to more drastic measures, such as pretending his car is broken down and he is late getting to the hospital to visit his dying mother. He will attempt to tug on your heart strings to get you to rescue him.

• **Mr. Rescuer:** He will come to your aid and do anything to assist you, whether it is helping you carry your groceries to the car or offering to share his umbrella in a rain storm. His intention is to buy time to speak with you and elicit information. He also wants you to feel obligated to somehow repay him for his services (usually by giving him more of your time and attention).

If you encounter any of these behaviors from strangers, consider them to be early warning signals and assess their significance to your situation and location. If you are alone with this person, you are probably in greater danger than if you have the safety net of a busy public location where you can find a way to break contact from this person. Obviously not every man using these techniques will fall into the predator category. Often men use some of the above techniques to try to meet you or get a date with you and they are perfectly harmless. What is important to remember when you are practicing situational awareness is that there are a multitude of possible truths for any given situation. Thus, when you see something it may or may not be actual danger. *What matters is that it may*, so you must train yourself to first recognize early warning signals of potential danger and then respond accordingly. Part of the denial process to which women succumb is that they focus too heavily on what we refer to as the potential "safe truths" versus the potential "threat truths" in a situation.

The following are examples of situations that contain early warning signals (EWS) and the possible safe truths, as well as the possible threat truths behind them. We also offer potential responses. You will notice that our responses exemplify taking the "threat truths" seriously and acting on the potential danger, rather than slipping into denial and complacency by prioritizing the possible safe truths.

EWS: A woman is walking to her car at a shopping mall parking lot at night and sees a man crouched behind a car several feet away.
Possible Safe Truths: He dropped his keys; he is fixing a flat tire; he is tying his shoe.
Possible Threat Truths: He is preparing to car jack her; he is a purse snatcher; he plans to abduct her.
Response: She goes back into the mall, reports the man, and asks a security guard to walk her to her car.

EWS: At a party, a high school girl notices a group of boys in a huddle discussing something secretive while looking at and pointing to a group of her girlfriends across the room.
Possible Safe Truth: They think the girls are attractive and are trying to work up the nerve to go talk to them.

Possible Threat Truth: They are planning to slip date rape drugs into one or more of the girls' drinks.

Response: The girl walks up to her group of girlfriends and discreetly warns them that the boys are obviously interested in them for some reason. She reminds them to keep careful control over their drinks just in case.

EWS: A woman who lives alone enters her home and notices the lock on the door appears to have been tampered with and is not working properly.

Possible Safe Truth: The lock is broken and she just did not notice it when she left the house.

Possible Threat Truth: Someone has broken into her home and may still be inside.

Response: She does not enter the home but relocks the door and drives out of the area to a safe location and notifies the police.

What you will notice about each of these scenarios is that the possible safe truths always tell us that there is no need for alarm. Women tend to latch on to these safe truths because we do not like to consider the potential danger. We also do not feel we have the time to hassle with the response to keep ourselves safe when, very likely, there is no need for concern. We fall into denial and allow our internal monologue to talk us out of the potential embarrassment of overreacting by assuming there is a real threat, thinking instead: "It's probably nothing and I'm just being paranoid."

Think about it this way: You are not privy to a potential attacker's intentions. Why not take the time and energy to err on the side of caution? The woman in the parking lot could be abducted. The girls at the party could be slipped a date rape drug. The woman who entered her home could be welcomed by an intruder who rapes her. Would you want to be any of these victims? Of course not, so pay attention to early warning signals and do not make emotional, subjective judgments about them. Use your situational awareness and consider the context of the particular threat so that you can question it and act on it appropriately. Train yourself to *always* respond with the safest option. In so doing you will exercise, strengthen, and refine your intuitive skills. You will also build your confidence and get better at putting your practice of situational awareness on auto-pilot.

Trust your mind to detect and interpret the early warning signals of potential danger. Your intuition is feeding your mind and your senses are its assets. Your body will follow its commands. Respect your intelligence, your analytical skills, and your instinct to survive. Your mental alertness to and awareness of early warning signals will allow you to respond appropriately to any given threat. Use your mind and heed the early warning signals; they are valuable assets for prevention.

Exercise 4: Early Warning Signals

Enter any public location where you can observe a lot of people. Sit down, if possible, and watch as people pass by you. Keep scanning the area and observe as many people as you can. Notice if anyone stands out or makes you feel uneasy (for any reason). Are you detecting any early warning signals of danger from this person? Is he or she doing anything specific that makes you uncomfortable? Are you intuitively feeling that this person's demeanor is potentially threatening? Is anyone behaving in an illogical manner? Is anyone focusing his or her attention on you? Do you sense any 'bad vibes' from anyone in the location?

If there is a person who, for any reason, makes you uncomfortable, does he or she do anything to escalate the situation and make you feel at greater risk? For example, you may first notice a man who gives you a bad vibe. This bad vibe is your early warning signal. He may then escalate the situation and add to your discomfort by approaching you to ask you the time. Notice how you react to any early warning signals from any of the people you are observing. Does your body freeze? Do you feel confused or embarrassed? Do you take action and remove yourself from the potential danger? It is very possible that no one will stand out as a threat during this exercise; what is important is that you are taking the time to notice people and their behaviors.

Creating a 'What If' Plan

Okay, you say, I am programmed to the hilt with awareness. What do I do with it all? We say: Use it to think ahead. Prevention involves foresight. Would you not rather live by the motto "Foresight is twenty-twenty" than "Hindsight is twenty-twenty"? It is not that difficult to do, but you must remember to create a 'what if' plan.

What if I am at the grocery store and a fire breaks out? What if my daughter comes home from school and tells me a strange man approached her on the playground that day? What if I am working out at the gym and a man enters the locker room while I am taking a shower? You do not need to sit around and obsess about all the possible 'what ifs' in life. Instead, begin to consider some of the potential 'what ifs' and take the next critical step to remind yourself that you can, even right there on the spot, create a 'what if' plan for any scenario you have not yet imagined. Situational awareness includes taking ownership of your readiness and willingness to survive in any given situation.

Here is how it works:

Amy takes a run with her dog in the park every morning at six. She is careful and does everything possible to mitigate her risks of being attacked or harmed. Often it is dark, so she wears reflective clothing. She only runs on well lit pathways where there are many other runners. Amy has considered some of her 'what ifs' and carries a personal alarm to signal for help if she feels threatened. She carries a small flashlight and has set her cell phone on speed dial for the local police. She has also identified and avoids high risk areas, such as poorly lit paths, ravines, and thickly wooded areas.

In addition to these basic precautions, Amy has also devised the following 'what if plans:

- *What if someone drags me into the bushes?* Solution: I will avoid running near overgrown areas and use my personal alarm if anyone closes in on me.

- *What if someone trips me and then tackles me to the ground?* Solution: I will avoid allowing anyone to close the distance on me.
- *What if someone points a gun at me?* Solution: I will keep running as fast as possible in a zigzag pattern and sound my personal alarm.
- *What if someone drives up along side of me on my way home from my run and throws me in a car?* Solution: I will run in the opposite direction of the flow of traffic and stay on the sidewalks as much as possible. If someone manages to get me into a car, I will sound my personal alarm and scream and fight so that other drivers will notice the struggle.

There was a time when all of these 'what ifs' almost made Amy stop running, but she realized running was just too important to her and early in the morning was the only time slot she had available for it. One morning while out on her run, a 'what if' she had never considered occurred.

Another runner passed Amy and his dog got into a fight with hers. She had noticed him on several such mornings and thought he was attractive. Plus, he had a dog, so that was a bonus. She had imagined meeting him someday, possibly while she was stretching out before her run. But on this particular morning, that fantasy turned into a nightmare.

Their dogs were snarling at each other viciously. Amy tried her hardest to pull her dog away. The man became very agitated with Amy for not controlling her dog. He suddenly became very aggressive and started coming towards her. Amy knew she was in trouble. Not only did she have two barking, angry dogs with which to contend, but she also had a man in her midst closing in on her physically and yelling at her. She needed a 'what if' plan on the spot in a big way.

Amy was at a fully heightened state of alertness and knew she had to respond right there in the moment. She was able to successfully improvise the perfect 'what if' plan because she had already rehearsed similar 'what if' plans in her mind. She sounded her personal alarm. The dogs went crazy. The man was stopped dead in his tracks because now several other people in the distance were attuned to his aggressive behavior. He muttered a few more scolding words, pulled his dog's leash, and ran along his way.

The moral of the story is this: If you take the time to consider even some of the possible 'what if' scenarios you will be preparing your mind, and therefore your body, with a survival response. That response can then be translated into a variety of situations and circumstances. Even if the situation is totally bizarre and completely removed from any of the 'what ifs' you have previously entertained in your mind, still you are mentally ready to function, no matter the reality of the 'what if.' Taking the time to mentally rehearse 'what if' plans significantly improves your ability to respond successfully in a threatening situation. Normally when under any kind of threat our limbic system will respond either by taking our most recent action associated with that skill set or by doing what we have trained ourselves to do the most. When we imagine 'what if' scenarios, we literally train our minds and bodies to respond automatically, thereby improving our chances of escaping the danger.

One great way to train yourself in 'what if' plans is to take stories you hear on the news or read in the newspaper and discuss them with a friend, co-worker, or family member. Discuss what each of you would do if such a thing happened to you. This is a great exercise to do with older kids if they watch the news with you or hear something on the radio. Of course you do not want to frighten them too much, but if you hear a story that pertains to a potential threat they may face someday, let them verbally rehearse their 'what if' plan. Most of us have participated in some type of 'what if' planning, whether through conducting fire drills at school or by scanning for the exits when we first sit down in a movie theater. The point is you have done this before to some extent, so allow yourself to develop this ability to think ahead and make it a habit to consider 'what if' scenarios.

Exercise 5: Creating a 'What If' Plan

Enter any public location and take a moment to imagine a dangerous scenario. Rehearse in your mind how you would respond. For example, you might imagine that the man sitting at the table next to you in a restaurant approaches you and asks if he can join you since you are both alone. Run it through your mind. What would you do? Would his looks and demeanor be the deciding factors? Would you automatically say "No, thank you"? If you invited him to sit down and he turned out to be an aggressive man whom you feared, could you get out of the location immediately? Would you know where the exits are located?

After you have allowed your scenario to play out in your mind, check in with your body and your emotions. Take as much time as you need to think about how each step affected your body and emotions. Did any intuitive word alarm you? Did you notice a greater level of awareness of time and space and the situation in general? Did you notice things about the location that surprised you or that you had never paid attention to before now? Did you feel a greater sense of control over your body and the situation? Were your emotions or body impacted in any positive or negative way? Did you feel yourself freeze when thinking about the threat?

How detailed was your 'what if' plan? Did any other possible dangers creep in to your scenario, causing you to create other 'what if' possibilities? Did you imagine yourself successfully avoiding the danger? Rehearsing 'what if' plans allows you to train your mind to visualize yourself successfully escaping the danger and avoiding being attacked or harmed. Use 'What if' plans to train your mind in prevention.

Situational awareness is about training yourself to tap into the big picture, the whole enchilada versus your tiny personal story in the universe. Imagine you are out with a friend on a beautiful hiking trail. The sun is warm, but the breeze cools and relaxes you as you and your close friend discuss your lives. You are feeling the safety and support of our amazing earth. You have a moment of feeling so connected to the planet and to life. No predators, animal or human, are in your midst, (none that you can see anyway). You are in a relatively safe area and your focus is on your enjoyment of this day and this time with your friend. Still, a small portion of your attention remembers that it is possible that someone may attack you on the trail. You have read stories and are an alert enough person to consider this remote possibility. It is a fleeting thought that wakes up your consciousness and keeps you in sync with your situation.

Now, switch the story. You are walking alone down a dark alley because you got lost trying to find where you parked your car after attending a concert. You suddenly find yourself negotiating this alley. Every strange noise is cause for alarm. The smell of urine and that familiar, repulsive dumpster stench add to your discomfort. A cat knocks over an empty liquor bottle, sending a chill up and down your spine. Your alertness and awareness of danger are peaked. Now ask yourself: Do you have some small level of awareness of the safety surrounding you (safe locations, surrounding homes, sources of light, avenues of escape, possible weapons you can use)? Are you allowing your focus to encompass the whole picture or are you fixating on the danger and forgetting the prospect of safety?

We live on a planet that is in constant flux between creation and destruction. All of our societies are comprised of populations that spread both goodness and evil. Our world fluctuates every moment between states of danger and security. Our small individual lives face this same ebb and flow. If we can tune in our awareness to the big picture, we stand a better chance of averting danger and locating security. On that hike, if a proportional amount of our awareness is focused on the potential threat of danger (given the context and the perceived threat) we are better prepared to respond to that threat effectively if it really happens. Likewise, in the dark alley if we focus some of our awareness on the potential for safety, we will more likely be able to locate that safety if we fall under attack than if our full attention is on the danger alone. We are each part of an entire universe, a complete planet, a whole world made up of both large established societies and the microcosms of our individual lives. Developing situational awareness requires that we remember to perceive ourselves as part of the big picture.

We now turn to our sixteen year old low threat character, Tammy, in order to illustrate just how simply all of the information you have read in this chapter fuses together. Even if you are considered at low risk of being attacked, just like Tammy is, you are still wise to integrate the practice of SA into your daily life.

The most dangerous part of Tammy's day is her walk home from where her school bus stops. Although she is sixteen years old, Tammy has no car. Her mother takes her to school in the morning, but then goes to work, leaving Tammy no alternative ride home save the bus. Tammy must walk four blocks from the bus stop to her home.

One afternoon when she got off the bus she had an intuitive feeling of danger. Tammy looked around but saw no one in the area. Still, she was pestered by this nudge of fear. As she began walking home, she opted to forego listening to her music on her MP3 player as she normally would. Instead, she paid close attention to everything happening around her.

One block into her walk she heard the sound of footsteps in the distance behind her. Afraid to turn around and take a look, she decided to stop instead for a moment to zip up her coat. The footsteps stopped when she did. Still afraid, Tammy began to use her peripheral vision and to focus on possible places she could run to for help. Since she was in a quiet, residential neighborhood, she began paying attention to houses that looked like someone was home. She looked for houses with lights on inside, with cars in the driveways, or for signs of anyone outside in their yards.

The sound of the footsteps behind her quickened so she crossed the street and, while looking both ways, caught a glimpse of the man behind her. He called out: "Excuse me, can you help me with directions? I'm lost."

Tammy recognized this as an early warning signal. She realized in a flash that, although the possible 'safe truth' was that this man only wanted directions, the possible threat truth is that he was after her. Other indicators that made Tammy sense danger related to the way he interacted with her. First, when she crossed the street, he followed her. Next, he engaged her in conversation by soliciting help from her. He even manipulated her by changing the sound of his voice to a rather pathetic tone when he said "I'm lost."

Savvy Tammy was too smart to drop her guard and fall for his potentially threatening antics. She made a hasty 'what if' plan and quickly assessed that the house next door looked occupied and she would run there for help if necessary. She turned around and held out her arm towards him, indicating he should back off and keep his distance.

"What are you trying to find," she asked in a friendly but firm voice. The man kept walking towards her. "I would be more comfortable if you would stop, please," she said as she took a few steps backwards. The man stopped.

"Hey, I'm not going to hurt you, sweetheart, I'm just lost. Do you know how to get to Olive Boulevard?"

Tammy recognized immediately that he was lying about being lost. Olive Boulevard was a busy street miles away from this secluded subdivision. It would take a lengthy description before he could find his way. Tammy recognized immediately that he was trying to buy time with her.

Her mind raced frantically to edit her 'what if' plan. Her internal monologue bombarded her with a keen assessment of the situation. "If I tell him I live at this nearby house, he may ask to come in. If I walk home, he will follow me and then he will know where I live."

In a flash she knew exactly what to say:

"No, I'm not sure where Olive is. Listen, I'm late for my babysitting job, so good luck!"

Tammy turned and walked swiftly towards the house she had identified. She rang the doorbell, and was relieved when a middle aged woman answered the door.

Tammy wasted no time: "Can you please help me? I live about two blocks from here. That man out on the street followed me from my bus stop to here. He is pretending to be lost. I told him I was babysitting here so that he wouldn't know where I lived."

The woman let Tammy come inside. They discreetly watched the man leave the neighborhood while the woman called the police. Tammy gave her report and the police drove her home. Tammy notified her mother about the incident. Her mother alerted the school and the bus driver. Tammy disseminated the information to her friends, including a description of the man and the details of the incident, just in case the man showed up at her school.

The next day, before Tammy disembarked from the school bus, she looked around to make sure the man was nowhere in sight. She used an alternate route to walk home from school.

Remember, Tammy is our low threat character. Still, one moment changed her low threat status and she was able to use situational awareness to adjust to the escalation in the level of threat. The salient point is that Tammy did not hesitate to activate and rely on her situational awareness. Very likely, even if you have never been attacked, you have had some situation like Tammy's. Making a conscious decision to practice and integrate SA into your daily life is what will allow you to perform well in future threatening situations and prevent the danger of being attacked.

Situational Awareness Pitfalls

By now we hope you are psyched to get out there and practice SA. Be warned of the following common pitfalls so that you can catch yourself when you are in some way compromising your situational awareness.

- **Laziness/Complacency:** SA enemy number one is laziness! Laziness causes us to become complacent about our own safety so we 'forget' about locking doors or checking the back seat of the car before getting in and starting the engine. In order to make your situational awareness practice a habit in your daily life, you must break through your laziness and complacency about its importance. Be systematic and take small steps towards improving your situational awareness. Acknowledge your successes and learn from your mistakes.
- **Denial:** We are often completely caught up in our own denial that nothing bad will ever happen to us. We see the world through rose colored glasses. We talk ourselves into believing that bad things only happen to those women you hear about on the news. On some level we convince ourselves: "Nothing bad will ever happen to me or someone I

love." When the voice of your denial creeps up, identify it and move through it. Challenge its authority. For example, you might think to yourself: "I could just as easily be raped as that woman on the news." Then the voice of your denial might creep in and reply: "No, you will never be that unlucky." You could then challenge the voice of your denial and retort: "Stop kidding yourself; she didn't get raped because she was unlucky."

- **Distraction:** We are always busy with whatever is at hand and we feel too overwhelmed to add anything else into the picture. We are constantly multi-tasking just to be able to keep up with all we feel we must accomplish on any given day. It is not uncommon to talk on the cell phone while you are rummaging through your purse or writing down appointments in your calendar. Even when we are walking or driving we are caught up in other small activities that demand some of our concentration, like reading directions or flipping through the radio stations looking for good music. Identify when you are distracting yourself unnecessarily. Remind yourself to practice situational awareness even while you are engaging in distracting activities. For example, when you are picking up your kids from school and are distracted by loading them in the car, getting them to buckle their seat belts, and making sure they have all of their belongings, take a moment to pause before you drive away. Breathe. Look around. Is anyone in the area watching you and your children intently? Perhaps you will, in that moment, see a man sitting in a parked car just outside the school grounds. It only takes a moment to direct yourself back into a heightened awareness of your surroundings and of potential danger, but if you deny yourself that moment, you may miss something important.

- **"Clear Skies Syndrome":** Pilots talk about the "clear skies syndrome" as a detractor from SA. Basically this means falling into a false sense of security because everything is hunky-dory, blue skies ahead. Turbulence of all kinds can affect our lives at any given moment. Life is in a constant state of flux between calm and storm. Carry an umbrella! You cannot count on security; it is not a given. Any situation can change for the worse in the blink of an eye. Situational awareness is what allows you to be ready to handle these changes. Do not assume that, because you are safe in one moment, you will continue to be safe in the next.

- **Daydreaming:** Our minds float away all the time into that abstract space where we are somewhere in between an alpha state and a scene from a romantic movie where we are making out with a handsome hero. You do not need to stop daydreaming or fantasizing in order to maintain situational awareness. You do, however, need to develop the ability to snap out of it when your intuition cautions you or you identify early warning signals of danger. For example, when you are driving in your car, engrossed in your thoughts, and another car pulls up beside you, press the pause button on the daydream and reconnect to reality for a moment and assess the situation. If the person in the car is a little old lady, you are probably in a position to continue your daydream. If he is a man who is leering at you, keep your daydream on pause and tune back into prevention mode.

The Benefits of Situational Awareness

If you practice our exercises, you are giving your body and mind the chance to acquire training. The intention behind training in situational awareness is to allow the cumulative effect to take hold. Your body and mind are like a sophisticated laboratory that specializes in one thing: you. When you train yourself in any new practice, you are programming your limbic system (the primitive, emotional part of your brain) to take over in an emergency. Practicing situational awareness (both through isolated exercises and in your daily life) will boost your reaction time to any threat and allow you to respond appropriately. The best time to practice using situational awareness in your daily life is during any transition time, when you are moving from one place to another. Also, use SA anytime you are in public locations, parking lots, or public restrooms (common attack locations).

At first, practicing SA may feel like a burden but very quickly you will see how much it empowers you. Give yourself the chance to get over that initial hump and let yourself arrive at the place where SA becomes a natural habit. The reward is a bolstered level of control over your own response to danger and your ability to survive. There are also wonderful perks that come along with practicing SA. Your very presence becomes more noticeable and more impressive. You will emit a self-confidence that is attractive to people and people will respond to you in a positive way. When practiced regularly, it will not be long before you make situational awareness a habit, one that does not require much energy. In the beginning, practicing SA may feel a bit stressful or distracting, but very soon it will become part of your daily life and you will not notice that you are doing it until the moment arrives when something or someone suspicious or threatening enters your sphere. At that moment, because you have been practicing situational awareness, your intuition and senses will be in a heightened state and you will easily detect danger. Remember: Situational awareness is your forgotten instinct. Instinct is instant.

When you take responsibility for yourself and make the practice of situational awareness a habit, you will reap the following rewards:

- Honed intuition skills.
- Heightened awareness level.
- Improved ability to sense any kind of danger or threat much more quickly.
- A sense of empowerment and greater control over your environment, your own safety, as well as your decisions and choices.
- A well-developed early warning system for prevention of crime and violence.
- The ability to develop clear boundaries.
- Greater self-confidence and connection with yourself and your perceptions.
- Enhanced ability to respond and function in the event you are attacked.

Developing strong situational awareness is really a matter of remembering your survival instinct. All animals in the wild have an awareness of their predators and develop natural, instinctive methods of avoiding danger from these predators. As we have become a more civilized species, in some ways women have dropped their guard. Remember, it is our nature to avoid conflict. Ironically, *avoiding conflict is what prevention is all about.* We should be skilled at prevention, yet we are not. Our nurturing nature sometimes works against us when it could so easily work for us. We have to reboot our survival instinct by learning some new survival tools and taking some we already have out of storage and shaking off the dust.

The truth is that predators are out there in abundance and they are sneaky. You may encounter several on any given day and they will be sizing you up as a potential victim. Having good situational awareness means developing a subtle alertness that allows you to tune in to the predator mindset. Train yourself to be in a state of mind where you are ready for trouble. This does not mean you should be on edge all day long, suspicious of every look you receive. It simply means allowing your basic survival instinct to guide you when you encounter others. And remember, predators can be strangers, co-workers, friends, family members, teachers, clergy, health care providers, anyone.

Many readers may initially object to living a life which incorporates situational awareness on the basis that they feel uncomfortable living in a way that makes them mistrustful of everyone. Unfortunately, predators are not going away. Reality dictates that we must defend and protect ourselves from potential threats. Yet, developing strong situational awareness is not equivalent to becoming mistrustful of everyone you meet. On the contrary, it means activating a comprehensive awareness about everyone you encounter so that you can assess all of their qualities, good and bad, and take them at face value in a non-emotional way. To some extent you are probably already practicing SA every day. For example, most of us drive somewhat defensively. This does not mean that we mistrust every other driver in our midst, but we are aware of those vehicles around us and we do not dismiss the potential for an accident if one of those drivers behaves unpredictably.

Imagine how beneficial the practice of SA becomes for the teenage girl who tends to overrate the boy she has a crush on and "can't live without." Before she jumps into the emotional, crush phase, it behooves her to simply size up this boy, bearing in mind that he could be a threat and then allowing her instinct and sensibility to guide her rather than the swooning effects of that adrenaline crush rush. This is not to say that she should not enjoy the crush rush; it is a terrific feeling and one of life's more dazzling experiences. But before she abandons herself, and in fact while she is abandoning herself to those emotions, she should maintain her SA mindset. That way, if crush boy becomes predator boy she will see the signals early on and be able to separate her SA self from her emotional self and take the appropriate actions to protect herself.

The reality is that we women owe nothing to any strange men who approach us or to anyone who intends us harm. We do not owe predators the courtesy of the benefit of the doubt about their intentions towards us. And we do not owe anyone the benefit of the doubt when it comes to our trust and personal safety. People need to prove their worth to us to gain our trust, just as we must prove our worth and intentions to them. But in our giving, trustful nature we often forget this tenet and we hand over our open, accommodating, trusting nature before discerning if the receiver might take advantage of or abuse our good intentions.

Somewhere along the evolutionary chain women seem to have lost touch with their instinct to survive. We have replaced this instinctive programming with denial, fear, and an excess of trust towards everyone we encounter. Were we still living in caves, defending our young and scrounging for food, this survival instinct would still be honed. Our civilized, evolved nature is noticeably lacking in basic survival tendencies. This is one reason we see so many women being victimized, even in sophisticated, western societies.

It is time to empower our species by replenishing the female gene pool with new ways of adapting and thriving. If behaviors, adaptation, and survival skills are handed down on a genetic level, how is it that we are losing touch with this key mechanism so relevant to the survival of our species? We believe that if women actively participate in their own evolution by developing situational awareness skills, practicing them, and handing them down to our younger generations we can reboot this forgotten instinct. By integrating situational awareness into our daily lives we remember and re-train our survival instinct, thereby *complementing* our innate nature to resolve conflict and create a happy ending. As we make a stand for ourselves, we contribute to decreasing the violence against us. Recovery from violent attacks takes a lot of time and emotional energy. Investing that time and energy in prevention is much more sensible. As every woman reboots and strengthens her innate survival instinct, she redeems the potential victim by replacing her with the empowered woman who uses prevention to take ownership of and responsibility for her own security.

At the crux of the matter, always this primordial desire to survive...

CHAPTER TWO

PRIVACY AND IDENTITY

There is the one who arrives suddenly
interrupts the sanctuary of self
and digs the hollow hole of danger

Your situational awareness practice can be seriously undermined if you do not also develop the habit of retaining your privacy and closely guarding any personal information that pertains to your identity. Privacy issues abound in our world today and identity theft has become a serious threat we all face. For women, a large part of our security relates directly to the amount of information we release to predators, both knowingly and unwittingly. We paint our own self-portrait every time we encounter someone new. Imagine yourself on an airplane flight talking to the person sitting next to you. How much personal information will you reveal? At what point do you decide that social courtesy and basic friendliness can become a liability? How do you know if you are putting yourself in danger? There is so much ambiguity surrounding these situations and, again, women have been conditioned to appease. We do not want to be rude, unfriendly, or unkind; yet we *must* shift our priority to staying safe. It is maddening trying to determine where to draw the line in terms of being "too friendly." The voice of our internal monologue cries out with resentment that we even have to consider protecting ourselves. We yearn to be able to relax and not be fearful of every stranger we meet. However, if we guard our personal information with the same level of attention we give to our practice of situational awareness, we can easily develop a working system of security that does not inhibit our ability to remain friendly, cordial, pleasant, and feminine.

Consider your privacy as a "need to know" policy. Only release the information you feel comfortable with and no more. Consider what others "need" to know about you and only extend this information if you feel safe doing so. This includes everything from using discretion when giving out your social security number to closing your blinds at night so that a predator cannot see in and collect information on your whereabouts in your home. Everyone wants our social security numbers these days, but only certain people truly "need to know" them. When you feel too lazy to close the blinds because you think no one is in the vicinity, imagine a predator with a pair of binoculars hiding out in the woods behind your home. Does he "need to know" you are undressing? Of course not!

In future chapters we will explore in depth how predators use the information they collect to plan their attacks. Cut them off from access to this information and you will very quickly minimize your chances of becoming a target. This is the heart of prevention; this is empowerment at work. Remember that the majority of predators know they will be committing a crime when they execute their hostile acts against you. In addition, the vast majority of criminals are recidivists. Regardless if they are new to crime or are repeat offenders, they do not want to be caught and punished; thus they will collect information in order to plan carefully so that they get away with their crimes.

If five different women are walking down the same street, each carrying a purse, a purse snatcher does not just randomly pick one to target. He will pick the target that best ensures a successful snatch. The target who walks by carrying her purse confidently and is obviously emboldened with a strong aura that she is aware of her surroundings and situation has just given this predator information about herself that will alter how he perceives her as a potential target. The woman who carries her purse half unzipped while she balances grocery bags and chats on her cell phone is giving the predator an entirely different set of information about herself. It is not simply that she exudes an aura of being spaced-out or scattered. It is also that the predator can look inside the purse, can see her hands are full, can hear her focus is on the phone call, and can watch her movements without being detected because she is otherwise engaged. This is all information. The predator can now plan the snatch because she has just handed over the critical information necessary for him to succeed in his attack.

You are in charge, for the most part, of the information you will release about yourself. Even if a predator collects information on you, you still have the ability to prevent him from using it against you. Why make things easy on him? Why put yourself at risk unnecessarily? One of the main reasons women give out so much information on themselves is that they do not want to be 'rude.' It is difficult; people put us on the spot all the time with their questions and we have to think quickly before we respond. The best defense against this is to train yourself to give certain types of responses to certain questions, no matter who is asking them. For example, you might always give out your P.O. Box information (if you have one) when anyone asks for your address. Or, if someone asks where you live you might habitually respond by naming a general part of the city, versus your street name. You can always elaborate on an answer or add more information later. Editing your responses to questions is the problem. Once you have said too much, you have said too much and you cannot take it back.

Below are some checklists you can use to train yourself to limit and control the amount of information you release when at home, out in public, at work, through the mail, and over the telephone. Make these habits that you practice regularly. Part of having situational awareness involves being tuned in to people who are trying to elicit private information about you. This is one of the early warning signals we discussed in the last chapter. Predators *need information about you* so that they can plan successful attacks. Do not give them this head start.

Privacy At Home

If you are targeted by any type of predator, he will likely try to determine where you live and collect information about the security of your home and your habits while you are there. He will watch for gaps in your residential security. For example, he may test how easily you will open the door when someone knocks or rings the bell. He may watch to see what service people are allowed to access your home. He may look for signs that you are out of town. If you are a college student living in a dorm or in your first apartment he may watch you in order to determine your class schedule or to verify if you live with a roommate.

In order to protect your identity and to guard your information, put yourself in his shoes and consider where and how he can collect information about you at your residence. Then take the following list of tips as your defenses against him.

- Answer the door to strangers from inside by using your voice and a peep hole. When you are close to the door, yell out "I'll get it, Jim!" (or any male name). Do not allow access to any service people unless you initiated an appointment. If someone appears at your door selling firewood or something you need, ask him to leave a business card so you can do due diligence on him first. Tell him you do not open the door for strangers. If he claims to be from one of the utility companies, ask for his name and badge number and call the company in question to ascertain that he is there legitimately. (One ploy used by burglars is the guise of a utility company service call. They may even present fake badges).

- If you have an appointment with a service provider, have a male friend or family member present. Close doors and limit access to rooms that do not relate to the service being provided. Be aware of what is laying out on tables and countertops. Put away any papers that contain personal information, such as bank statements, information on any organizations or clubs you belong to, invitations to parties, etc. Turn around calendars if you normally indicate your schedule and appointments on them. Do not dress in provocative clothing. Designate a bathroom for them to use and do not leave anything in it, such as tampons, birth control pills, or prescription drugs. These intimate details should be kept private. Be aware of what books are in sight. Any self-help books, for example, may reveal information about you that a predator can exploit. Sterilize the environment so that your identity and personality are not written all over the walls and surfaces.

- Do not allow your computer to be repaired out of your line of sight, unless you mail it in to the manufacturer.

- Instruct your bank not to mail your new checks or credit cards to your home. Instead, request that you pick them up at the bank. Do not put personal information on the check. If you have a P.O. Box, use that as your address. Do not have your phone number or driver's license number preprinted on your checks. *Never ever* preprint your social security number on checks!

- When you travel, stop deliveries of newspapers and have the post office hold your mail. Arrange for lawn care if you will be gone a long time. Leave some lights on, preferably by using timers.

- On trash collection day put out the trash that morning, not the night before. (In some counties it is legal for people to take trash that is left out on the street. People who want to steal your identity may begin by taking your trash and sifting through it for useful information).

- If you are dating, for the first few date Always keep doors locked. Keep blinds and curtains closed after dark, especially in the bedroom. Do not be lazy about this (even if you live in a rural area). If you have a home alarm system, use it both when you are at home and when you are away.

- Shred or burn any documents that contain your private information, such as new credit card offers that come in the mail, old statements from any accounts (including utilities, bank accounts, insurance policies, etc.).

- Do not leave bills with checks in the envelopes in your mailbox (you make it too easy for someone to steal your checks and forge blank ones). Mail all bills at the post office yourself.
- Instruct your friends that, if they intend to drop by with a friend, they need your permission first.
- s drive yourself and meet in a public place so your date will not know where you live. Although this may sound extreme, consider that if the date goes terribly wrong you will have prevented allowing this man to know where you live. If he asks, just say the general area, not the street name.
- If you are dating someone you trust and have given him your address, clarify that he must first get your permission before bringing over anyone to your home, even if it is a trusted friend of his.
- Always have dates and new male friends call before they come over, instead of just dropping by the house unannounced. When you have your date drop by, call a friend to let her know so that someone else is aware this person is coming to your home.

Privacy in Public

Whenever you are out in public you subject yourself to the potential that a predator may focus his attention on you. Since predators study their targets, if one focuses on you he will be interested in gathering as much information about you as he can. He will likely try to close in on you either by eavesdropping or by initiating some type of contact with you. He will also be watching your appearance, including your dress, mannerisms, vehicle, any accessories you are carrying, and anyone who is accompanying you. He may follow you or lurk around in your vicinity to pick up any tidbit of information he can use against you.

The following tips will help you to guard your information closely so that he cannot access it and harm you as a result.

- Do not broadcast personal information about yourself (such as travel plans, personal problems, where you live and work) when in earshot of others.
- Do not discuss your schedule for the day with strangers (including any appointments, meetings, places you might go to shop, modes of transportation you will use).
- If you are discussing where you live or work, talk about general areas of town, not specific streets or company names.
- Do not display your name on anything, such as your keychain. If you wear a nametag at work, put it inside your purse when out in public.
- Cover up the Vehicle Identification Number (VIN) on your vehicle windshield (this number can be used in a fraudulent scheme to sell another vehicle that is identical to yours).
- Keep parking decals or permits hidden in your vehicle (especially if they indicate anything about where you live, work, go to school), unless you are using them at a specific location.
- Do not display information about organizations to which you belong, as this will give predators an "in" for approaching you or for determining your habits and potential whereabouts.
- Do not use bumper stickers that associate you with any particular cause or organization. Sometimes these can agitate a predator and cause him to consider you as a target just because he disagrees with your viewpoint. Or, he now knows he can strike up a conversation with you and feign alignment with your viewpoint as a way to manipulate you.
- Be aware of any data you release to store clerks, especially phone numbers. Always be aware of those in earshot when you release any information. Request that you write down the information on a form

versus giving it out verbally with strangers standing in line right beside you.

- At the bank, ask to sit down with a representative when you need to discuss any personal information regarding your accounts.
- Do not fill out contest information sheets, unless you are willing to put that information into the hands of strangers.
- Consider getting a P.O. Box so that you can give out that address instead of your home address.

Privacy at Work

The potential for work related violence and harassment is reason enough for protecting your privacy and identity at work. Given that people change jobs so frequently, your workplace may be a source of change that brings with it the potential for new threats. Your co-workers have the opportunity to learn a lot about you and your private life if you let them. If one of them turns out to be a predator who is interested in targeting you, you may be at a major disadvantage if you have not been careful to guard your privacy and identity.

The following tips can be applied if you are beginning a new job or have been working at the same place for years:

- Until you have established trust with co-workers, guard your personal information and do not display photos of loved ones (in particular, children).
- Realize that the workplace is often a breeding ground for gossip. Even if you are very close to some co-workers and not others, the information you release to any of them is out of your control and may become fodder for office gossip. Any private information you share with a co-worker is now out of your hands and may be given to a third party whom you do not know. Distinguish between co-

workers who actually become friends and those who remain colleagues.

- When a newly hired co-worker arrives, take the time to establish trust with this person before revealing personal information to him/her.
- Shred or burn any documents containing private information that you no longer need.
- Do not leave personal items unattended when you are away from your workspace or cubicle. Take your purse with you wherever you go.
- Avoid giving out private information over the phone or through e-mails when at work. Be aware of who is in earshot when you are making any personal calls over the phone. E-mail at work is often unsecured and may be monitored by your employer.
- If you wear any type of identification badge, do not wear it out in public on your lunch break or when running errands. Never leave your ID badge unsecured at work.
- If you have a designated parking spot, vary your routine and park elsewhere on randomly designated days. If your parking space has a placard with your name on it, remove it if you are an executive, hold a high position, or are under high threat.
- Be alert to anyone trying to elicit specific information about your job. Keep it general and vague. Maintain a low profile with strangers regarding your work.
- Do not use the same passwords for your work computers or e-mail as the ones you use at home. Do not specify your gender in your e-mail address. It is best if you can have a generic e-mail address for work, such as "administration@mycompanyname.com."

Telephone and Mail Privacy

Predators intending to steal your identity will often target you by telephone or will attempt to steal your mail. Their objective is to collect information on your personal accounts. They are particularly interested in your social security number and any financial account and pin numbers they can access. Other predators may be using the phone or mail as a way of contacting you. Stalkers often use the phone and leave threatening messages or send unsolicited gifts or correspondences through the mail.

Depending on the threat level you are facing, use the following tips to protect yourself and your identity:

- If you can afford it, have an unlisted phone number.
- If you live alone and want a listed number, only use your first initial and last name in the listing. You can also use a male name; that way when someone calls and asks for that person, you will know he/she got the number out of the telephone book. Do not list your address.
- Have a male family member or friend record the message on your answering machine or voice mail. If you want to record one in your voice, do not say your name or number. Say something general such as: "We are not available. Please leave a message." Even if you live alone, saying "we" is advised.
- Get on "No Call Lists" to avoid unsolicited calls from telemarketers.
- Have caller ID and do not answer calls from numbers you do not recognize. Let the machine or voice mail take the call.
- Be aware of calls (especially at work) from "Social Engineers" who will try to elicit specific private information, such as computer passwords and social security numbers.
- Do not give out your social security number over the phone unless you initiated the call or you are giving it to a trusted party, such as your bank, health care professional, or insurance agent.
- When someone calls and asks for an unfamiliar person, ask them what number they dialed. If they recite your number, simply say: "No one lives here by that name." If they recite the wrong number, tell them they dialed incorrectly. Never tell them your number or name.

- Use discretion about giving out your phone number. If you are single and a man asks for your number, get his instead so that you get to control the phone calls. When you know him better and if you trust him, then give him your number. You can also get an inexpensive 'pay as you go' cell phone (with phone cards for minutes) and give out that number instead.

- Instruct telemarketers or charities to mail you the information (if you are interested). Tell them you do not do anything over the phone. If they ask for your address, only give it out if you know the organization and feel comfortable (often the caller will already have your address).

- Contact your bank for information on how to be taken off any lists for unsolicited materials from credit bureaus.

- Do not open any suspicious packages if you are in a high threat situation (for example, if you suspect you have a stalker).

- Stop mail delivery when you go out of town.

- Take outgoing mail to the post office rather than leaving it in your mailbox. When standing in line at the post office make sure your return address is not visible to others who are waiting next to you (there is no reason to advertise where you live).

We provide these suggestions to help you stay safe. We realize that not everyone will follow all of them at all times. We often make mistakes ourselves. It can be difficult to keep track of protecting one's identity these days. The basic idea, however, is to combine your situational awareness with a degree of sensitivity about the information you are releasing about yourself.

One way to accomplish retaining your privacy and identity is to have a plan for that aspect of your life. For example, you might decide that your plan for dealing with solicitors who come to your home is that you will never open the door to a stranger. That way when a solicitor knocks on your door you will have programmed a set response, such as calling out: "Please leave a brochure; we do not answer the door to strangers." Part of your plan might include posting a small sign on your door that reads: "No solicitors please." Once you establish your plan, you will be more likely to respond appropriately. However, even with a plan, you might succumb and open the door one day. If so, recognize you violated your intended response and remind yourself to practice your plan in the future.

You will make mistakes and have setbacks; we all do. If you make a mistake and walk away from a conversation with a stranger feeling as though you said too much, you probably said too much. Learn from the experience. Check yourself emotionally. What was it that caused you to say too much? Were you afraid of being rude? Was it just carelessness? Did you feel awkward keeping the information to a minimum? Were there any awkward moments in the conversation that you did not know how to handle? Review the incident and ask yourself, "How could I have handled that better?" Take the lessons learned for use in the future.

If you feel you might have put yourself in danger with whatever information you released, take the necessary steps to protect yourself. For example, if you told a man where you live on a first date, watch for his vehicle in the area of your home. If you announced to your neighbor that you are going out of town tomorrow and her tree trimmer was in earshot, write down the information on his truck (license plate number, his description, the date) just in case you return and your home was burglarized (we mean no offense to tree trimmers here). The point is, if you make a mistake by releasing information that puts you at risk, heighten your situational awareness around the incident, as warranted by the threat, and use back-up methods to help you do damage control.

Empowerment includes taking ownership of your personal information. This means that you get to be the person in charge of your privacy and identity. As we learn to respect and protect our own privacy and identity, we become role models for the other women and girls in our lives. We train one another and support one another in preventing danger. We also train the men in our lives to respect our boundaries and not encroach on our privacy. By practicing over time and allowing ourselves the process of trial and error we can learn to prevent our privacy and identity from becoming exploited by predators. Protecting your identity and maintaining situational awareness are daily methods of proactive prevention. Every time you take a proactive prevention measure you nudge one tooth in the cogwheel of your personal security forward, thereby moving the corresponding cogwheel of all women's security forward as well. Your security matters to you and to all women.

CHAPTER THREE

DETERMINING THE DANGER: RISK/THREAT ASSESSMENT

*Life's big scary
is that anything can happen
at anytime*

You can easily take a proactive look at your life from the standpoint of assessing the possible threats you face and then determining the risk level you are willing to accept. One of the best ways to assess your own personal security is to create what is known as a risk/threat assessment for yourself and your family. It is very easy to conduct a risk/threat assessment and it will not take up much of your time. We advise updating it whenever you have a significant change in your schedule or routine, or any life change that alters your patterns. The idea is to list or chart the changing risk level you face, based on the changing threats against you. In this chapter we will walk you through one and provide you with a basic model to follow. Once you learn the process, you can even conduct a risk/threat assessment mentally, on the spot if need be.

The overall idea behind conducting a risk/threat assessment is simple: In order to identify, evaluate, and mitigate your risks, you must first identify the potential threats against you and then determine your level of vulnerability. Since you may not work in any security related field, we are providing you with the same type of tool security professionals use successfully every day. Before beginning your formal risk/threat assessment we suggest you answer the following questions:

- **Current Events:** What is happening in your life currently that puts you at risk of becoming a victim? For example: Do you engage in any activities that involve risk, such as walking your dog after dark, going out on blind dates, parking in a poorly lit garage, etc.? Do you live or work in a dangerous area?
- **Recent Events:** What has happened recently that may be affecting your risk level? For example: Have you gone through a bad break up or divorce; a sexual harassment encounter; a recent move, etc.?
- **Past Events:** What has happened in the past that might cause you to be at risk? For example: Did you fire a disgruntled employee or have an argument with a volatile person?
- **Crimes in My Area:** What has been happening recently in the geographical areas you frequent, such as near your residence and workplace, (rapes; home intrusions; car jackings; muggings, etc.)?
- **Fears:** What fears do you have, no matter how irrational they may seem, about hypothetical attacks that could happen to you (being stalked, raped, or the victim of a terrorist attack)?

We begin with these questions because every woman has her own unique set of experiences and circumstances. Your personal security is just that: personal. The best way for you to stay safe is to look at your life and analyze the risks you face due to your unique set of circumstances.

Before beginning your risk assessment, we suggest you fill out the Personal Security Profile in Appendix B. Doing this will bring your attention to your personal routines and activities, thereby allowing you to assess the risks against you more realistically. Attackers and criminals will try to exploit your habits and routines. They will collect information on you in order to do so. If you take a fresh look at your own habits and routines, you will see what predators see. Be sure that you are careful with this document. Whether you fill it out in this book, on paper or on your computer, guard your personal information!

Risk Assessment

Your risk assessment will enable you to answer the following questions:

1.   Have you received any implied and/or expressed threats?
2.   Do any of these threats put you at high risk of danger? Medium risk? Low risk?
3.   What factors determine your risk level? Do certain circumstances that affect your life contribute to increasing the threats against you, such as where you live or where you park your car at work?
4.   What preventative courses of action can you take to mitigate the risks? What can you do to minimize your risk for each threat you face, given your financial means, time restraints, and your physical capabilities and limitations?
5.   What level of risk will you face after implementing these preventative courses of action? (The objective is, of course, to take actions that will substantially lower your level of risk).

When conducting your risk assessment you are considering where, when, why, and how much you are at risk. You can either use a laundry list format or a chart format. We are using a chart because it is really the easiest way to look at the big picture all at once.   When you make your risk/threat assessment chart be sure to keep it in a safe place so that you protect your private information.

Risk/Threat Assessment Chart

Column One: You will begin your chart by determining and listing what threats you have against you. Your threats consist of the types of potential crimes and attacks that could occur to you. Start by listing any specific threats, such as from a disgruntled employee or an estranged husband. These threats could be implied as well as expressed. For example, an angry ex-husband who has argued with his ex-wife might make an ambiguous comment like: "Don't expect me to just walk away from this." Because of the heated argument he might be implying that he could cause trouble for his ex-wife. She, therefore, will determine that she might be at risk of being harmed by him. However, she might determine that the risk is low since he is not a drinker, does not use drugs, and has no history of being violent with her or anyone else. On the contrary, if he did have an alcohol or drug abuse problem or any history of violence she might determine the risk is high that he will become physically abusive to her. In addition, if he expressly stated a threat, such as: "I'm going to make sure you pay for all the misery you caused me," the ex-wife will have greater reason to assume she is at high risk of being harmed by him.

Next on your list should be attacks that occur in your immediate geographical area. Since crime is often very widespread and not necessarily limited to "bad areas," you should include attacks that are possible regardless of where you are. Car jacking is an example; it can occur practically anywhere, especially to women.

We will use our medium threat character, Victoria, to teach you how to fill out a risk/threat assessment.

Victoria is a dental assistant. She works part time for a dentist in San Francisco. His office is located downtown near the financial district. She drives to work and usually stops at a neighborhood café for an espresso on her way to work. She parks in a parking garage at the office building where she works. After work she drives to the nearby Marina district to pick up her twelve year old son, Jake, from school. They drive home to their small apartment in a suburb outside of the city. Jake spends the weekends with his father. Victoria normally stays home on Friday nights because her ex-husband comes to pick up Jake for the weekend. On Saturday afternoons Victoria rides her bike alone through Golden Gate Park. On Saturday nights she either goes out with her girlfriends or has a date.

After her divorce, Victoria became much more aware of security. Living with her son without the protection of her husband made her feel very vulnerable. Victoria decided to take charge of the situation and do everything possible to protect herself and her son from danger. She decided to begin by conducting a risk/threat assessment.

Victoria began her chart with the list of threats she and her son face, including threats that are based on particular circumstances about their lives, on recent crimes in geographical areas that are significant to them, and on hypothetical fears.

	Threat
1.	**Current Events:** I ride my bike alone through Golden Gate Park every Saturday.
2.	**Recent Events:** Man at café stares at me every morning and has asked me for personal information. There is something creepy about him and I feel fear whenever I see him.
3.	**Past events:** Former boyfriend threatened to "never give up" on winning me back after I broke it off with him.
4.	**Crimes in my area:** Sexual Assault, Rape and Home Intrusion
5.	**Crimes in my area:** Children kidnapped
6.	**Crimes in my area:**

	Car Jacking	
7.	**Crimes in my area:** Vandalism to home or auto	
8.	**Fears:** Terrorist Attack	

Column Two: Now that she has listed the threats she and Jake face, she will estimate the risk level of each threat, rating them as either low, medium, or high.

Column Three: She will also add a column where she can list the factors that affect the risk level. In other words, how did she determine she was at low risk for one threat and at high risk for another? What factors influence the risk level?

	Threat	Estimated Risk	Risk Factors
1	**Current Events:** I ride my bike alone through Golden Gate Park every Saturday.	Medium	There are many wooded and overgrown areas. Rapes have been reported.
2.	**Recent Events:** Man at café stares at me every morning and has asked me for personal information. There is something creepy about him and I feel fear whenever I see him.	High	I saw him recently sitting on a bench outside my place of work. I intuitively felt I was in danger.
3.	**Past events:** Former boyfriend threatened to "never give up" on winning me back after I broke off our relationship.	Low	I haven't seen any sign of him since our break up 15 years ago and I heard from his best friend that he moved out of state.

4.	**Crimes in my area:** Sexual Assault or Rape and Home Intrusion.	Medium	There have been two rapes of women in my area of town in the last year. The attacks occurred in the home.

Frequent articles have appeared in the newspapers recently about attacks on women in parking garages in the financial district. |
5.	**Crimes in my area:** Children kidnapped	Medium	There have been children kidnapped, raped, and murdered in my city 6 times in the last year.
6.	**Crimes in my area:** Car Jacking	Medium	In the past 8 months several women in my city have been car jacked from grocery or convenience store parking lots.
7.	**Crimes in my area:** Vandalism to home or auto	Medium	It occurs frequently all over the city, but not especially in my neighborhood.
8.	**Fears:** Terrorist Attack	Low	I'm just a single mother living a normal life with a regular job.

Column Four: Victoria has listed her threats, the risk level, and the risk factors. Now it is time for her to take action and determine what she can do to protect herself and her child. She now adds a column where she can list the preventative courses of action she can take to mitigate these threats.

You will notice that Victoria mentions one preventative measure several times: surveillance detection. After reading Chapter Five you will see why she opts for this highly effective measure. She also mentions something called a "route review," which we discuss at length in Chapter Six.

Column Five: It is important that Victoria take another look at the risk level, once she has implemented her preventative courses of action. Did she substantially reduce the risk? If not, perhaps she should add more courses of action. You will notice that some of her threats required no preventative courses of action, while others required she take some strong actions to reduce her risk.

	Threat	Estimat -ed Risk	Risk Factors	Preventative Course of Action	Estimated Residual Risk
1	Current Events: I ride my bike alone through Golden Gate Park every Saturday	Medium	There are many wooded and overgrown areas. Rapes have been reported.	Avoid secluded areas. Ride with friends or close to other cyclists. Carry a whistle around my neck and attach an air horn to my bicycle.	Low
2	Recent Events: Man at café stares at me every morning and has asked me for personal infor- mation. There is some- thing creepy about him and I feel fear whenever I see him.	High	I saw him recently sitting on a bench outside my place of work. I intuitively felt I was in danger.	Inform my family, nearby neighbors and key work associates. Give them his description and ask them to watch for him and record any pertinent information. Improve my home and vehicle security by keeping doors locked at all times. Install a home alarm. Conduct route reviews of all of my typical travel. Use basic surveillance detection to determine if he is watching me, my home, or my family. Practice using my cell phone.	Medium

				camera so that I am ready to discreetly obtain a photo of him if I see him again. If the situation escalates, stop going to the café.	
3	Past events: Former boy-friend threat-ened to "never give up" on winning me back after I broke off our relation-ship.	Low	I haven't seen any sign of him since our break up 8 months ago and I heard from his best friend that he moved out of state.	No additional preventative courses of action required.	Low

| 4 | Crimes in my area: Sexual Assault or Rape | Medium | There have been two rapes of women in my area of town in the last year. The attacks occurred in the home.

Frequent articles have appeared in the newspapers recently about attacks on women in parking garages in the financial district. | Ask the local police department about any specific techniques used in the home intrusions and any specific information about the rapes that was not released to the public.

Inspect the security status of my home.

Install a home alarm or get a dog.

Give basic home surveillance detection and response guidance to Jake and my ex-husband.

Carry a flashlight and personal alarm when walking in any parking garage. | Low |
| 5 | Crimes in my area: Children Kid-napped | Medium | There have been children kidnapped, raped, and murdered in my city 6 times in the last year. | Ask the local police department about any information on specific techniques or patterns in the past attacks that was not released to the public. | Low |

| | | | | Provide guidance and training to my son about emergency communication, basic surveillance detection, and basic home security procedures, such as not answering the door to strangers.

Coordinate with local police and Jake's school to get surveillance detection training for teachers and security guards.

Start a Neighborhood Watch program on my street.

My ex-husband and I can use basic surveillance detection measures at home and when dropping off Jake at school or activities. | |
|---|---|---|---|---|---|
| 6 | Crimes in my area: Car Jacking | Medium | In the past 8 months several women in my city have been car jacked from grocery or convenience store parking | Research car jacking counter-measures.

Use situational awareness and surveillance detection when driving and | Low |

			lots.	parking my vehicle.	
				Ask for evasive driving training course for my next birthday present.	
				Carry a cell phone at all times.	
				Keep my vehicle doors locked at all times.	
				Practice using the remote on my keychain to sound my car alarm.	
7	Crimes in my area: Vandalism to home or auto	Medium	It occurs frequently all over the city, but not especially in my neighborhood.	Conduct a home security inspection and make necessary changes. Coordinate with local law enforcement to give Neighborhood Watch and surveillance detection instruction to myself and other residents. Use basic surveillance detection around my home and on my street to look	Low

				for indicators of vandalism attempts.	
8	Fears: Terror- ist Attack	Low	I'm just a single mother living a normal life with a regular job.	Use situational awareness and surveillance detection techniques when in public places that may be targeted by terrorists.

If I travel abroad, choose places to visit that are not appealing targets for terrorists.

Put myself at ease by becoming more informed about the likelihood that terrorists would strike in my city and the locations they would choose to attack. | Low |

Do not sugar-coat this assessment. Keep it real. Risk assessment is a process that needs to be conducted with an objective mindset. It must also be reviewed periodically to be viable. Your initial assessment is the beginning of that process, but the element of risk changes as the level of threat evolves. As you can see, creating a risk assessment for yourself in the same way Victoria did is not terribly complex, but it is wonderfully effective. Taking the appropriate measures to reduce your risk is highly beneficial in that it will:

- Empower you to take the lead with your own security.
- Reduce your fears about being attacked and keep you conscious of the *reality* of the threats you face.
- Enhance your situational awareness by virtue of the fact that you are analyzing your risk level and are thereby placing it at the forefront of your mind.
- Prevent security gaps which will place you at greater risk.
- Provide you with a comprehensive security plan for all aspects of your life. Having a plan will enable you to take away the element of surprise from your attacker and to avoid being caught off guard (so that if you are attacked you can function and respond).

If this process seems like a daunting task or a huge hassle, consider that you nudge the cogwheel forward every day in many ways in order to mitigate risks in your life and the lives of your children. Perhaps you keep track of your diet, take vitamins or birth control pills. Maybe you keep up with getting shots for your small children. At work you follow up by writing memos and keeping files of correspondences. Every day you spend time protecting yourself in other areas of your life. Why not spend some of that time on your security? It will only take you an hour or so to create a risk/threat assessment chart and, once you have done so, it is easy to update it as changes occur which impact the risks you face.

Risks and threats evolve constantly, so we have to remain aware of the reality of the current threats we face and respond to them in ways we can accept and afford. The process of evolution includes adaptation. As the threats against women increase, we must adapt our responses to those threats by focusing our efforts on prevention. We encourage you to take an active role in this adaptation process by creating a risk assessment for yourself and your loved ones. If you are married or are in a relationship, do this with your partner. If you have children, you may want to conduct a separate assessment for them. This is a powerful tool because it puts you on the same playing field as potential aggressors. *You will begin the process of analyzing the very same information about yourself that they analyze when they study you as a target.* This is why security professionals conduct risk/threat assessments on a regular basis when protecting important people. You are as important as any politician, celebrity, or corporate executive. You deserve to know how to use this process to keep yourself and your family safe.

Once you have created your risk/threat assessment you will be in a much better position to develop a well-rounded personal security response. In the next chapter you will learn how to bolster your personal security by putting as many people in your corner as possible from whom you can receive some type of support in order to face the threats against you.

CHAPTER FOUR

YOU ARE NOT ALONE: ESTABLISHING A SUPPORT NETWORK

"Even in the worst of times I give my best to you."

--Sheryl Crow

One of the most powerful tools we have in our survival toolbox is our SUPNET (support network). When we involve other people, be they friends, family, professionals, or authorities, we increase our chances of avoiding becoming victims because we are stocking our box of tools with people who can help protect us from harm. Creating a SUPNET is an inexpensive way of immediately and exponentially bolstering your personal security. The more people we have out there reinforcing our safety the better. Think of all you do for others and do not hesitate to let them help you when you are in need.

If you are ever under threat or even attack, you must: take action to mitigate or escape the threat; commit to being decisive and following through on any actions you take; and then communicate to people in your SUPNET in order to receive guidance, encouragement, and the appropriate professional help. This advice is just common sense, but it is amazing how crippling fear can obscure your ability to think straight. The more you can take control and prepare yourself in advance to get help, the better able you will be to function and know where and when help is available.

Predators are often interested in soft, easy targets. Women who are physically and/or emotionally isolated in their lives make themselves softer targets because no one is around to help defend them. Predators have an uncanny ability to spot vulnerabilities in your demeanor. If they sense you have low self-esteem or are an isolated woman, they will capitalize on your weaknesses. Your compromised demeanor will trigger them to tune in and further scrutinize you as a potential target. You never need to feel embarrassed about becoming a potential target or victim of a crime, but on some level many women fall prey to feelings of inferiority about needing to ask for help. Many of us feel we will be burdening others if we ask for assistance or we feel we are inadequate for doing so. Shift your paradigm. Shake up your mental template. You are never alone.

Creating a SUPNET is one of the healthiest, most stabilizing actions women can take. Women tend to isolate themselves and fall easily into the mode of "not wanting to bother people" with their problems. This is a mistake. If someone you approach for help is hesitant, they can always refuse to help you. They may, however, point you in the direction of someone else who can help you, such as an organization with which you are unfamiliar. Social advocacy and community programs exist in most parts of our country. Emergency hotlines, law enforcement, legal aid, and other professionals such as therapists provide additional avenues of support. It never hurts to ask for help, but it may hurt terribly not to ask. Part of the reason women isolate themselves is that they do not want to involve too many people in what they might perceive to be private, possibly embarrassing situations. This is understandable, especially if any kind of abuse or domestic violence is involved. The shame that can go along with these incidences is a valid emotion. But personal security is not based on emotions; it is based on objectivity, practicality, and prevention.

One exercise we recommend is called "Netting." The idea is to create a large net for yourself which begins with a list of people you intend to include in your SUPNET. You can start simply by making a list of people you know who, in some way, can offer you support. This could be anything from babysitting support to someone you can call to come over to your house if you are afraid of being bothered by a menacing landlord. You have friends, family, church members, co-workers, neighbors, and even some peripheral people in your life who may become valuable resources if you are ever in trouble. You can also access professional support groups in your area for all kinds of problems, such as domestic abuse, molestation, and rape (see Appendix E).

The second part of the Netting exercise involves listing all the safe locations in your area. Imagine you are being followed to work. Where along your route can you seek safety? Are there any police stations, hospitals, crowded public locations, banks with security cameras, homes of people you know along your route? Consider the operating hours so that, if you are traveling at night, you are aware of which of these safe locations will be open.

Now turn to communications. Do you have OnStar in your vehicle, a cell phone in your purse, or any other way to communicate to get help? If you are endangered, create a communications support network. Make sure phone numbers of people in your SUPNET are readily available in your purse and your vehicle and are clearly posted in your home (you can make an emergency cheat sheet that you always carry on your person wherever you go). Get your SUPNET members on speed dial in your cell phone, home phone, and work phone.

Your SUPNET will permeate all of your personal security plans for all aspects of your life. You are programming your internal survival mechanism by making these SUPNET lists and by taking the simple action of bringing the people in your SUPNET into the forefront of your mind. By listing them and defining the ways in which they can help you, you are giving yourself some mental preparation training as well as a practical way of getting yourself ready to seek help. It is also a kind of affirmation process for your psychology. You are basically saying to yourself: "I am a survivor; I will do everything I can to ready myself to ask for and seek help in the moment I need it." This has power! Readiness during any kind of an attack is the key to living through it (see Chapter Thirteen).

In the following example, you will see how the Netting exercise works:

Grace is in an abusive relationship with her boyfriend, Brian. He has, on multiple occasions, been verbally abusive with her and he hit her in the arm once, bruising her badly. Brian threatened to beat Grace if she told anyone about it. Brian made this threat because he wanted control over Grace. Brian's need for control is actually his weakness, but Grace has taken it on as her own and is too afraid to confront him or leave him. She is completely embarrassed by the turmoil in her relationship. Brian calmed down after the incident and was embarrassed that he hit her and threatened her. He became quiet and introverted for awhile, but over time his behavior escalated when he began verbally abusing her again.

Grace is a college graduate, has a respectable job at a law firm, and is a talented, competitive tennis player. She decided to make a list of all the people she can include in her support network. This does not mean she has to tell each of them about her circumstances, though in her situation the more people she tells the better (see Chapter Eight). What is important is that Grace realizes that, if it comes down to it, she could elicit some type of needed support from the people in her list. As afraid as she is, Grace knows deep down that she must protect herself, thus she discreetly takes action by establishing her SUPNET.

Grace's List

Person	Type of Support
1. Mom	Love; Advice; Spare Room.
2. Ralph	Big Brother; Rescuer; Alternate vehicle; Love; Physical Protection.
3. Penny	Best Friend; Great Listener; Safe Location; Will accompany me to support group meetings.

4. Mr. Hobbs   Most qualified lawyer in our firm; Will maintain confidentiality; Comforting, like a father figure who gives great advice.

5. Coach Keener   Will be there for me no matter what. Even though I'm embarrassed to tell her about this, she would stand by me.

6. Community Advocacy   Local chapter of Association for Abused Women is located close to my home. Their 24/7 emergency hotline is on my speed dial. I can go there for help in an emergency or call them for advice.

7. St. Mary's Church   Father Matthews is a great person to talk with if I am feeling lost and do not know how to break off the relationship safely.

8. Police Station   Closest is 5 minutes from my home.

9. Greg Sanderson   My accountant. Can provide financial advice if I need to relocate or seek the help of experts if Brian were to stalk me in the future after we break up.

Note: Obviously Grace would also add all the contact phone numbers of the people she listed above and so should you when completing your Netting exercise. She will also handle this document with discretion and so should you with your SUPNET list.

You do not know Grace, but reading her list probably makes you want to scream: "Wake up and smell the dysfunctional relationship!" The very fact that she has so many emergency contingency plans in her list is an early warning signal that she is in serious danger. If she read back all that she wrote, she might look at it more objectively and be able to more clearly see how unsafe a life she is living with Brian. One of the most powerful benefits of listing your support network and safe locations is that it forces you to face the truth about your threats. You are taking your risk assessment (Chapter Three) and are adding a safety buffer by identifying your sources of help. Often this process will be just the thing to make you step back and take a hard look at the risks you face and how you could mitigate them if you had the courage to make changes in your life.

You might discover when you create your own support network list that you are focused on a particular threat you face. Imagine a college girl whose list focuses on her friends and how they can help her prevent being slipped a date rape drug. Obviously if this girl requires a lot of support for this particular threat, that alone should be a wake up call to her that she is placing herself in danger from this threat too often. She can make a choice to change this.

Sometimes women have no choice but to put themselves in harm's way. If their place of employment is in a dangerous neighborhood, for example, they may not be able to make changes to avoid the threats they face. For these women, identifying and listing a support network and safe locations is critical because it places their attention on getting help should the threat catch up with them some day. When you create your SUPNET, you present opportunities for other women in your life to bolster their security as well. For example, imagine you work in a high threat area for crime. If you and the women with whom you work were to get together and make a collective effort, you could influence the policies and procedures at your place of employment. You stand a better chance of convincing your employer if you collectively approach him/her about adding more lights in the parking lot or having more guards on the night shift to escort women to their vehicles. You also form a bond with other women when you work together to demand that your security be taken seriously. This is powerful. It is the very reason women now have the right to vote; our ancestors worked together to make it so.

Think also of other ways you find support. You can support yourself by surrounding yourself with people who care about you and who are willing to help you. You can also surround yourself with support you glean from other aspects of your life, such as activities in which you participate that contribute to helping you feel supported. You may support yourself through your religious or spiritual practices, be they prayer or meditation. Perhaps being in nature is a source of support for you or engaging in some physical activity or sport. Our approach to your personal security is a holistic one in that we want you to know yourself well and be honest with yourself about both the external SUPNET you already have in place (through others) as well as the internal SUPNET you can and should create. Your internal SUPNET will include all of your sources of self-confidence and self-esteem, as well as your sources of inspiration and calming influences. The more balanced an individual you are, the better you will be able to support yourself internally, should your life be turned upside-down by a predator. The purposes behind creating your SUPNET include building self-confidence, self-esteem, and strengthening your security.

On the next page you will see something called a mind map (to learn more about mind maps see *Notes* section). The basic idea is to place a word in the center of the page and then draw images and write words that expound on the central idea. You can use different colored pens or pencils to make it vibrant. Our mind map is a sample we created by using the word SUPNET in the center. You will notice that many sources of support are included on the net, not just other people. If you make your own mind map as a starting point for creating your internal as well as external SUPNET, you may be able to approach this part of your personal security creatively and with a more expansive outlook. Mind maps are great fun and the best part is you need no artistic skill.

One of the most important reasons for having others in your corner to support you is that, if you are currently facing a threatening situation or end up in one in the future, your SUPNET can assist you with many of the new techniques you are about to learn by reading the rest of this book, in particular one called surveillance detection.

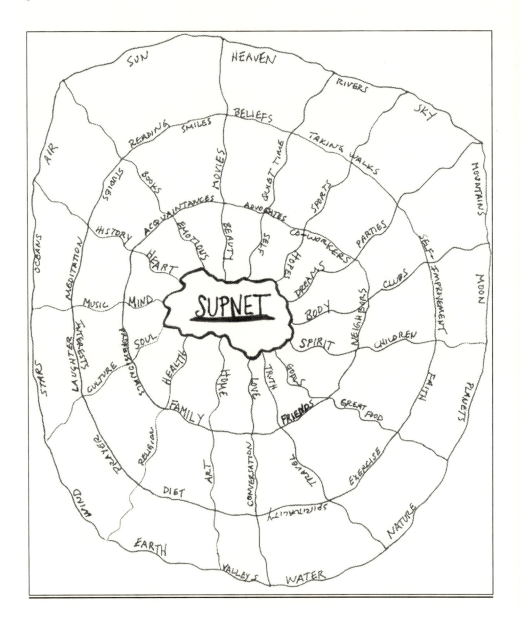

CHAPTER FIVE

SURVEILLANCE DETECTION:
THE CUTTING EDGE
OF PREVENTION

*"I was looking back to see if you were looking back at me
to see me looking back at you."*

--Massive Attack

Imagine what it would be like if a predator was watching you without your knowledge. What if he was studying your child's daily schedule and routine? How would you feel if you discovered you were secretly being photographed while out jogging or partying with your friends or going to your weekly manicure appointment? What would you do to protect yourself and your child?

You are about to be introduced to one of the most effective measures in existence for preventing both criminal and terrorist acts: Surveillance Detection (SD). Our intention is to introduce this practice into the mainstream so that women are informed about this powerful technique which, up until now, has been reserved for use primarily by security professionals protecting heads of state, government facilities, and elite corporate executives. After years of training surveillance detection operators all over the world, we know with certainty that average citizens are fully capable of utilizing this legal prevention method to bolster their personal security. (Our book: *Surveillance Detection: The Art of Prevention* explores the subject of SD in great detail. If you are in a high threat situation or are simply interested in learning more about SD see Appendix A).

The premise behind the practice of SD is that all crimes and terrorist attacks are stories. All stories have a beginning, middle, and end. Often people think that the story begins the moment the crime or attack is committed. This is a misconception; the actual crime or attack is the middle of the story. The beginning of the story is the planning phase carried out by the criminal or terrorist, which almost always involves surveillance. The end of the story includes the aftermath and repercussions of the crime/attack.

SD focuses on the beginning of the story because the common element in planning the vast majority of crimes and terrorist attacks is surveillance.

In order to be successful in committing a crime/attack, a predator (or someone associated with him) must get out there to collect information on his target. In order to do so, he must position himself within line of sight to his target. Thus, if the target is a person the predator must choose a location from which he can observe this person (either by using optics or the naked eye). If the target is a building, the predator must choose a location which offers him line of sight to the parts of the building that interest him (for example, he will want to watch any security procedures at the building and the entrances and exits will be important for him to study).

When potential victims are trained in surveillance detection they learn where to find these predators, what to look for, and when to look for it. Thus, they can detect the predators while they are in the early stages of their planning. Predators have an Achilles heel: their need to go on site to collect information in order to plan successfully. Practicing SD enables potential victims to legally and easily exploit this part of the predator's process. In this book we will elaborate on SD techniques that relate directly to the threats women face. We will teach you how to use this powerful prevention method to overcome these various threats.

First, a lesson in some basic terminology so that you learn to distinguish between the three groups of players in this game: Surveillance (SV); Surveillance Detection (SD); and Counter Surveillance (CS).

Rick parks his car down the street so that he can see Hadley's driveway. He situates his vehicle so that he is in a ready position to pull out and follow her. He uses his side mirror to look behind at her driveway entrance. He will follow her and, if the opportunity arises he is going to "get that bitch." Hadley is at the house now, so he parks and waits for her to depart. Rick is conducting <u>*surveillance.*</u>

Hadley, a single mom, living in the suburbs, works as a sales rep for a pharmaceutical company. Three months ago she filed a sexual harassment claim against Rick, one of the stock clerks working at the company. The end result was that Rick was fired and, as far as Hadley knows, he skipped town. Sometimes she lies awake at night worrying about retribution, but since three months have gone by without incident, she feels she and her two children are probably safe. Nonetheless, before she departs from her house, she always looks out from the upstairs window discreetly, through the Venetian blinds, to see if any strange vehicles are within line of sight to her driveway. Hadley is conducting <u>*surveillance detection*</u>.

Mary overheard her husband Bob talking to his friend Rick one night. Rick was divulging his plan to get revenge on Hadley. Rick explained to Bob that he had followed Hadley after she left work one day so that he could determine where she lives. Now that he knows where Hadley lives, he intends to watch her and make her pay for getting him fired. Mary could tell he was serious. She never liked Rick and did not want Bob to hang out with him. Mary called the local police and told them of Rick's plan. Officer Johnson was put on the case and began following Rick. Officer Johnson positioned his vehicle on a side street next to Hadley's street so that he could observe Rick as he put Hadley under surveillance. Officer Johnson is conducting <u>*counter surveillance*</u>.

Who Conducts Surveillance and Why?

Almost every crime story includes surveillance. Surveillance (SV) with a hostile intention can be conducted by pickpockets, carjackers, thieves, rapists, stalkers, murderers, and terrorists, to name a few. In this chapter and throughout the book you will see that we name them all 'surveillance' because it is easier to categorize them by this activity which normally precedes all of the above crimes. Also, we are trying to get you to focus on them at this early stage, so if you think about them as 'surveillance' you will be programming your mind to see them in action.

Hostile surveillance conducts purposeful observation of people, places, vehicles, and locations with the intention of collecting information which can be used in planning any type of hostile action, be it criminal or terrorist, against a specific target. Surveillance is also used as a method of collecting information on a variety of potential targets in order to eliminate target options and choose a target which satisfies the objectives of the attacker. For example, a rapist may put several women under surveillance at a particular location, such as a grocery store parking lot. His objective is to select the woman who is easiest and 'safest' for him to attack successfully (meaning he gets away with it because he is not caught). Criminals conduct surveillance because they want to plan carefully so that they do not get hurt or caught when committing their crimes.

Surveillance is a logical step for criminals to take. Put yourself in the shoes of a criminal for a moment. If you were planning to abduct a woman, what kinds of information would you need to collect to do so successfully? Obviously you would need to know where she lives, with whom she lives, what car she drives, where she works, what her schedule is, and so on. To collect this information, you would have to come out and be within line of sight to her home and workplace and other locations she frequents regularly. It would take you some time to study her. If you intended to snatch her while she was in her car driving to work, you would have to learn and study the routes she travels in order to determine the best location along her routes to abduct her. All of this takes time and puts the bad guys out in plain sight. Criminals are vulnerable during the surveillance stage because their victims can detect them.

Even attackers who strike in the moment and commit random crimes of opportunity are detectable. If you are SASD (meaning you are practicing both situational awareness and surveillance detection) you will spot a predator's suspicious behavior. The combination of your awareness and his wariness of being caught will likely cause him to avoid you. He will likely defer to a softer, easier target if he notices that you are SASD and are aware of his presence.

What is Surveillance Detection and How Will it Help Me?

Surveillance detection (SD) can be conducted by housewives, security personnel, executives, government agencies, and the military, again to name just a few. We will name all of these people 'surveillance detection' or 'SD' so that they are identified by their activity. Surveillance detection conducts purposeful observation of people, places, vehicles, and locations with the express purpose of determining whether or not surveillance is being conducted against a potential target. Conducting surveillance detection means watching the watcher.

You can either enlist the help from someone in your SUPNET to practice 'Buddy SD' or you can conduct 'Self SD' (meaning you can discreetly watch the surveillance and collect information on him yourself rather than employing someone in your SUPNET to conduct SD for you). You can also combine buddy SD with self SD. Regardless if you are conducting buddy SD or self SD, it is important that you never let on to the surveillance that you know you are being watched by him or that you are watching him. Likewise, your SD support should never let the surveillance be aware of his/her presence and surveillance detection activities. There are several important reasons for remaining discreet about your SD practice:

- You do not want to spook the surveillance or cause him to retreat and use tactics that are harder to detect.

- You do not want to trigger a confrontation or instigate an attack by putting him under pressure.

- Giving him a false sense of security and allowing him to relax (because he is unaware he is being watched) will cause him to drop his guard and make mistakes that you can detect.

- The longer he is out there watching you, the more evidence you can collect against him.

- You will gain time to plan and prepare to keep yourself safe and you will have more information to report to the authorities.

- The authorities will have more time and evidence to use to identify, apprehend, and prosecute the predator.

The focus of SD's observation (buddy or self SD) is to distinguish types of behavior and indicators of possible surveillance (discussed later in this chapter). SD practitioners report any such suspicious behaviors or indicators to the appropriate authorities. These reports are analyzed by the proper authorities, who will then determine an appropriate response to the threat. This response may include an investigation, an arrest, or a counter surveillance operation (meaning the authorities will put the people who are conducting surveillance under surveillance in order to learn more about them before taking further action).

As a basic overview, surveillance detection can be used by anyone who feels under threat for any reason. Surveillance detection can be applied as a prevention method against all crimes against women, including rape, abuse, stalking, abduction, molestation, mugging, robbery, car jacking; the list goes on.

If you are under threat or just want to make it a habit to practice SD, you can do it yourself or you can enlist the help of trusted family, friends, neighbors, or co-workers. The beauty of SD is that you get to take charge of your own security by becoming proactive and incorporating prevention into your life in an easy, legal way. You will nip the threat in the bud by using SD because you will see the surveillance early on and be able to involve the authorities in a timely manner. So many crimes against women occur because the victim has no idea she is being watched and studied as a target. Once the actual crime or attack occurs, she is totally caught off guard and only has seconds to react. Practicing SD puts you ahead of the attacker, on the offense, so to speak. SD gives you time to prepare, plan, and be ready to act on early warning signals of danger.

If women begin to practice surveillance detection on a regular basis, the end result will be that more predators will be caught and prosecuted. This is a huge step in the evolution of our empowerment, one that we can achieve both as individuals and collectively in our communities. Imagine how we can influence our security by using this simple, but powerful practice. Think of the impact we could have on fighting crime if all women learned to practice surveillance detection, thereby allowing them to spot predators early on and report them to the authorities.

What is Counter Surveillance and How is it Different from Surveillance Detection?

The only reason we want you to know about counter surveillance is that *we do not want you to practice it!* Counter surveillance (CS) is commonly conducted by professionals who are trying to exploit the hostile surveillance. Generally speaking, counter surveillance is an operational measure taken once it is determined that surveillance is being conducted. CS then places the surveillance operators under surveillance and uses the information they collect to manipulate, exploit, or apprehend them. Normally CS is conducted by intelligence agencies, law enforcement, and the military.

It is important to understand that counter surveillance is *not* an option for the average woman/citizen facing a threat. It is illegal for you to follow and conduct surveillance on anyone whom you detect conducting surveillance on you (unless you hire a licensed private investigator). You must remain a passive observer of them, out there simply to detect them and report them to the authorities. You cannot become an aggressor towards them by following them or pursuing them in any way. Confusing surveillance detection with counter surveillance can result in disaster. CS is a more aggressive, often illegal tactic that would put an untrained person at high risk of being seen by the surveillance or arrested by the police. We *only* recommend utilizing SD and *only* in a manner which is legal!

How do I Begin Practicing Surveillance Detection?

When conducting surveillance detection you will look for *types and indicators of surveillance*. When people conduct surveillance, they use specific techniques. If you learn about the basic methodology used by surveillance operators, you can easily begin to detect them.

Types and Indicators of Surveillance

It is important that you keep in mind that a predator working alone will normally conduct the surveillance himself. However, some predators will work with a partner. In addition, for more complex crimes such as abductions, the predators may work in teams. The surveillance team may be different from the actual attack team (this is also common in terrorist attacks).

STATIC SURVEILLANCE

Rick used a static position (parked in his car on Hadley's street) to watch Hadley as she left for work each day.

Static surveillance is the method wherein surveillance finds a static location (sitting on a park bench; sitting in a parked car; positioned behind a curtain on a window with a camera, etc.) and conducts the job while remaining in a fixed position.

When surveillance takes the time to use static positions they are able to collect a lot of information over a period of time. Try just sitting still and watching the world go by and you will be amazed at how much information you can collect simply by paying attention. However, the surveillance operators also put themselves at risk by remaining static; unless they are concealed, camouflaged, or have something to do which helps them to blend in well to the area (known as *cover*), they are very detectable. It is easy to spot them when they are static because you have ample time to study their behaviors.

Indicators of Static Surveillance:

- Any stranger sitting or parking at a location which gives him/her a good visual vantage point (line of sight) to the target.
- Anyone loitering in a position within line of sight to the target.
- Writing notes or drawing diagrams while fixating on the target.
- Behavior that correlates with or relates to the movement of the target or some security procedure that is significant (such as the shift change of the guards at a bank).
- Using a cell phone to call in to report movement of the target.
- Use of optics, cameras, or any recording devices.
- Staring or fixating on the target.
- Avoiding eye contact.
- Being nervous and worried about being noticed.
- Peeking over one's shoulder or from behind a newspaper at the target.
- Using car mirrors for viewing enhancement.
- Anyone who stays too long in one spot with no apparent reason.
- Repeated sightings of the same or different persons in one or many significant locations.

In order to detect static surveillance you have to think like the bad guy. If you were the one watching yourself, where could you go to find static positions near your home or workplace, from which you could collect information? If you discreetly identify and scan the areas from which someone could watch you and you observe these areas you will easily notice anyone in a static location who is exhibiting one or more of the above indicators.

MOBILE SURVEILLANCE

Imagine how long it would take Rick to determine Hadley's travel routines if he only remained in static positions to collect the information. He can determine her routes much more quickly by following her in his vehicle. Although he uses a static position in order to 'pick up' her vehicle, once she drives past him he will use mobile surveillance to follow her so that he, in essence, moves with her and learns her travel patterns.

Surveillance can operate by moving in any number of ways including, but not limited to: motorcycle, automobile, public transportation, boat, bicycle, or on foot, depending on the focus of the mission and the movement of the target.

Moving while conducting the surveillance works to surveillance's advantage in that they can cover a large amount of ground in a short time and determine the movement patterns of their target. One disadvantage of moving is that the surveillance operators must now split their concentration between studying their target and moving safely and discreetly. Unless the surveillance is extremely proficient in moving discreetly, they are easily detectable when mobile. Normally when people conduct mobile surveillance, unless they are highly trained professionals, they will follow the target too closely. In addition, mobile surveillance involves more resources and cost. Plus, unless they are using phony license plates, the surveillance now reveals identifying information (a plate number) which can be used to catch them.

Indicators of Mobile Surveillance:

- Following on foot or in a vehicle at a safe distance but stopping and starting with target.
- Making multiple passes, either on foot or in a vehicle, around the potential target (office, residence, etc.).
- Driving erratically while following.
- Mimicking the driving patterns of the potential target.
- Flashing lights to signal other surveillance vehicles.
- Alternating speed or matching speed of the target's vehicle.
- Using mirrors excessively.
- Target fixation.
- Catching glimpses of the target's vehicle at traffic lights.
- Using their vehicle as a way to blend into an area (e.g. an ice cream truck).
- Correlation, such as repeated sightings of the same or different persons or vehicles in one or many significant locations that relate to the target (more on correlation later in this chapter).

Again, put yourself in the bad guy's position. If you were the target, how could someone follow you discreetly? What kinds of information could he collect about you while moving with you? Certainly a predator who follows you can learn what routes you normally travel. He can collect information about your vehicle, the times you move, and with whom you move (e.g. if you carpool to work or drive your children to school, etc.).

In order to discreetly detect someone following you, you must again combine situational awareness with surveillance detection. In Chapter Six we will discuss at length how to detect mobile surveillance. For now, suffice it to say that if you notice any of the above indicators, you should pay attention and discreetly record any information you can get about the description of the vehicle. Continue with your normal routine but note any safe locations where you can seek help along your routes (such as police stations, hospitals, or any busy public location). Notify people in your SUPNET about your observations so that, if need be, they will be ready to come to your assistance and practice buddy SD for you.

TECHNICAL SURVEILLANCE

When Rick is in his car watching Hadley's house, he may need to use a small pair of binoculars to get a closer look. He also may decide to use a camera to take photographs of Hadley. His use of both of these pieces of equipment actually puts him at greater risk of being detected by Hadley or one of her neighbors if he is not discreet.

The range of technical devices available to surveillance is far-reaching and includes everything from simple technical equipment like binoculars and cameras, to moderately complex equipment like listening devices and phone taps, to more complex tactics like installing Trojan Horse or malicious software programs on computers. Women should be concerned with both the basic technical surveillance methods, as well as more high tech methods involving the use of computers.

Whenever surveillance uses any kind of camera equipment or recording device they collect a permanent record for themselves which they can spend time analyzing and reviewing in a safe location. Therefore, it is common to see surveillance using basic technical equipment for the purposes of enhancing their view and for creating a record of information (either by still or video camera).

Since more women are using computers, both at work and at home, computer surveillance is something to consider. At work, consider your computer an open source. This means, whenever you are away from it, anyone can potentially access it. You may be able to protect it with a password, but then you must guard the password. At home, your computer is also at risk if the man with whom you are living decides to poke around in your files or if a computer repair person has unsupervised access. Remember to deny access to people who may have the intention of putting you under surveillance using any technical means. But most of all, consult a professional to help deter any high-tech surveillance. Whenever you use your e-mail or if you have a blog be cautious about the information that you release about yourself that could be used against you. If you have photos of yourself and personal information on your blog, you could be asking for trouble from a predator. Remember that surveillance focuses on collecting information in order to plan successful attacks.

For most of us, our concern is with basic technical surveillance. This means that the predator is using basic technical equipment, such as cameras, binoculars, and basic communication devices such as cell phones to assist him in collecting information on his target. Although surveillance can use the internet to garner some information, in order to plan any type of crime or attack against a woman, they must get out there and collect *real time* information on her. This is precisely why surveillance detection is such an effective preventative measure. Luckily for SD, surveillance more often than not *must* go on site to collect the information they need to plan a successful attack.

When surveillance enters an area and conducts either static or mobile surveillance while using basic technical equipment, they immediately make themselves more detectable. Of course this does not mean that everyone in the area using this equipment is conducting surveillance. However, anyone's use of this equipment should catch your attention and merit further study for correlating behaviors or other indicators of surveillance.

Indicators of Basic Technical Surveillance

Pay attention to anyone who is:

- Photographing or videotaping with the target in the background.
- Excessively photographing or videotaping.
- Using any technical equipment in an inappropriate location.
- Using a voice recorder.

- Using binoculars.
- Behind window curtains with a camera lens poking out.
- Using a cell phone camera.
- Making contact via the internet and attempting to elicit information from you.
- Tampering with your exterior phone box (check your phone box regularly).
- Using your computer without your permission.

When you begin practicing surveillance detection, use your situational awareness to notice anyone who is using either static or mobile surveillance techniques in conjunction with technical equipment. If you see someone in your neighborhood or near your workplace photographing you, this is an indicator.

High Tech Surveillance

If you are a celebrity or a high profile business woman, politician or diplomat, more complex technical means of surveillance may be a legitimate threat for you. Using bugs or tapping a telephone, although a bit more high-tech, are methods of surveillance which may be used against you. If you are a potential victim of industrial espionage or if you are in a high threat situation, look for listening devices attached to the bottom of furniture. Sometimes they can even be sewn into curtains or upholstery. Keep your exterior phone box locked (usually attached to the side or back of your house). If you detect any bugs, do not attempt to remove them. Rather, consult a professional and inform the authorities immediately. You can also hire a professional to conduct a "sweep" of your location for listening devices.

Pay attention to any signs of tampering with your technical equipment. Remember that predators must gain access in order to emplace their technical surveillance devices. Social engineering is an example of access: you answer the phone and they attempt to trick you into giving out company passwords.

Any unsolicited approaches or attempts to access your information or property should cause you to become aware of potential misconduct. Likewise, any correlation with changes in your technical service (such as your phone, cable, or internet services) should also raise your level of alertness to possible technical surveillance. For example, if you allow access to a service provider for your computer and the next day a virus appears, consider that this person may have had a nefarious intention.

MIXED METHODS SURVEILLANCE

If Rick parks in the same spot every morning to watch Hadley, he makes himself predictable and she will quickly spot him in his habitual location. However, if Rick varies his surveillance methods and sometimes follows her from a different starting point, he decreases his risk of being detected.

The most sophisticated surveillance knows that utilizing a combination of the above methods makes them the least detectable because they become less predictable. In addition, surveillance enhances their operation when they use a variety of methods because they then collect a variety of information which allows them a more comprehensive study of their target.

The important lesson is to *assume* surveillance will mix their methods and to continue to be aware of the many indicators of the various types of surveillance. Put another way, if you are using SD and you observe a man sitting on a bench one day staring at the front door of your house and you focus too narrowly on that position and indicator, you may miss the very same man driving around your neighborhood the next day or photographing you as you are walking into work. When practicing SD you must broaden your perspective and open your mind to all of the possibilities.

Correlation

Rick parks in front of Mrs. Weisman's house each morning to watch Hadley depart for work and follow her. Mrs. Weisman sits in her kitchen each morning watching the birds come to the feeder. Her kitchen window faces the street. Every morning for the past week she has noticed a man parked in his car. She has seen him start his engine shortly before her neighbor, Hadley, drives by. Mrs. Weisman has also seen that the man pulls out about fifteen seconds after Hadley drives past his car. Mrs. Weisman has seen two examples of correlation: Rick starting his engine and pulling out after Hadley's car. Both of these actions relate to the movement of Rick's target.

Keep in mind that, if you are the target, anyone conducting surveillance on you will be correlating with your movements and activities. Correlation means that there will be a relationship between your movement and/or actions and the movement and/or actions of the person watching you. Any correlation is a key indicator in and of itself. For example, if someone parked in front of your house makes a call on his cell phone as you are pulling out of your driveway his action has just correlated with yours. Perhaps he is calling his partner to let him know you just left the house. You might see indicators from the lists above, but if those indicators do not directly correlate to you in some way, then probably that person is not putting you under surveillance. We recommend, however, that you trust your intuition. You may feel as though you are being watched, even if you have not observed a very specific indicator of surveillance or incident of correlation. Trust your instincts and keep looking.

Now That I Know About Indicators and Types of Surveillance, How Do I Develop My Surveillance Detection Plan?

Your surveillance detection plan will be a reflection of the threat level you face. Since Victoria is our medium threat character and she has already conducted a risk/threat assessment, we will use her example to illustrate the steps you must take in order to develop an effective SD plan.

Conducting SD means doing the following:

1. **Determining the Threats:** You will first assess the threats against you, your family, your home, your workplace, your vehicle, or anything related to you. You will conduct a risk/threat assessment in order to identify these threats (see Chapter Three). For example, a woman may feel under threat of being attacked or raped as she walks to her car in the parking garage at work everyday. Or, a corporate executive may feel under threat of abduction. A government building may be a target for terrorists.

Victoria's recent threat (listed in her assessment) is the man at the café who pays too much attention to her and has tried to get personal information about her. She saw him one day sitting on a bench outside her workplace. This is significant. True, it could be a coincidence, but given his expressed interest in her, she is wise to take steps to confirm if he is conducting surveillance on her. She has indicated that he gives her a creepy feeling. He could be a prospective stalker, rapist, abductor, or even murderer. Perhaps her inner monologue will try to talk her out of being suspicious of him: "Maybe he is just a homeless man and is lonely. I shouldn't be so heartless. Maybe if I'm friendly to him I won't have this creepy feeling."

Victoria will identify that her internal monologue could be denial and she will proceed with developing an SD plan in order to confirm or deny if this man is actually following her. Her plan will take into consideration that the man may also be interested in her son, Jake.

2. **Developing and Implementing an SD Plan:** You will formulate a plan to conduct SD with the purpose of determining whether or not someone is watching you (or the target). The threat level will dictate the parameters of your plan. If you are in a low threat situation, your SD plan will not need to be too elaborate. If you face a serious, immediate threat you will need to develop a detailed, comprehensive SD plan (we will show you how to do both). Regardless of your threat level, your SD plan will include the following:

- Surveillance detection for your routine travel (see Chapter Six).
- Surveillance detection around your home, workplace and any other location you frequent regularly (see Chapter Seven).
- A means of recording incidents of surveillance.
- Your strategy for reporting discovery of surveillance to the appropriate authorities.

Victoria's preventative courses of action for this particular threat include:

- ***Inform my family, nearby neighbors, and key work associates. Give them his description and ask them to watch for him and record any pertinent information.***

First and foremost, Victoria must not isolate herself where this threat is concerned. She must immediately bring on board her support network of friends, family, neighbors, and co-workers. These people can assist her by conducting buddy SD to help her watch for this man. For example, Victoria could have a friend go to the café she visits each morning and arrive a half an hour before she normally arrives. This friend can conduct buddy SD by watching for the man in question. If the man is at the café, the friend can notice what, if any, action the man takes when Victoria arrives, while she is in the café, and after she leaves the café. Does he get up and follow her out? Does he record any information, such as the time? Does he fix his attention on Victoria? Does he do anything to correlate with Victoria's movements or actions?

Likewise, Victoria can provide her neighbors with the man's description and ask them to watch for him in her neighborhood. Since he has been seen near her workplace, she should definitely enlist the help of co-workers. Whenever her co-workers go out on break or to lunch, they can scan the area to see if the man is hanging out anywhere in the vicinity. Victoria too can find a window inside the office building that faces the bench where he was seen, or any other key locations from which he could watch her movements. She can look to see if he is present before exiting the building.

- *Install a home alarm.*

If Victoria can afford to install a home alarm system, now might be the time to actually take care of this. Unfortunately women often put off taking such measures until a real threat causes them great concern. She could also get a dog, if her landlord will allow it. She should keep the alarm activated both while inside and away from her home.

- *Conduct route reviews of all my typical travel.*

Victoria will study her routes and habits. She may want to add alternative routes she can use. She must pay attention when she travels. Somehow this man went from the café to her workplace. How did he know where she works unless he followed her there from the café one morning? She never gave him that information and no one at the café knows where she works. When she examines her routes she will identify locations where the man could position himself to watch her and collect information on her routine travel patterns. (See Chapter Six for an explanation on conducting route reviews).

- *Use basic surveillance detection to determine if he is watching me, my home, or my family.*

Victoria will use basic surveillance detection measures to determine if he knows where she lives and is watching her or her son, Jake. Victoria will take the time to discreetly look out of her window before she leaves for work each morning to see if anyone is within line of sight to her driveway and is watching her. As she travels along her route, she will pay attention to see if anyone is following her or if she sees the man sitting anywhere along her route watching her drive by. She will also pay attention at Jake's school to be sure that the man is not loitering in the area or hanging out in a vehicle and driving by the school when she drops off or picks up Jake.

- *Practice using my cell phone camera so that I can discreetly obtain a photograph of him if I see him again.*

By practicing using her cell phone camera, she will be ready to discreetly photograph the man if he appears again. If she can discreetly take a photo of him, she can show it to her neighbors and others in her SUPNET who are assisting her so they have more than just a description of the man. It would be smart for Victoria to give the administrators at Jake's school a description or photo of the man. She can also show the photograph to the police if the situation escalates and she determines that the man is indeed following her or her son.

- *If the situation escalates, stop going to the café.*

She has already determined that she may have to stop going to her regular café each morning. She is ready and willing to make this change if the situation dictates. Rather than approaching the threat with a defiant attitude ("He can't scare me!"), she accepts that this man could be a stalker and is willing to take action to prevent any confrontations with him.

3. **Maintaining Discretion and Keeping it Legal:** You must conduct surveillance detection in a discreet and legal manner in order to verify whether or not surveillance is present. The whole idea is for you to detect surveillance without them ever knowing you are watching them. If they know you are watching them, they will retreat and may resort to using methods to study you that are more difficult for you to detect. Or, they may pull a surprise attack if they feel pressured by you. Surveillance detection is normally a viable, legal option. However, you must pay attention to the local laws when practicing it. For example, if you live in a place where it is illegal to photograph someone without their knowledge or consent, then we do not recommend using photography in your SD practice.

Victoria will use great discretion whenever she attempts to detect this man in the act of watching her or her son. If she uses binoculars from inside her home, she will turn off the lights so that he cannot see her. If she takes his photo, she will do so only if she can obtain the photo without him seeing her. If she does spot the man, she will not react overtly so that he knows he has been detected. Rather, she will record the information, including the date and time of the incident, and will report him to the police as soon as possible.

Victoria will not break the law by following this man or encountering him in any way. Nor will she use any third party to threaten him. She will allow the authorities to determine what actions should be taken towards this man, should she detect him watching her.

4. **Detecting and Reporting Surveillance:** If surveillance is observed, you must discreetly record the details, inform your SUPNET, and report pertinent details to the appropriate authorities in a timely manner. Your response to the discovery of surveillance will depend on the situation and the potential threat at the moment of discovery. You may opt to simply record the incident and wait for further proof that you are being watched or a call to 911 may be warranted if you deem the surveillance is an immediate threat to you or your family.

You might be questioning if Victoria is overreacting, given it could just be a coincidence that this man was seen near her workplace. True, Victoria will want to look for other indicators that he is following her before contacting the authorities. If her threat level increases with more sightings of this man, so too should her response to the increase in threat. However, she is wise to immediately err on the side of caution and practice basic situational awareness and surveillance detection techniques to either confirm or deny her suspicions. The total time required for Victoria to take her preventative courses of action is minimal compared to the peace of mind she will obtain from doing so.

If Victoria sees no further indicators that the man is watching her, then she can breathe a sigh of relief knowing that she has been proactive about her own personal security, rather than acting like a sitting duck waiting for a predator to surprise and attack her. She will feel empowered and will have reduced her fear because she took the lead by focusing on prevention early in the game. On the other hand, if she does confirm future indicators of surveillance, she then has more information to take to the authorities when she asks them for help. Again, she will be in a more empowered position because she will have collected evidence that this man is targeting her. She can take action by providing the authorities with what they need to be able to question and possibly arrest this man.

She can also help protect herself by changing her routines, alternating the times she leaves for work in the morning, varying the routes she travels, and bolstering her personal security by staying one step ahead of this potential attacker. Because Victoria conducted a risk/threat assessment and identified her threats, she was able to get SASD (situational awareness and surveillance detection) and capitalize on implementing preventative measures before it was too late.

What Do I Do If I Discover I Am Under Surveillance?

Your response to the discovery of surveillance will be situation and threat specific. In some circumstances, you may want to wait and collect several incidences of reported data on the presence of surveillance before taking any action. In other cases, you may decide to contact the appropriate authorities immediately. Do not shy away from contacting the authorities; in fact, err on the side of caution and report it anyway. If you are correct, this early contact with the authorities may make all the difference if it turns out you truly need their support. Plus, you will have established a contact person with whom you can communicate should the threat turn out to be legitimate.

In general, do not tip your hand and let the surveillance know you are onto them. Again, you do not want to chase them into hiding or provoke an attack. Inform your SUPNET and identify safe locations where you can go to for help. Document any incidents of surveillance and collect any evidence. Maintain your discretion so that predators are none the wiser that you have detected them. However, if you feel an attack is imminent, you must move out of the attack zone and take appropriate measures to protect yourself (see Chapter Thirteen).

Remember that SD is an early warning/prevention system so, in most cases, the surveillance you observe will be out there with the express purpose of collecting information. But remember also (and this is important) that when you see them out there, you cannot be certain how far along they are in their surveillance process. Maybe they are only a day away from the attack and the people you are observing are out there to take one last look before implementing their plan or to conduct a "dry run" (rehearsal) of the attack. Trust your intuition and the early warning signals, record and report your observations, and notify the proper authorities.

By implementing a basic surveillance detection plan, Victoria is able to design her response and defend herself early on by detecting the predator during the planning phase of his attack. This puts her in a powerful position from which she can assert her ability to handle this potentially threatening situation. If Victoria confirms one more sighting of this man anywhere along her routes, near her home, near her workplace, or near her son's school, she will immediately file a report with the local police.

In the event that this man were to attack her, the very fact that Victoria is concentrating on his surveillance activities means she is already aware she faces a potentially serious threat. If he does manage to attack her before she can get the help she needs, she will at the very least be better able to escape and defend herself because she is already of the mindset to pay attention and be prepared for danger. That element of surprise upon which the attacker so relies in order to attack successfully has now been compromised by Victoria's astute posturing against this man who threatens her safety.

What are the Benefits of Implementing a Surveillance Detection Plan?

Implementing a surveillance detection plan will benefit you by:

- Giving you the opportunity to do your due diligence to protect yourself from any threat.

- Helping you to reduce the crippling fear that you may experience when you worry about becoming a victim of violence.

- Allowing you to take the lead in preventing crime against you and those you love.

- Allowing you to think like the bad guy. You will ask yourself: "If I wanted to attack a target such as myself, where would I go to watch her? What kind of information would I need to collect? How can I blend in to the area so she will not notice me watching her?" By asking yourself these questions, you begin to study yourself as a target. In so doing you train yourself to notice if anyone with a hostile intention might be studying you as a target.

As we progress in this book we will give you very specific SD methods that you can implement in all aspects of your life. In the next two chapters we will discuss in depth the specific information that surveillance must collect in order to plan an attack on an individual during routine travel or an attack on any type of structure, and how you can detect them doing so. If you are under any serious threat, these next two chapters will be of great value. Even if you have no immediate threat, reading and understanding the surveillance detection and analytical skills in both chapters will heighten your awareness and help you identify where, when, and how someone would watch you, either as you travel along your daily routes or while you are at home or at work. Our objective is to teach you to ready yourself to stay a step ahead of anyone who might be targeting you for any reason. Remember that your life can change in one moment should a predator decide to make you his target. It makes sense to learn now how to prepare yourself to spot him and prevent him from harming you.

CHAPTER SIX

VEHICLE SECURITY: ROUTE REVIEWS

*"There's a stranger in a car
Driving down your street
Acts like he knows who you are…
Just a stranger in a car"*

--Marc Cohn

Another powerful prevention tool and an extension of your SD plan is what we call a route review. Now that you have a better understanding of what surveillance detection is we will focus on how you can use it to protect yourself as you move from place to place. Regardless of how you travel (on foot, by bicycle, using public transportation, or in your car) you can apply this prevention process on a daily basis. Route reviews allow you to fuse your practice of situational awareness with your surveillance detection plan in order to keep you safe when you are mobile. The reward of learning to conduct route reviews is peace of mind. Even if you would categorize yourself as being at low risk of any serious threats, knowing how to conduct route reviews will empower you to immediately adjust should your threat level increase for any reason. In addition, this system will work for defending yourself against other potential threats about which you may feel concern (for example, if you are worried that your child might be targeted for a kidnapping or if you are concerned that a disgruntled employee whom you recently fired might come after you).

The main premise behind conducting route reviews is actually quite simple and easy to grasp. When we move between locations, we are more vulnerable to attacks because it is easier for predators to access targets who are not protected inside a structure (such as a home with locked doors and an alarm system or a workplace with security guards and cameras). Predators have certain advantages when they plan to attack us while we move. First, when in transition we are normally preoccupied and distracted. When we drive we often fall into a 'drone zone' and are moving on autopilot, not paying attention to our surroundings except to follow the rules of the road. Second, attack locations along routes are terrain dictated. This means that predators can take advantage of parts of our routes that provide them with the elements they need to attack us successfully. They can study our movements and designate attack locations ahead of time. Once they decide where to attack us, they can then select locations from which to watch us as we approach and enter their chosen attack locations. When predators take the time to study us as targets, they will be very interested in collecting information about how we move, when we move, with whom we move (e.g., if we drive our children to school), and where we move.

When attackers want to determine your routine travel times and routes they (or surveillance working for them) will try to watch you move between your home and your place of employment first. Generally speaking, we are at our most predictable when moving between these two locations. They may follow you from your home in the morning, perhaps just a short distance initially, to determine your habitual routes. Or they may opt to follow you home when you leave work at the end of the day in order to determine where you live. Predators have an advantage when they study our routes: our predictability. Human beings are creatures of habit; we tend to seek out the path of least resistance when we travel by settling into routine routes and taking the shortest and fastest route between locations. Seldom do we change our routes because it is easier to cruise along on autopilot when we are comfortable in our patterns.

At our homes and workplaces, we are protected by walls, alarms, fences, and locked doors. When we are in our vehicles, we are generally more vulnerable to attack. When we are moving in our vehicles, anyone who is out there studying our movement patterns can ascertain a good place to attack us successfully. A stalker, for example, can sit back and watch you leave your home in the morning and follow you from a distance to determine how and when you go to work, where you park your vehicle, and what route you use for your return trip home. There may be a narrow, secluded street you travel on each day. He will collect this information and may intend to stop you in your vehicle and attack you there because you are secluded and vulnerable in this spot. If you study your travel patterns and routes, from the perspective of an attacker, you will quickly see your vulnerabilities. Since you know that attack locations are terrain driven, you will be able to study your routes and determine where they would attempt to attack you. Once you identify these locations, you will know where to look for anyone who would be watching you move through these dangerous areas.

Aside from your home and place of employment, predators may also try to observe you at any other known or predictable locations you frequent, such as child care, church, the bank, the health club, or at any routine appointments. Therefore, if you are under high threat it is wise to study and analyze all of your routine travel. If your schedule is made public it is even easier for predators to find you. For example, celebrities and politicians have many appearances that are publicized, making their schedules readily available to anyone interested in watching them.

Predators use their planning phase and the information they collect during their surveillance phase to outsmart us and surprise us. If we want to stay safe, we need to use discretion and outsmart them early on while they are out there in plain sight collecting information on us.

How Do I Begin the Route Review Process?

In order to stay one step ahead of them and to predict where the surveillance will go, you must analyze your own patterns by simply paying attention to your own routines. This is the first step towards safeguarding yourself and your family while traveling. Without changing your habits, observe and pay attention to the routes you travel. Keeping a log of your routes is an easy way to do this. Just write down your routes in a simple format each day for a week or, even better, mark your routes on a map. No matter how you travel along these routes (in a car, on foot, using public transportation) be sure to map out your routes in detail.

Perhaps you travel to work by taking a two lane road to an inner beltway and you exit close to your office, where you park in the same parking lot at the same spot every day. When you return home you may follow the same route in reverse or you may use an entirely different route because you stop by the gym. When traffic is bad perhaps you try a different route. You are more apt to be punctual in the morning because you have to be at work on time. Your afternoon travel is probably less predictable because sometimes you stay late at work or stop on your way home to do errands or go to daycare to pick up your children. As part of your initial route log, note your time patterns as well. Your predictability pertains to both time and location. Where and when can a predator be certain to find you?

Creating My Route Review:

Once you have completed this initial log, we recommend you conduct a formal route review in order to:

- Determine your own patterns.
- Determine which parts of your routes overlap (meaning where the surveillance can be sure to find you each day).
- Assess where surveillance will go to watch you.

- Speculate as to what they can use for "cover" (a way to blend in) or where they can conceal themselves while they are out watching you.
- Determine where and how you can conduct SD to watch for the presence of surveillance.
- Analyze where along your routes they may opt to attack you.
- Verify how they can escape after attacking you (since they will choose an attack site that offers them a good avenue of escape).
- Determine safe locations along your routes where you can get help.

Because we want to teach you how to use this material to its fullest potential, we are introducing Kate in this chapter (our character who is in a high threat situation). Kate has a stalker. Once you learn how a woman under serious threat can use these techniques to keep herself safe, you will be able to see how you can apply the same techniques in a more simplified way if you are in a medium or low threat situation. Trust the techniques used by security professionals. It is well worth your effort to read through this chapter and make sure you comprehend the material. Once you put forth this effort towards understanding, you will be able to begin applying this process and the end result could very likely be that, someday, you detect a threat in its earliest stages.

Part of the reason we are using Kate's story in this chapter is that she is catching on to her predator very late in the game. Kate will learn that, had she conducted route reviews before she ever had a stalker, she would have seen her stalker sooner and would have been able to take action very early on to mitigate the threat. Since she did not use these techniques early on, her threat escalated and is much harder to control.

At the end of each step we include a sample map for Kate. Looking at Kate's maps will help you to determine if you are on the right track when you make your maps. Kate will create route reviews so that she can identify exactly where her stalker might go to watch her and collect information on her, especially information that would help him to identify a good place to attack her. Kate has already spotted her stalker twice at her workplace and once in the park near her neighborhood. Her stalker has sent her flowers at work, several cards to her home address, and even approached her for a date while she was at the cafeteria on her lunch break at work. Kate has been avoiding him as best she can, but he recently left a threatening message on her home voicemail. Although Kate is conducting her route review late in the game, it still behooves her to do so to mitigate the chances of being attacked by her stalker while she is en route. She intends to stay one step ahead of him so that she can involve the authorities and give them specific proof that this man is indeed stalking her. She will practice SD along her routes so that she can collect evidence that her stalker is putting her under surveillance.

Prevention is the name of the game. We are asking you to have the courage to sink your teeth into this somewhat technical but highly effective material so that you do not become a victim. You can do this! You do not need to feel intimidated by the diagrams in this chapter. Even if you do not normally learn well using visual aides, we encourage you to take the time to look at each diagram so that you can grasp how this process works. One way to make this process more enjoyable and insightful is to team up with a friend. Not only will you have fun, but you will also gain an objective view of your travel patterns and vulnerabilities. You can then offer your friend the same help with her routes. As you conduct your route reviews, assume that you are already under surveillance (because you may be) and operate discreetly so that the surveillance does not realize you are onto them. This is a good way to practice being aware of anyone who may be watching you (even if no one is).

Conducting a route review is a simple four step process. We suggest that you buy some large paper such as easel size paper or poster boards and use a variety of colored pens for labeling different features. Note: We are breaking down this process into steps, thus we are creating several maps and building on them as we go. You only need to create one large map for each route which will include all of the steps below.

Step One: Predictable Travel Locations (PTL)

The first step in conducting a route review is to use your enlarged paper to map out your route(s) from your residence to your workplace. Once your routes are drawn on your map you can locate your *Predictable Travel Locations (PTL)*. Predictable travel locations are the common roads and intersections you *must* go through or by, no matter which route you take that day. The first PTL is always going to be your home driveway unless you have another way into your home that you use. If you only use one route, you will complete this process by noting each intersection and indicating how you are brought to a stop there (light or stop sign). Your major disadvantage in using only one route is that you make it too easy on your attacker. He now gets to choose exactly where along this route to go after you and he can be well assured that you will appear when he is ready for the attack.

If you use more than one route and vary your routes randomly (highly recommended), you help make yourself less predictable to your attacker and you force him into smaller areas where you can be certain he will be watching you. In order to do this you will examine all of your routes for overlaps. For example, if you have three routes you can choose from to go to work each day and all of them go through the same traffic circle, this traffic circle is a key location from which the predator can put you under surveillance and potentially attack you. He knows he can find you at that traffic circle, no matter which of your three routes you travel that day, because all three routes pass through it. This traffic circle should be labeled as a PTL. Unless your predator is working in a large team, he will have limited manpower (or womanpower), so you can assume he will not have the capability of watching all portions of your routes. Determine and note all locations where your predator can confirm your presence each day and be sure to find you based on your patterns and your particular route choices. Label these predictable travel locations (PTL) on your map. Make sure to indicate any traffic lights or stop signs.

One note on using multiple routes: make sure they are all safe routes. Do not vary your routes just for the sake of it. If you choose three routes to make yourself less predictable but one of those routes is a secluded, narrow side street, you are endangering yourself. Stay on busy, fast moving routes if at all possible. Also, pay attention to any restrictions along your routes, such as a road construction sites or poorly lit areas. Where can the bad guy conceal himself and wait for you to arrive so that he can pull a surprise attack on you?

Step One: Kate

Example *(See Diagram 1)*

Kate uses two alternate routes to travel from her home to her work, (represented by the solid arrow and the hollow arrow). As you can see in the diagram below, the circled areas are the places where both of Kate's two routes overlap. This means that, if her stalker were to follow her along either of these two routes, he could be sure to find her in any of these circled and labeled predictable travel locations (PTL) because, no matter which route she takes on any particular day, she surely will travel through all of these PTL.

When she exits her garage, she must drive down Poppy Lane and up Cedar Drive. Her stalker can determine this by watching her leave in the morning. The next place she is predictable is on Maple Street between Lincoln and Pine. Finally, her stalker will learn that she always enters the parking garage off Market Street. Kate has four locations where she is predictable in her travel (indicated by the dotted circles):

- **PTL 1** = From out of her garage all the way to the end of Poppy Lane
- **PTL 2** = From the bottom of Cedar Drive to the intersection of Cedar Drive and Mulberry Street
- **PTL 3** = From the intersection of Pine Street and Maple Street to the intersection of Lincoln Boulevard and

Maple Street
- **PTL 4** = From the point on Market Street that leads into the entrance ramp of the Parking Garage

It is very important for you to realize that Kate must make a separate diagram or map for her routes from work to home. They could be totally different routes from the ones she travels from home to work. Perhaps she goes to a health club every day after work or runs errands at various locations. When making your own route reviews, make sure you use as many maps as you need to complete this process correctly for each direction of your daily travel. Think of the attention to detail you can muster when planning a party or juggling your children's schedules and be equally thorough with this process.

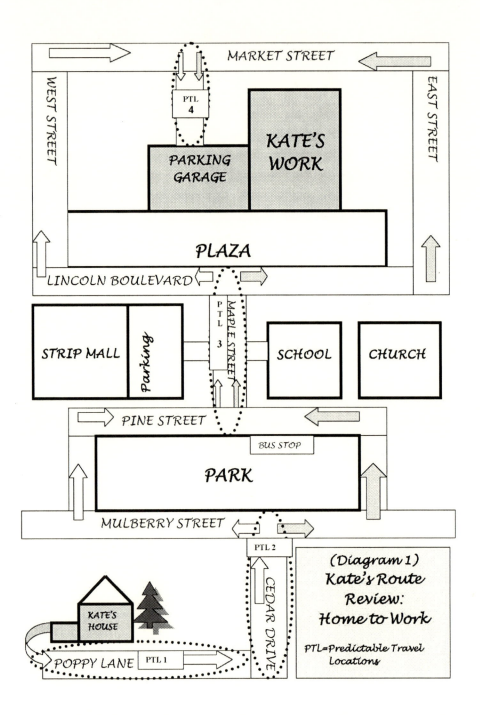

MARKET STREET

WEST STREET

EAST STREET

PTL
4

PARKING
GARAGE

KATE'S
WORK

PLAZA

LINCOLN BOULEVARD

STRIP MALL

Parking

P
T
L
3

MAPLE STREET

SCHOOL

CHURCH

PINE STREET

BUS STOP

PARK

MULBERRY STREET

PTL 2

CEDAR DRIVE

KATE'S
HOUSE

POPPY LANE   PTL 1

(Diagram 1)
Kate's Route
Review:
Home to Work

PTL=Predictable Travel
Locations

Step Two: Surveillance Locations (SVL)

Your next step in the route review process is to locate probable surveillance locations (SVL). Surveillance locations can either be specific locations or larger areas; they are defined as anywhere the surveillance can be to have line of sight to the target. Indicate on your map any specific locations or areas where you think surveillance operators can situate themselves to watch you travel through your PTL. Remember:

- They will seek out a spot that is within line of sight of your PTL so they can observe you traversing it.
- They will use a location where they can blend in with the normal surroundings, conceal themselves, or not attract too much attention.
- They will choose a location to which they have access so they can quickly and naturally arrive and depart (especially in your direction of travel) without arising suspicion.
- They may place surveillance along other portions of your routes that are outside of your PTL, if they deem there is a good attack location worth watching (such as a secluded portion of your route or a narrow road with a hairpin turn that forces you to slow down).

Label and number these SVL on your map and also label what the surveillance might use as cover (a way to blend in) or concealment (a way to hide) while they are there. For example, one SVL may be a bus stop. Possible cover at this spot would be waiting for a bus. Once you have indicated this on your map, you now know to pay attention to the behavior of people waiting at this bus stop each day when you drive by on your way to work or home. Does anyone at the bus stop correlate with your movement or display any indicators of the various types of surveillance? If there are any landmarks or billboards near the SVL you identified, put these on your map as well so that, when you are approaching an SVL, the landmark or billboard will remind you to be on the lookout for signs of surveillance.

Step Two: Kate

Example (See *Diagram 2*)

Kate will now examine her predictable travel locations (PTL) and determine the surveillance locations (SVL) where her stalker could watch her traverse each of her predictable travel locations. She will also indicate on her map (or on a separate page) what her stalker can do to blend in or hide at each SVL.

As you can see, Kate has identified her first SVL at the intersection of Cedar Drive and Mulberry Street. Her stalker would choose to watch her at this location because it is the best place to learn which way she will turn. Also, since Kate has to come to this intersection each morning, perhaps her stalker will choose to attack her there. He does not need to risk standing out on Poppy Lane or Cedar Drive where he has no cover or way of blending in or hiding. He can, however, find good cover options in the park (such as throwing a ball to his dog) and wait to watch her when she comes up to the intersection.

The following are the surveillance locations Kate labeled and options for cover in each of those locations. She will think like her stalker so that she can identify ways he might attempt to blend in to these areas.

Surveillance Locations and Cover

SVL 1: PARK: Park activities such as picnicking; reading; walking dog.
    SVL 1 offers line of sight to PTL 2.
SVL 2: PARK: Park activities.
    SVL 2 offers line of sight to PTL 3.
SVL 3: SITTING IN PARKED CAR: Reading newspaper; talking on cell phone.
    SVL 3 offers line of sight to PTL 3.
SVL 4: PLAZA: Reading newspaper; eating lunch; drinking coffee; talking on cell phone.
    SVL 4 offers line of sight to PTL 4.

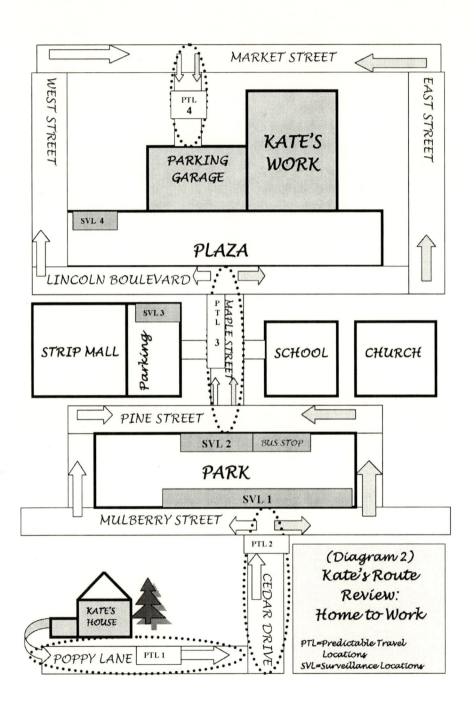

MARKET STREET

WEST STREET

EAST STREET

PTL 4

PARKING GARAGE

KATE'S WORK

SVL 4

PLAZA

LINCOLN BOULEVARD

SVL 3

STRIP MALL

Parking

PTL 3

MAPLE STREET

SCHOOL

CHURCH

PINE STREET

SVL 2   BUS STOP

PARK

SVL 1

MULBERRY STREET

PTL 2

CEDAR DRIVE

KATE'S HOUSE

POPPY LANE   PTL 1

(Diagram 2)
Kate's Route Review:
Home to Work

PTL=Predictable Travel Locations
SVL=Surveillance Locations

Step Three: Surveillance Detection Locations (SDL)

Your next step is to locate your SD locations (SDL). These are the places where you or your security support can conduct SD discreetly. These positions will be used if the threat level escalates, as Kate's has. If you determine someone is following you or watching you as you travel, you could enlist the help of family, friends, or co-workers to support you in your SD efforts. If you are driving yourself, you cannot be the one to position yourself in an SD location. However, you can train yourself to practice SD from inside your vehicle. Obviously you must pay attention to driving, but you can still catch a glimpse of anyone conducting surveillance on you once you identify where they will be positioned.

Surveillance detection locations (SDL) must be within line of sight to the probable surveillance locations (SVL) you identified near or in your predictable travel locations (PTL) or near a likely attack location (AL) that you will identify on your route (see Step Four). Anyone conducting surveillance detection on your behalf must be able to see the surveillance but does not necessarily need to be within line of sight to the target (although it is usually best if that person can see both in order to detect correlation between the surveillance and the target's movements). Remember also that anyone conducting surveillance detection must also have a way to blend in or be concealed so that the surveillance is unaware they are being watched. Label and number these surveillance detection locations (SDL) on your map as well as ideas for cover anyone supporting you by conducting SD could use in those locations.

Even if you are not experiencing any serious threats right now, learning to study your routes will give you the ability to make a very quick mental assessment of locations a predator could use to watch you. If your threat level heightens, you can then immediately implement a surveillance detection plan because you will know how to identify SD locations that people in your SUPNET can use to help you spot the surveillance.

Step Three: Kate

Example *(See Diagram 3)*

Now that Kate has figured out and labeled on her map where her stalker will go to watch her, she will determine the surveillance detection locations that are available for her SD support to use to watch her stalker at the same time he is watching her. Ideally it should look something like the diagram below. Note that the surveillance detection is positioned *behind* the surveillance, whose focus and attention is forward, towards the target.

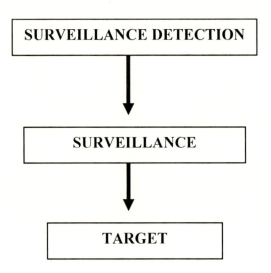

Remember, Kate will be driving herself to work, so even though she has identified where her potential stalker can watch her, she has limited ability to see him doing so because she must concentrate on driving. By identifying locations where someone in her SUPNET can conduct surveillance detection, Kate expands her options for protection. Kate's next move will be to add an ounce of prevention by enlisting help from at least one person in her SUPNET, such as a family member, neighbor, friend, or co-worker. This person will alternate using these surveillance detection locations shortly before Kate leaves for work in the morning for a period of several days. Kate's buddy will conduct SD, watch her stalker in action, and prepare a report for each incident of surveillance (possibly including a photograph). Her buddy will also communicate with Kate by cell phone so that Kate is notified of her stalker's whereabouts whenever possible.

Kate will be as creative as possible when considering what surveillance detection locations (SDL) will work. In some cases she will achieve the ideal by placing her surveillance detection support behind her stalker. In other cases, her SD support will be forced into the same area as her stalker. If they are forced to share the location with her stalker, then Kate will provide them with an effective cover or way to blend in to the area so that they are not noticed by her stalker.

Kate has identified and labeled three possible surveillance detection locations and has listed some cover options anyone helping her could use in each of these locations.

Surveillance Detection Locations and Cover

SDL 1: PARK: Park activities such as playing Frisbee; picnicking; walking dog; playing with children.
SDL 1 offers line of sight to SVL 1&2.

SDL 2: INSIDE STORE OR PARKED IN A CAR: Concealed inside store pretending to shop; reading newspaper in vehicle.
SDL 2 offers line of sight to SVL 3.

SDL 3: PLAZA: Sitting on bench reading newspaper; talking with a friend; drinking coffee; eating lunch; talking on cell phone.
SDL 3 offers line of sight to SVL 4.

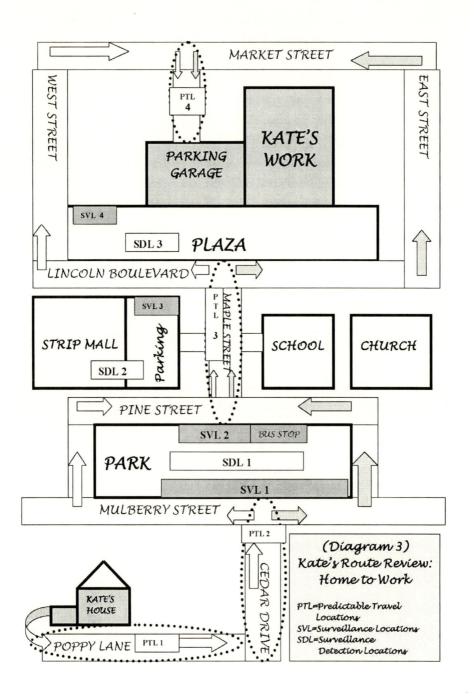

(Diagram 3)
Kate's Route Review:
Home to Work

PTL=Predictable Travel
Locations
SVL=Surveillance Locations
SDL=Surveillance
Detection Locations

Step Four: Attack Locations (AL) and Safe Locations

Attack Locations:

Now you must locate likely attack locations (AL). These are locations that make it easier for an attacker simply because of what is at the location. Your attacker will choose a spot that will help ensure his attack will be successful. First he will need to stop you, slow you down, or control your vehicle. He can do this by using existing traffic lights, sharp curves in the road, stop signs, or he can create a plausible reason for you to stop or slow down, such as a road block, a broken down car, or some type of barricade. He may opt to use a ruse such as approaching your vehicle ostensibly to collect money for a bogus charity or to sell newspapers. He will want a location where he can blend into the normal setting or can hide from view. He will need easy access to the attack location and an escape route.

Ask yourself two questions:

1. Do any of my predictable travel locations make a good attack site? (This is important because if any of your PTL makes a good attack site then the predator has a greater advantage because he knows for sure that you will travel through his chosen attack site).

2. Do any locations *outside* my predictable travel locations make a good attack site? (This is important so that you know to be more alert when traveling through these locations, even if you do not go through them on days you use alternate routes).

Indicate all attack locations (AL) on your map and pay special attention to anything particular along your routes that provides the attacker with an easy way to control your vehicle, such as road construction or a very sharp turn. It is also helpful to make a mental note of the attacker's potential escape routes, bearing in mind that he will not likely follow normal traffic laws or patterns when escaping. Thinking about his potential escape routes will help you become aware of his presence in the event that he enters and escapes from the same place.

Safe Locations:

Finally, it is very important for you to label any safe locations that exist along your routes. Safe locations include police stations, fire stations, hospitals, crowded public locations, gas stations, or any place where you can enlist the help of others in an emergency. Identifying these safe locations and labeling them on your map will allow you to think clearly and know exactly where to go in the event that someone tries to control your vehicle or attack you.

If you are in a high threat situation, it is extremely important to go take a look at these locations and determine when they are open and where exactly inside the location you could access help. You should become completely familiar with the roads leading to these locations and all possible means of accessing them (entrances and exits). If you are currently in a high threat situation, go into your safe locations and establish rapport with as many of the personnel as possible; become a familiar face and name to them. Remember that security professionals routinely identify and determine safe locations along all of the routes traveled by their most important clients. Give yourself the same degree of protection.

Step Four: Kate

Example *(See Diagram 4)*

Kate will now complete her map by labeling any attack locations (AL) and safe locations along her routes. First, she will look at her predictable travel locations (PTL) to see if any of these locations makes a good place to attack her. It makes sense that her stalker would choose to attack her inside one of her PTL because he can predict with relative certainty when she will be there.

Next she will look at other places on her routes that for any reason would make a good attack site. She will consider areas of her routes where her stalker could be concealed or where she is somehow restricted by the flow of traffic or road conditions. She will also consider lighting, given that she leaves while it is still dark some mornings. Now she knows to pay particular attention when traveling through these areas and she can identify if her stalker is watching her there.

Although there are many possibilities for attack locations, Kate's stalker will want to choose a location where he is sure to find her and one he can access easily, blend in while he is there waiting for Kate, and escape after his attack. The terrain will dictate his choice of an attack site. Perhaps it will be inside a PTL or perhaps it will be on some portion of one of Kate's routes that affords her stalker a concealed position from which to surprise her. Kate will analyze all portions of her routes, keeping in mind her stalker's perspective. For example, he could come down and attack her as she pulls out of her garage, but his escape route there is not great. A much better location is at the intersection of Cedar Drive and Mulberry Street. He has good cover in the park while he waits for Kate's vehicle to arrive. He can control her vehicle at the stop sign. He can escape in either direction in his vehicle or by foot through the park and then into a vehicle parked on Pine Street. It is unwise for him to attack Kate anywhere in her PTL 3 because the school and strip mall traffic provide too many witnesses and it would be difficult for him to escape, since Pine Street and Lincoln Boulevard do not offer him a quick way out of the area. He might, however, opt to attack her at PTL 4 as she enters the parking garage, but then he is caught in a small area and may have difficulty escaping down the busy Market Street. In addition, there may be security cameras near the parking garage entrance that would catch him on tape.

Kate has many safe locations she can use in the middle of her routes (the school, church, strip mall). She does not have any safe locations to use near the park, thus this is a dangerous location for her. Since she has identified this as the best location for an attack, she will be very careful when approaching and traversing this part of her route. She will also be mentally prepared to respond, should she come under attack by her stalker. She can think ahead and create 'what if' plans to prepare herself for the possibility of an attack. One of her 'what if' plans might be to put her car in reverse and back down Cedar Drive if she feels it is too unsafe to approach the intersection. She can also plan to run to a neighbor's house for help if necessary, but she would be wise to choose a neighbor who is home that time of day and who would be willing to help her. She and this neighbor could even develop some type of distress signal to use in the event of an emergency. Kate must remember to keep her awareness heightened any time she is passing through any of her predictable travel locations. She is at risk for attack in any of them by virtue of the fact that her stalker knows he can find her in any of these locations at a predictable time each morning.

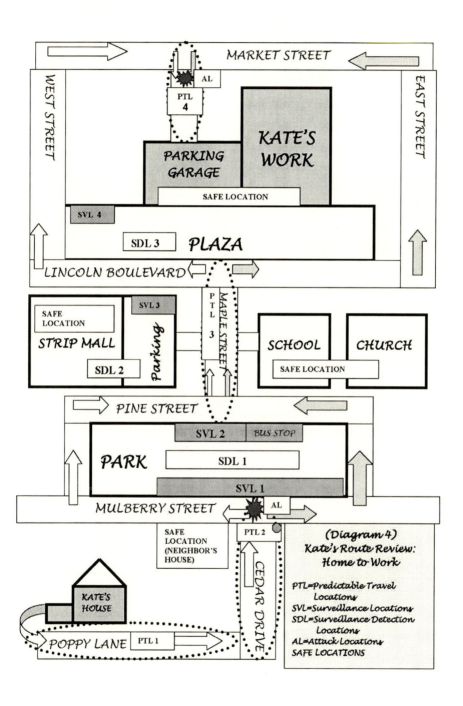

(Diagram 4)
Kate's Route Review:
Home to Work

PTL=Predictable Travel
Locations
SVL=Surveillance Locations
SDL=Surveillance Detection
Locations
AL=Attack Locations
SAFE LOCATIONS

In summary, each route review will include a map labeled with the following:

- PTL (your Predictable Travel Locations, indicating any traffic lights or stop signs at these locations).
- SVL (Surveillance Locations, indicating what predators can use for cover or concealment in each location).
- SDL (Surveillance Detection Locations, indicating what someone practicing SD can use for cover or concealment in these locations).
- AL (Attack Locations, which are conducive to an attack because an attacker can stop/entrap/control his target, blend in to the area, and escape after the attack) and Safe Locations (such as, police stations, hospitals, crowded public locations, or anywhere you could seek outside help in the event of an attack).

Your final routes portfolio, which includes all your route reviews, can be as in-depth and specific as you deem necessary for your particular situation. If you are a dignitary living overseas you may have your security detail produce an extensive portfolio for all your travel, which might include dozens of route reviews. If you are a corporate executive you may have a routes portfolio that is a few pages in length and consists of two or three maps. If you are a working woman with kids and two jobs, you will have route reviews for each of the routes you use, including the routes you take when driving your kids to school. If you are a college student walking from your dorm to classes you can apply this same route review process to analyze your daily routes.

Create the maps, label them, and analyze all of your routes thoroughly. Even if you will not have SD support out along your routes, you will still conduct SD to some extent from within your vehicle. This process will inform you as to where to look for surveillance and where you could be attacked. If the threat against you increases, creating route reviews will enable you to be ready in the event that you need to get a friend or family member to come out along an area of your routes to confirm the presence of surveillance.

How To Conduct Surveillance Detection Yourself While Moving

You yourself can employ some basic SD methods to bolster your personal security while you conduct your routine travel. The following is a simple but effective solution for implementing SD based on your route reviews:

A. Study your route reviews before you travel and review your identified likely surveillance and attack locations, as well as other dangerous locations so you are prepared and extra alert when you approach those areas. To avoid being predictable, change your schedule, alternate your departure and arrival times, and remain on the lookout for signs of surveillance or an attack. Never hesitate to call for help!

B. Before departing, look out from your residence discreetly to see if there are any vehicles parked within line of sight to your driveway or your parked vehicle. If so, do you recognize them? Are there people in them? Do you recognize anyone? Do you see any indicators that the occupant(s) of the vehicle are conducting surveillance? What is your intuition telling you? Are you receiving any early warning signals of trouble?

If a vehicle is parked with someone in it, write down any information you can obtain discreetly (license plate number, make, model, color, description of vehicle and person) and report it to the police or appropriate authorities if you feel you are in danger. Do not depart if you see anyone out there waiting for you. Trust your intuition and err on the side of caution.

C. If there are no vehicles, once you depart stay alert to any vehicles that immediately come into line of sight to your vehicle (or if you are on foot, anyone who begins walking behind you). There may be a vehicle parked (or a person positioned) just out of view of your residence but at a key location through which you have to pass. Have a notebook and pen handy and write down whatever information you can collect discreetly. If you have a cell phone, keep it on and accessible in case you need to call for help. Do not panic, but remain alert to this vehicle (or person). Do not let the person following you know you are aware of his presence. Doing so may prompt him to use tactics in the future that make him less detectable to you. You want to take away his ability to surprise you, so if you tip him off that you are aware he is following you, he learns to be sneakier.

D. If you suspect any vehicles are following you (or anyone is following you on foot), make sure to avoid narrow or secluded roads and stay in public areas where you are visible. Do not hesitate to go into a safe location or call the police if you feel threatened.

E. If you suspect you have a vehicle following you, one way you can confirm or deny your suspicions is by incorporating specified stops along your route for the purpose of drawing the suspected surveillance into an area where you can watch him respond. For example, if you stop at a coffee shop on the way to work, you can see if anyone stops with you, follows you inside, or waits for you and then continues to follow you after you leave the coffee shop. You need to be careful using this technique. Make sure your stops are plausible and are in safe, public locations. Also, be very discreet when watching to see if anyone is following you. Do not tip him off or cause him to feel he is being lured into a trap. Remember, you want to keep it legal and you do not want to put yourself in harm's way by instigating a confrontation. There is more than one way to play a hand of cards. Avoid compromising your superior position. Evolve into an empowered woman who is successful at aiding the authorities in bringing predators to justice (by collecting evidence against them to be used during prosecution).

F. If you suspect someone is following you, you can also confirm this by making a series of turns. However, you will alert the driver of the vehicle that you are aware of him if you make a full 360 degree turn. Make your turns logical and do not put yourself in an unknown or isolated location where you have no help if you need it.

G. If you suspect you are being followed, call someone in your SUPNET or someone who is at your current destination to let them know about the situation. That way, if you are very late arriving they can contact you to check up on you.

H. If you are being followed, go to a safe location (you will have identified these during your route reviews). Notice if the person follows you into the safe location or waits for you outside in his vehicle.

I. If any vehicle makes an attempt to control your vehicle, do whatever you can to drive out of the situation. Use your instincts and trust your intuition. If you feel threatened, take it seriously. Quickly, yet safely, drive away and break contact. If you cannot move away and you are certain you are under attack, realize that you have at least two tons of steel under your control. Realize also that your vehicle is expendable; you are not.

We strongly advise you get evasive driving training if you are in a high threat situation so that you learn how to correctly maneuver your vehicle in an attack situation. We believe every woman would benefit from receiving evasive driving training. We learn other useful emergency procedures, such as how to perform CPR and the Heimlich maneuver. Evasive driving training is helpful regardless if you are threatened by a predator. Negotiating weather, bad road conditions, and dangerous drivers are reasons enough to get training (See Appendix E).

The above mentioned SD solutions are applicable to anyone facing a threat during routine travel. Perhaps you are an attorney who has had several heated lawsuits or criminal trials you won. Or perhaps you are the judge who presided over the cases, or the deputy sheriff who escorted the convicted violent criminal to jail (Were you wearing a name tag? Were you ever threatened directly or indirectly?). Perhaps you filed a sexual harassment claim against a co-worker and are concerned about retribution. Or maybe you are in a high risk category due to a heated divorce or because you have a stalker. Be creative and conduct route reviews for your unique situation and circumstances.

The whole point of conducting route reviews is to help you get SASD while you move. To review, being SASD means first having situational awareness. This means staying in the present, observing your current situation, and retaining your composure so that you can function if your threat level escalates or you are attacked. By taking the time and making the effort to go out and study your routes, you are giving yourself the advantage of processing a large amount of information so that when you are conducting your routine travel you will have already assimilated important data. Having this data and maintaining situational awareness as you travel will help you respond to any changes more effectively and efficiently. You will be more relaxed and focused because you will have a plan. Maintaining situational awareness means paying attention and avoiding distractions. If you are under threat, listening to music or talking on your cell phone as you drive are ways of detracting from your situational awareness. If you are being driven and you are a passenger reading the newspaper, your situational awareness is compromised and you are putting all of your personal safety into the hands of your driver.

The second part of staying SASD as you move is integrating a surveillance detection practice into your daily travel routines. Even if you are in a low threat category, it is still wise to practice basic SD by completing your route reviews and paying extra attention in the areas that you have identified as potential surveillance locations or attack sites. If you stay SASD as you move, you stand a better chance of detecting a predator early on and being able to prevent becoming a victim.

Other common sense tips for staying safe in your vehicle include:

- Keeping your vehicle locked at all times.

- Being prepared and alert when you transition from your vehicle to a location. When you arrive at any location, do not immediately turn off your engine. Take a moment to first scan the area for danger.

- Maintaining your vehicle so that it remains in good running order.

- Having a working, charged cell phone in your vehicle at all times.

- Keep a small notebook and pen in your vehicle for recording information on anyone who is watching you, harassing you, or following you.

- Having an emergency road repair service membership.

- Keeping your vehicle filled with gas. Never allow the tank to fall below half-filled.

- Using a car alarm system with a panic button on the key remote.

- Using good situational awareness when approaching and exiting your vehicle.

- Looking for indicators that someone is tampering with your vehicle.

- Limiting what people can see in your windows, such as valuables and personal information.

- Looking in the area underneath and around your car and in the back seat before approaching and entering your vehicle.

- Taking evasive driving training if you are under high threat.

- When driving on a multilane road and approaching either a traffic light or stop sign, do not come up beside the driver in the next lane. If possible, position your vehicle a car length's distance from the car next to yours. If you can see the rear wheels of the other car it means you will have room to maneuver.

- Do not instigate a possible road rage incident. For example, if another driver cuts off your vehicle or aggressively tailgates you, do not sneer, scowl, or flip him off; you would be asking for a road rage incident. Just ignore him and keep going. You can also put your cell phone to your ear so that he sees you have a way to call for help.

- If you are car jacked, drive away from the attack if you can do so safely (meaning the car jacker is outside of the vehicle and you are able to break contact). If this is not possible, abandon your vehicle and allow him to take it. Keeping your house keys separate from your car keys is advised, so that your car jacker cannot get into your home.

- If you are abducted and are a passenger in a vehicle, if possible grab the wheel and wreck the car (without harming innocent bystanders). Your objective is to avoid being taken to a second location. If you cause a minor accident, your attacker now must contend with the witnesses (he cannot abduct all of them as well). You must act early on, be decisive, and do as much as possible to make noise and create a raucous in order to draw attention to yourself and your abductors so that you attract witnesses and get help.

- If you are abducted and are thrown into the trunk of a car, try to punch out the tail lights and wave for help.

If you are a target, give yourself the advantage of preparation. Have a plan for your routine travel. You have the power to reverse the attacker's element of surprise by being ready for it. Giving yourself a plan to follow as you travel also allows you to develop better reactions to anything out of the ordinary. This preparation may save your life. Often, after a successful attack, people who know the victim will speculate as to how it could have been prevented. They will ponder and offer the adage "Hindsight is twenty-twenty," as if to say that it would have been impossible to predict the actions of the attacker. Actually, it is more accurate to say that foresight is twenty-twenty. If you have determined you are at serious risk of being attacked, then have the foresight to implement preventative measures immediately. Why put your friends and family in the position of "armchair quarterbacking" the situation in a desperate search for answers, when answers are already available?

The following story is an example of a woman who had no training in conducting route reviews or in conducting surveillance detection. She, like the majority of women in her situation, would not have known how to access this type of training (hence, a big part of our mission is to introduce these prevention methods into the mainstream so that woman *can* access them). We use her story because it clearly exemplifies a woman whose domestic situation left her entirely disempowered. The tragedy here is that women do not (until now) have the information about where they can receive training that will save their lives. It is our sincere hope that any woman in her type of situation will read our book and contact us for help.

After many troubled years of marriage, Sally decided to separate from her husband, Bob. He was against their separation and probable divorce. He was perceived by virtually everyone who knew him as a hot-tempered individual who had anger management issues. Sally had a court protection order prohibiting him from coming near her. Sally's close friend, Margaret, invited Sally and her children to move in with Margaret and her family to help keep them safe.

A few days before a hearing was scheduled to determine if Bob would be required to be supervised during visitations with their children, Bob murdered Sally and Margaret. Bob had a prearranged meeting with his children at a school event. Margaret was to chaperone this visit so that Sally would not need to be there. Unfortunately, Bob intercepted Sally's vehicle as she was on her way to rendezvous with Margaret to drop off the children.

Bob knew which route Sally would be traveling so he parked in a neighborhood which afforded him line of sight to her predictable travel location (his chosen attack location) and waited for Sally to arrive. When Sally approached his chosen attack location he pulled in front of her car blocking her forward progress. Sally, who was traveling with the children in her vehicle, got out of her car. Bob then exited his vehicle and shot both Sally and Margaret, (who had approached in her vehicle to come meet Sally to pick up the children). Shortly thereafter Bob died in an automobile accident while trying to escape during a high-speed chase with the police.

Bob chose his attack time because he knew when and where to find Sally that day. He chose his attack location based on his ability to sit and wait for her arrival and then control her vehicle. When she arrived on the quiet, residential two lane street, he controlled her vehicle by pulling out perpendicular to her vehicle and blocking her from the front. Witnesses reported that Sally did not try any evasive maneuvers to drive away from his vehicle or ram into it. Instead she got out of her car and was now directly in the kill-zone. We will never know if the escape element was significant to Bob, though his high-speed attempt at escaping leads us to assume it was.

After this tragedy police discovered that Bob had made appearances in the neighborhood where Sally and her children were staying, but no one reported him at the time. Bob was watching Sally. He knew her habits and he used their children as his excuse to lure her into his trap. He was able to stage the attack on his terms by planning according to her travel routine for that event. He knew where she would be and when she would be there.

Sally and Bob's situation ended tragically for both of them, their children, and Margaret and her family. When you read Sally's story, you might have an understandably defeatist perspective regarding Sally's chance of survival given Bob's determination to harm her and his predisposition towards rage. A similar throw up our hands perspective is evident when people talk about terrorist attacks. It goes something like this: "If they really want to get you, they will." In Sally's case, even domestic violence, legal, and law enforcement experts remain at a loss for what more she could have done to protect herself. Perhaps we can shed some light on this darkened perspective and hopefully help other victims of domestic violence.

First, given that so many people who knew Bob indicated that he was like a time bomb waiting to explode, Sally might have opted to go into hiding through a women's shelter. This is not always a clear, easy choice to make, but if we looked at a risk/threat assessment for Sally, we could easily see that drastic prevention measures were required. Let us review the early warning signals:

- Bob was known to be aggressive and hot-tempered.
- They had an upcoming court hearing to discuss child custody issues.

- Sally had a court protection order filed against him.
- Bob knew her routines and travel patterns.
- Bob was seen in the neighborhood where Sally was staying, but neighbors were not informed about the threat.
- Even though Bob telegraphed the attack by blocking her car, Sally did not attempt to drive out of the attack (she was very likely taken by surprise, even though Bob's hostile behavior was highly predictable).

Sally knew she was faced with certain danger from Bob and had expressed this to the courts when obtaining the protection order. Preventative measures had to be taken, but Sally likely felt very powerless even with the court protection order. If Sally had been trained in conducting route reviews and in basic surveillance detection, she might have been able to avoid or at least survive the attack. Her assessments would have, at the very least, helped her to recognize that he was about to attack her and she could have attempted to drive out of the kill-zone once she saw him get out of his vehicle brandishing a handgun.

If you are involved in any similar hostile domestic situation or are under threat by someone for any reason, you can employ some basic SD measures to help ensure your safety and peace of mind. You can also seek out affordable training in surveillance detection and evasive driving skills (find the time for training if your life is at stake). You should not be concerned that these skills are beyond your reach. On the contrary, they are accessible and you do have the ability to change your situation so that you are sitting in the advantaged position. You are not and do not have to remain a sitting duck waiting to be shot to death. The police can only do so much to help those in domestic violence situations, but there are ways we can take our personal safety into our own hands. Taking threats seriously means changing our ordinary routines and taking definitive measures for protection. These changes in our ordinary routines will quickly become habits if we practice them and take them seriously.

Getting SASD, conducting a risk/threat assessment, and creating a SUPNET are the beginning steps to preventing being victimized. Creating a routes portfolio which contains separate reviews and labeled maps for each of your routes is a powerful preventative measure which complements these personal security practices so that you can stay safe while you move. Next we will look at another preventative measure you can take to avoid being attacked while in or around any static location, such as your residence and workplace. Just as you can conduct route reviews to assess your vulnerabilities while you travel, you can also conduct building reviews in order to determine the vulnerabilities in and around any structure you spend time in on a regular basis.

CHAPTER SEVEN

HOME AND WORK SECURTIY: BUILDING REVIEWS

*"Why is a woman still not safe
when she's in her home"*

--Tracy Chapman

"Home sweet home." Even the maxim helps us breathe a sigh of relief at the prospect of being safe and sheltered. Of course, when we analyze how safe we really are at home, this comforting phrase takes on a new twist. Our safety while ensconced in the sweetness of our homes is not guaranteed and we usually have to pay a little attention and often a fair amount of money to secure ourselves inside our primary domain. Regardless if we do everything we can to secure our home or do nothing at all, most of us, when at home, drop our guard and relax. This relaxed state of mind is part of the bliss of home.

Predators study their victims' homes and workplaces. In most cases, they are attempting to collect information on how to gain entry into these structures. They are also interested in learning about the existing security measures and procedures at these locations so that they can devise ways to bypass the security. In this chapter we teach you how to assess the security you have at home and at work, how to improve it, and where to look for signs of surveillance. It is easy to conduct a building review and your rewards for doing so are many: You will improve your security; you will feel greater ease knowing that you can recognize a predator early on if you are ever targeted; and you will know how to mitigate your risk of being attacked in or around any of these buildings.

Before we get into the mechanics of conducting building reviews, take a moment to assess your habits. When at home, are you conscientious about security? Do you always keep doors locked, even while inside your home? Do you activate your alarm system both when in the house and when you go out? Do you have a dog? Do you keep your blinds drawn at night and use a peep hole at the front door? Have you installed fences around your property? Do you lock gates, secure basement entrances with bars, and keep your home well lit? Study your home security and be honest about your habits. Notice any gaps that exist. For example, perhaps you are consistent about keeping doors locked, but often are so relaxed when at home that you forget to close the blinds or curtains at night. Remember that, if a predator is studying you, he is looking for these gaps in your security procedures.

If you study your habits, you will realize that it is not difficult or expensive to improve your security. Make sure you are actually using your existing resources. For example, if you have deadbolts, are you actually locking them? Think of creative and inexpensive ways to improve your home security. For example, you can improvise a home alarm system quickly by purchasing inexpensive stick-on alarms that sound if a door or window is opened. At a minimum you can stack something in front of your door that would make a sound and awaken you should anyone try to break in to your home. Or, if you do not have a dog, you can at least buy a "Beware of Dog" sign or a water bowl that you fill and leave on the porch to create the illusion that you have a big dog. Your home security is versatile. If you are in a low threat situation, taking basic security measures is usually enough. If your threat level suddenly escalates, you might need to spend more money on a home alarm system or surveillance cameras.

By learning to conduct building reviews, you will easily and quickly bolster your security, both at your residence and your place of work. You will also learn to apply surveillance detection methods to ascertain if someone is watching you at your home or workplace. You can apply the building review process to any type of structure (for example, perhaps you go to the same gym five days a week). Remember that predators study your habits, thus patterns you set while in any buildings will be of interest to them.

RESIDENCE AND WORKPLACE REVIEW

If a predator intends on attacking you either in your home or at your workplace, he must study these facilities and learn certain information in order to plan a successful attack against you. When collecting information on a building he must assess a host of features about the structure. In turn, as you conduct your building reviews, you will look at the same features and determine the most vulnerable areas of your structure. Since predators are doing the same, once they determine where you are most vulnerable in and around your structure, they will then watch those areas more carefully to collect the information that will become necessary for the attack.

The area must support an attack in that the attackers must be able to:

- Obtain access to the building and discreetly bring in the appropriate weapon.
- Blend into the area easily without arising suspicion while they are conducting the surveillance and waiting to make the attack.
- Escape after the attack (both physically and without being filmed or witnessed).

Basic Building Security

You can improve your security and privacy in any building by simply analyzing the layers of security it has, and then by identifying how and from where surveillance will watch the building. All buildings have varied layers of security that people must pass through in order to enter. Some security layers are visible to predators and some are not. At a minimum, one visible security layer all buildings have in common is the exterior walls of the building itself. The exterior walls act as a physical barrier to the elements of weather, wild animals, and predators with an illegal intent. Other common physical barriers for buildings include fences, gates, walls, and blockades such as concrete planters.

However, since all buildings have to be accessed there will be entrances such as doors and windows (referred to as 'portals' by security professionals) which allow someone to pass through those physical barriers. All building portals are important because predators tend to initially focus on them. For example, a stalker will watch the door from which his victim enters and departs the building and the windows to see where the victim goes when inside the building. Burglars may focus their surveillance on other building portals, such as rear windows or utility access-ways through which they hope to gain surreptitious entry. A rapist intent on attacking a woman in a parking garage may initially focus his surveillance on the entryway to a parking garage and the secluded areas, such as corners or stairwells. Then he will watch to see if the garage is patrolled by security guards or if surveillance cameras are positioned in his potential attack locations.

Aside from barriers and portals, buildings may have security procedures which create yet another layer of security. This layer may include technical, procedural, environmental, and informative security measures. Examples of technical layers of security are door locks, alarm systems, motion detectors, surveillance cameras, and lighting. Sometimes technical layers of security are not visible and other times they are made visible to act as a deterrent, such as prominently posting a home alarm system placard at a residence. Procedural layers of security include measures like using an identification card or badge system to control access to a building. Having a parking permit system or a sign-in desk are other examples of procedural layers of security. Basically any procedure that is used to screen people entering the building will help deter predators. Environmental layers of security are created by the terrain and activity around the building. A home located in a cul-de-sac of an exclusive and well police patrolled residential area is considered a good layer of security for crime, just by virtue of its location in that environment. Landscaping, such as a berm or vegetation which limits visibility of the building, can also function as an environmental layer of security. Informative layers of security include any source that provides you with information regarding potential threats. Surveillance detection is the most powerful informative layer of security if it is done correctly because it is invisible to the predator. SD is a powerful technique for helping you know how to collect information on predators and where to look for them. Other examples of informative security layers are police warnings alerting you to specific threats and neighbors or service people living and working in the area who provide information about suspicious people or activities.

Building Review

To begin this process you will again need some easel size paper or poster board and different colored pens. You will make a diagram for each building where you spend time on a regular basis; at a minimum this will be for your home and workplace. If there are any other buildings you spend time in regularly, such as a health club or educational institution, you can apply the same process for those. At the end of each step we provide Kate's example so that you can see exactly how it is done. We will study both Kate's residence and her workplace.

Note: We are breaking down this process into steps, thus we are creating several maps and building on them as we go. You will only create one large map for each building which will include all of the steps below.

Step One: Existing Layers of Security

Draw a diagram of the building in the center of the piece of paper. Draw everything around the building, such as other homes or structures, significant landscaping features, parks, bus stops, stores, and parking areas. Indicate all of the existing layers of security in and around your building, such as alarm systems, gates, surveillance cameras, and locks. Including these pre-existing security measures will help you to become more aware of any gaps (areas where you are missing security layers) and how you can improve the security that is already in place.

Step One: Kate

Residence Example: (see Diagram 1A)

Kate's residence has very little in the way of existing security. She does have deadbolts on the primary doors. She also keeps her garage door closed, except when in use. She has decent lighting around the house, though no motion-activated lights. Although the woods in her back yard offer privacy, she has no fences, gates, or barriers of any kind between her home and the woods. She also has no alarm system.

Kate keeps the blinds closed at night, but during the day the windows in her office and bedroom afford a view into her house to anyone parked out on the street within line of sight. Because the woods behind Kate's house are thick, it would be easy for her stalker to watch her when she is out on her deck or in her kitchen.

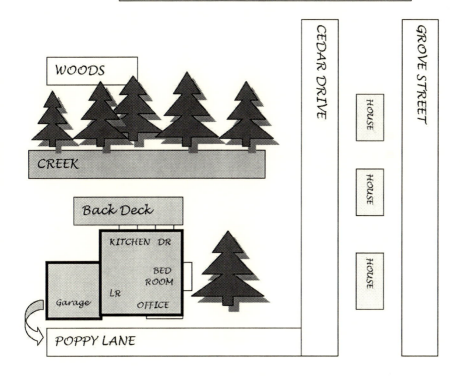

(Diagram 1A)
KATE'S HOUSE

Existing Layers of Security: Kate has deadbolts on her front and back doors. Her garage door is remote controlled and she keeps it closed at all times, unless in use. All her windows have Venetian blinds. She has a light over her front door and on her back wall near the deck. The areas surrounding the walls of her home are open and are not obstructed by hedges or overgrown shrubbery.

Gaps: Kate has no fences or gates around her yard, no outdoor motion-activated lights, and no home alarm system. Kate also does not have a dog.

Workplace Example: (see Diagram 1B)

Kate's workplace is a much better secured facility. The parking garage is permit only parking and any vehicle entering must display a parking sticker. Armed security guards work in and around her office building. Both the garage and the building have an extensive surveillance camera system. Kate's stalker could sit at the plaza to learn what times she arrives to and departs from work each day. However, gaining access to Kate both inside the parking garage and in her office is more risky due to the security presence and surveillance cameras. Still, Kate's stalker can access the building through the main lobby and it is possible he can follow her into the parking garage on foot.

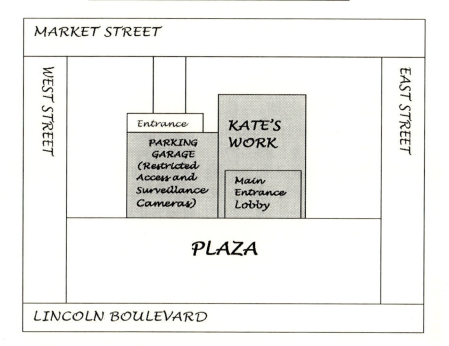

(Diagram 1B)
KATE'S WORK

MARKET STREET

WEST STREET

EAST STREET

Entrance

PARKING
GARAGE
(Restricted
Access and
Surveillance
Cameras)

KATE'S
WORK

Main
Entrance
Lobby

PLAZA

LINCOLN BOULEVARD

Existing Security Layers: The parking garage has restricted access and only vehicles with parking stickers can gain entry. Armed security guards monitor the garage and an extensive surveillance camera system is in place. The building itself has a surveillance camera system, though only the entrance lobby, elevators, and hallways are monitored. Security guards have a booth in the main entrance lobby where they watch the surveillance camera footage in real time. The guards patrol inside the building and the parameters of the building during operating hours.

Gaps: The building is open to the public and anyone can enter the main lobby and move throughout the various floors and hallways of the building, using both the elevators and the staircases. The parking garage can be accessed on foot from inside of the building. The building cafeteria is also open to the public.

Step Two: Surveillance Locations (SVL)

Determine, label, and number the surveillance locations (SVL). You may need to actually get outside and walk around the building in order to do this. Stand or sit in these locations before you label them on your diagram. You may realize that the surveillance cannot see anything of significance in a particular spot. Then again, you may get out there and realize there is a hidden spot that offers them a great view into your living room or office. Remember to consider how the seasons affect these locations. In winter, trees are bare, affording views that are unattainable during the rest of the year.

It is also important to indicate what surveillance might use for cover in each location. Most people will try to be discreet when conducting surveillance. That means they will come up with some plausible story so that they can stay in an area for a certain length of time without arousing suspicion. This is not necessarily a verbal story; rather their "story" will be evident when you see them. For example, if you see a man in a jogging suit, stretching his legs in an area of a public park, his "story" is that he is a jogger who is either warming up before or cooling down after his run. You do not have to go up and ask him why he is there; you can see his story for yourself.

When determining the surveillance locations (SVL), remember what types of information someone might try to collect on you. If a predator wants to determine what time you leave for work each morning, he will position himself someplace where he has line of sight to your driveway so that he can see you exiting. If he wants to watch you sunbathing in your backyard, he will find a position that affords him line of sight to your chaise lounge. Or perhaps he wants to follow you on your lunch break at work so he must choose a position where he can see you exit the building.

Step Two: Kate

Residence Example: (see Diagram 2A)

When Kate labels the surveillance locations at her residence she will consider what is realistic. For example, her stalker will probably not choose to sit on the front porch of her neighbor's house unless he can come up with a plausible way to access and use that position for any length of time. However, he would easily be able find a spot tucked away in the woods behind her house near the creek from which to hide and watch her. Or he can sit in a parked car in a location where he is afforded a view of her home.

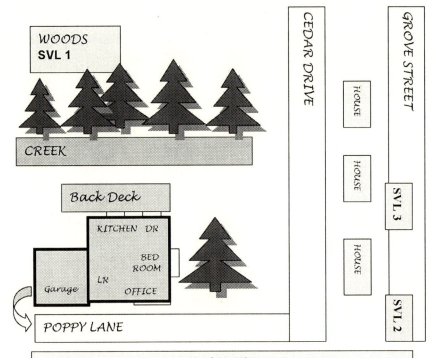

SVL=Surveillance Locations

(Diagram 2A)
KATE'S HOUSE

WOODS
SVL 1

CREEK

Back Deck

KITCHEN   DR

BED
ROOM

LR

Garage   OFFICE

POPPY LANE

CEDAR DRIVE

GROVE STREET

HOUSE

HOUSE

HOUSE

SVL 3

SVL 2

OPEN FIELD

SVL 1: Gives line of sight to her backyard and kitchen.
Cover: Probably attempts to remain concealed, since it is private property. He may use camouflage clothing or create a dugout from which he can position himself discreetly.

SVL 2: Gives line of sight to the front of her house so he can see her coming and going.

SVL 3: Gives line of sight into her backyard and a partial view into her bedroom window.

SVL 2&3 Cover: Sitting in a parked car, reading the newspaper; sitting in some type of service vehicle as though he were working in the neighborhood. Because he is one street away, he may use binoculars. During winter when the trees are bare these are better positions than the woods.

Note: Because Cedar Drive is a private street with no thru-traffic, it is unlikely her stalker will park and watch her anywhere on the street because he would be too exposed. Still, Kate is wise to consider he might be so bold. Also, the open field across the street offers no cover for her stalker, thus he would not use this area to conduct surveillance.

Workplace Example: (see Diagram 2B)

At Kate's workplace her stalker is denied vehicle access to the parking garage, though he can sneak into the garage on foot and he has access to the building. However, he puts himself at risk of being caught on film inside the building and potentially having to contend with the security guards. He does have access to a public location (the plaza) from which he can observe the main entrance to the building in the event that Kate leaves on foot to take a break or to go out to lunch. If Kate, like most employees in the building, sits in the plaza area during her breaks, her stalker can position himself there and watch her.

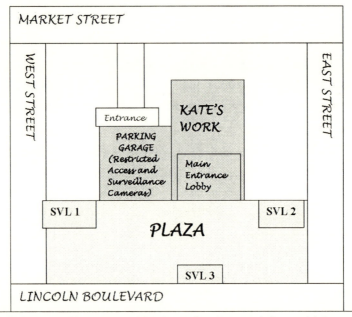

SVL=Surveillance Locations

(Diagram 2B)
KATE'S WORK

MARKET STREET

WEST STREET

EAST STREET

Entrance

KATE'S WORK

PARKING GARAGE (Restricted Access and Surveillance Cameras)

Main Entrance Lobby

SVL 1

SVL 2

PLAZA

SVL 3

LINCOLN BOULEVARD

SVL 1: This position allows Kate's stalker to watch her vehicle as she arrives and departs from the parking garage.

SVL 2: This position allows the stalker to watch her enter and exit the main entrance of the building. If he intends to follow her, this position allows him to get behind her when she exits the building, without her noticing him.

SVL 3: This position allows her stalker to see the main entrance as well as the entire plaza. He can use any part of the plaza if Kate is out there on break.

SVL 1, 2, & 3 Cover: Regardless of his position, his options could include: reading a book or newspaper; eating lunch; drinking coffee; chatting or playing chess with someone; talking on a cell phone.

Step Three: Interior Surveillance Detection Locations (ISDL)

Determine, label, and number your interior surveillance detection locations (ISDL). These are the locations inside your building that afford you line of sight to the surveillance locations you identified. Imagine that you labeled SVL 1 as a park bench that faces your entrance to your workplace. You will find an interior surveillance detection location that affords you line of sight to this park bench. It may be at a window which faces out to the park from which you can discreetly watch that bench with a small pair of binoculars.

In general, your interior surveillance detection locations are the safest bet. They keep you at a physical distance from the predator, while at the same time allowing you the freedom to watch him discreetly. Be creative when determining these ISDL. Remember that you can use optics to help increase your range of vision and you can turn off lights and close curtains or blinds to improve your ability to remain unseen. You will use your ISDL before and after you transition into and out of the building. For example, someone at your office might use buddy SD and position her/himself at your designated ISDL fifteen minutes before you arrive to work to see if anyone is in a surveillance location exhibiting indicators of surveillance that correlate with your arrival to work. Likewise, you can use this ISDL yourself before you leave work at the end of the day to see if anyone is out in a surveillance location waiting for you to exit the building.

Step Three: Kate

Residence Example: (see Diagram 3A)

Kate will now spend time discovering places inside her home and workplace that afford her views of the surveillance locations she identified and labeled on her map. At her home she will take her small pair of binoculars and will determine which windows offer her the best view of each surveillance location she identified. Kate knows she needs to be discreet as she watches each location, so she will adjust her curtains or blinds so that she can use these windows without being seen by her stalker.

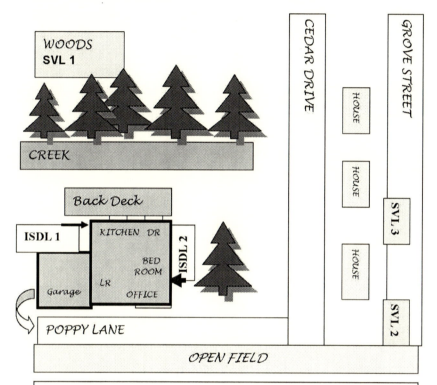

SVL=Surveillance Locations
ISDL=Interior Surveillance Detection Locations

(Diagram 3A)
KATE'S HOUSE

ISDL 1: From her kitchen window Kate has line of sight to her backyard and the woods (SVL 1).

Cover: Kate must adjust her blinds to be able to discreetly observe the woods. She should have a camera positioned here so that she can record any sightings. She will have to turn out any lights so that her stalker cannot see her. She will position a pen and paper allowing her to record the date, time, and details.

ISDL 2: Kate's bedroom window affords her line of sight to SVL 2 & 3.

Cover: Kate will remain concealed behind the curtains. She will position binoculars and recording materials and be discreet while observing.

Workplace Example: (see Diagram 3B)

At Kate's workplace, she has a greater challenge because her access to parts of the office building is limited. Since her office does not face the plaza (where she has identified her stalker will be), she must find a window from either a hallway or the lobby that she can use, (or she must enlist the help of someone in the building whose office does have a view of the plaza). Her stalker is not trying to watch her inside her office, rather at the locations where she enters and exits her office. The back entrance to the building is too unsafe for Kate to use. It is situated in a back alley with high brick walls. She would have no way to escape back there or get help. It is safer for her to stick with the more visible and busy area of the plaza.

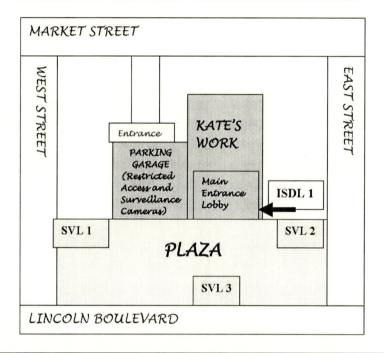

SVL=Surveillance Locations
ISDL=Interior Surveillance
Detection Locations

(Diagram 3B)
KATE'S WORK

MARKET STREET

WEST STREET

EAST STREET

Entrance

KATE'S WORK

PARKING GARAGE
(Restricted Access and Surveillance Cameras)

Main Entrance Lobby

ISDL 1

SVL 1

SVL 2

PLAZA

SVL 3

LINCOLN BOULEVARD

ISDL 1: Kate's office window does not face the plaza; thus, her best option to look out onto the plaza from inside the building is from inside the main entrance lobby. The entrance has tall glass windows and doors. Kate can sit away from the windows so that she is not visible but can see out onto the entire plaza. Since her stalker can access this entrance lobby, she must first scan the lobby to make sure he is not there before choosing a position from which to view the plaza.

Cover: Kate will be concealed because she will position herself back from the glass. She will have her recording materials ready, though she may not be able to take a photograph unless she has a good digital camera.

Step Four: Exterior Surveillance Detection Locations (ESDL)

Determine, label, and number your exterior surveillance detection locations (ESDL). These are any exterior locations that give you line of sight to the surveillance locations. Remember, it is best to be behind the surveillance when outside. If you are in front of them, they can see you watching them. You are less likely to use these positions, unless you are in a high threat situation, but it is extremely valuable and worth your time to identify them. If you need extra support from family or friends to help you detect surveillance, they can use your exterior surveillance detection locations. For example, if you had determined a man was stalking you at your home, you could have a friend set up in one of these ESDL and photograph the stalker while you created a distraction by moving inside of your home with the blinds open so that the stalker's attention is focused on you rather than on what is going on behind him.

Make sure to indicate what you, or anyone using these ESDL, can use as cover. Remember that surveillance detection works best as a discreet method. Thus, if someone in your SUPNET is outside in public conducting SD, he/she needs to either be concealed somehow or have very good cover, meaning an excellent way of blending in to the environment. If we take your friend who is photographing the stalker as an example, this friend must have a plausible story for being in the area, one that is visible to anyone passing by. Walking a dog or sitting on a bench reading the newspaper are examples. When determining cover options, see what is appropriate and normal for the specific area and notice what options are already available. Perhaps there is a newsstand that affords line of sight to the surveillance location where your friend could spend time browsing through magazines as his/her cover.

Step Four: Kate

Residence Example: (see Diagram 4A)

At Kate's residence the exterior surveillance detection locations (ESDL) are limited. She can be out doing yard work or reading on the back deck. Note: If Kate can get her neighbors to help her, they could also conduct SD from either inside their homes or outside in their yards.

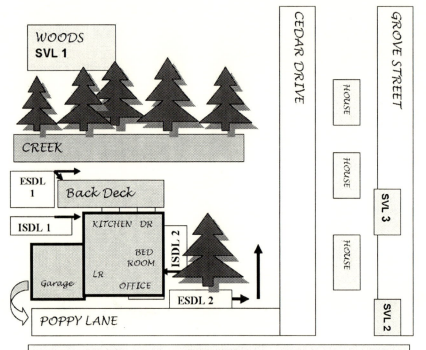

SVL=Surveillance Locations
ISDL=Interior Surveillance
        Detection Locations
ESDL=Exterior Surveillance
        Detection Locations

(Diagram 4A)
KATE'S HOUSE

WOODS
SVL 1

CEDAR DRIVE

GROVE STREET

HOUSE

HOUSE

HOUSE

SVL 3

SVL 2

CREEK

ESDL
1

Back Deck

ISDL 1

KITCHEN DR

ISDL 2

BED
ROOM

LR

Garage

OFFICE

ESDL 2

POPPY LANE

OPEN FIELD

ESDL 1: Kate can either spend time on her deck or in her backyard in order to conduct surveillance detection for her stalker's **SVL 1** in the woods.

Cover: Kate can do yard work or landscaping projects; sit on the deck and read or talk on the phone. It will be impossible for Kate to take photos discreetly because her stalker will be able to see her actions. Plus, Kate risks danger if her stalker is indeed in the woods, so she must be prepared to move inside quickly and lock her doors.

ESDL 2: Kate can see both **SVL 2 & 3** if she is out working in her side yard. She is safer out here because she is in sight of her neighbors' homes and her stalker would be farther away.

Cover: Yard work or landscaping.

Workplace Example: (see Diagram 4B)

At Kate's workplace, she has many options for exterior surveillance detection locations. The plaza area is large enough that she can find locations where she or someone supporting her could sit to watch her stalker arrive and select his surveillance location. Kate, or her support person, will need to use some kind of cover or way to blend in to the area, for example drinking a cup of coffee while reading a newspaper on a bench. She will need to consider how long this particular cover choice will work. What is the normal amount of time it takes for someone to do the activity? She also needs to behave naturally and not call attention to herself whenever she is out on the plaza (and her support SD must do the same).

SVL=Surveillance Locations
ISDL=Interior Surveillance Detection
    Locations
ESDL=Exterior Surveillance Detection
    Locations

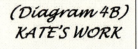

(Diagram 4B)
KATE'S WORK

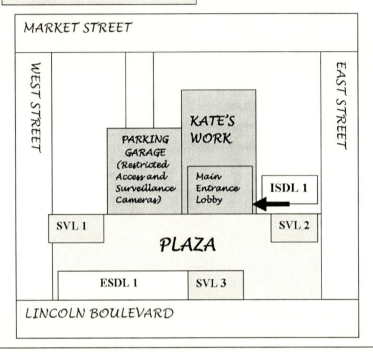

ESDL 1: Kate's best exterior SD location is anywhere along the south end of the Plaza (near Lincoln Boulevard). This location allows her to see the entire plaza without having to turn around and thereby possibly signaling to her stalker that she is aware she is under surveillance. She can also observe the building's main entrance. If her stalker follows her inside as she approaches the entrance, she has a better chance of detecting him through the reflection in the glass doors.

Cover: Kate or her support SD can eat lunch; drink coffee; read the paper; chat with a friend; talk on her cell phone; enjoy the sun. Her cover options are similar to her stalker's. She must be very discreet when recording any information.

Step Five: Attack Locations (AL) and Safe Locations

Determine, label, and number any attack locations (AL). These include any locations where attackers can gain access to your buildings, (even if they do so illegally) and any locations in the vicinity of your building that allow them to attack you without being observed, such as an enclosed pathway near where you park which you will walk through to your front door. If you conducted a risk/threat assessment, you may have already implemented preventative courses of action that will bolster the security of your home and workplace. Still, it is important for you to assess where you are vulnerable to attacks, either inside or around your buildings.

Perhaps you own a home which has a carport at the front entrance and someone could easily hide in there waiting for you to return home. Perhaps you park in a lot adjacent to your office and have to walk past an alley entrance in order to get into the building. Be thorough in identifying the places you are vulnerable in and around your buildings. Include areas where the attacker can be concealed, such as behind bushes, or where you could be restricted, such as in a narrow passageway. Also consider areas with poor lighting. If your home or workplace is in a bad area of town (meaning one with a high crime rate), take this into consideration as a factor that will work to your attacker's advantage. Remember, the predator is watching any areas where you are vulnerable because those vulnerable locations are his ticket to a successful attack scenario.

Once you have determined these vulnerabilities, go back and double check your surveillance locations. Did you miss any locations where surveillance can go to watch these vulnerable places in and around your building? You may now need to add more SVL to your diagram. If you add any more SVL, do not forget to then add any interior or exterior SDL that provide you with a view of the surveillance locations for each attack site.

Next add any safe locations you can use in and around your building. Perhaps there is a room inside where you can lock yourself in, should anyone break in and attempt to attack you. Make sure you have a telephone inside this room. Perhaps in the area around your building or home you have access to a public location or a nearby neighbor's home where you could retreat for help. Label these safe locations on your map.

Step Five: Kate

Residence Example: (see Diagram 5A)

At Kate's home she can identify the obvious attack sites that offer a way for her stalker to hide before the attack and escape afterwards. A more audacious attacker might not bother to hide and might just wait in his car for her to come home. Kate knows to pay careful attention around the attack locations she labeled and also to any unfamiliar cars parked in the area.

Kate has few options for safe locations, as she lives on a dead end street. Her own home or her nearest neighbors are her safest locations.

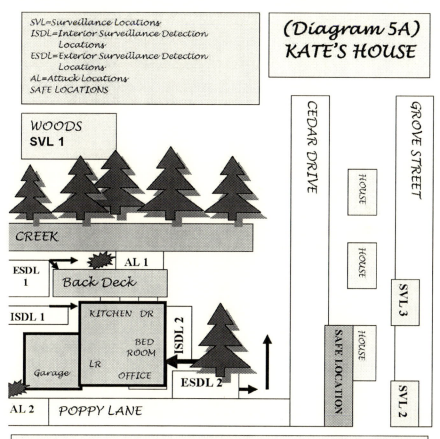

SVL=Surveillance Locations
ISDL=Interior Surveillance Detection
          Locations
ESDL=Exterior Surveillance Detection
          Locations
AL=Attack Locations
SAFE LOCATIONS

(Diagram 5A)
KATE'S HOUSE

WOODS
SVL 1

CEDAR DRIVE

GROVE STREET

HOUSE

HOUSE

CREEK

ESDL 1

AL 1

Back Deck

ISDL 1

KITCHEN DR

ISDL 2

BED
ROOM

LR

Garage

OFFICE

ESDL 2

SAFE LOCATION

HOUSE

SVL 3

SVL 2

AL 2

POPPY LANE

OPEN FIELD

AL 1: Kate is most vulnerable to attack in her back yard or on her back deck. Her stalker can either attack her there or drag her into the woods.

AL 2: Kate is also vulnerable to attack as she pulls out from or into her garage. Her stalker can be hiding beside the garage because the dead end street allows him to approach unseen from the woods and sneak over to the side of the garage.

Safe Location: Kate's nearest neighbor is her established safe location.

Note: If Kate is not extremely careful, she can also be attacked inside her home. She must strengthen her home security either by installing an alarm system or getting a dog. Installing motion lights is another wise move. She must keep her doors and windows locked at all times.

Workplace Example: (see Diagram 5B)

At her workplace, Kate has to be very discerning when identifying possible attack locations. Certainly, she is vulnerable in the parking garage. Even though there are security cameras and some uniformed guards, not every area is protected. Because of the danger, Kate carries a TASER ™ device (see Chapter Twelve) when she walks from her car to the building. Other isolated locations inside her building pose a threat, such as stairwells, so she avoids them. If she is alone in the elevator and a man gets on, she immediately gets off and waits for another elevator, unless it is a man she recognizes from her office.

Kate will also indicate any safe locations on her map. If she were to be attacked, where could she flee for help? She has identified all the security guard booths in the area surrounding the building. She knows where all of the major exits are and she has developed a 'what if' plan in the event that her stalker somehow confronts her in the building. She carries a panic button and cell phone with her at all times and she has shown her co-workers and the security staff a photo of her stalker.

SVL=Surveillance Locations
ISDL=Interior Surveillance Detection Locations
ESDL=Exterior Surveillance Detection Locations
AL=Attack Locations
SAFE LOCATIONS

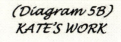

(Diagram 5B)
KATE'S WORK

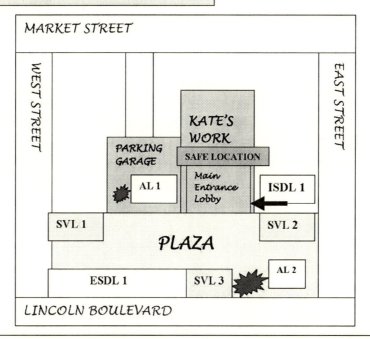

AL 1: Despite the security at the parking garage, Kate knows that her stalker could potentially access the garage on foot by entering through the building. Since the guards and security cameras are not positioned everywhere, Kate is very alert and always carries her **TASER** device when inside the garage. She also keeps her vehicle doors locked at all times. She knows her stalker could escape the same way he got into the garage and possibly avoid being recorded by the surveillance cameras.

AL 2: If her stalker were to become violent and reckless, he might opt to attack her at the plaza. Therefore, since incidents of surveillance confirm that she is being stalked, Kate now avoids the plaza, unless she is accompanied by a co-worker. Her stalker would likely choose to attack her at the south end of the plaza (near Lincoln Boulevard) because it offers him the easiest escape routes away from the building security.

SAFE LOCATION: Kate is safest inside the office building at the security booth in the main entrance lobby.

In summary, each building review will include a large diagram labeled with the following:

- Existing security measures (including technical, procedural, environmental, and informative).
- SVL (Surveillance Locations, indicating what they can use for cover or concealment in each location).
- ISDL (Interior Surveillance Detection Locations you can use to discreetly detect surveillance while safe inside your building).
- ESDL (Exterior Surveillance Detection Locations where you or your SD support can detect surveillance while outside in the surrounding area of your building. You or your SD support must use cover or be concealed in each of these locations so that the surveillance is not aware anyone is watching them).
- AL (Attack Locations are vulnerable areas in and around your structures that are conducive to an attack).
- Safe Locations are areas where you can retreat if you fall under attack or need immediate help.

Each building will be different based on the terrain, building design, and activity in the area. However, we always recommend beginning with at least limited SD from inside the building because you are most secure when you are looking out from property to which you control access. Surveillance will not be expecting you to be watching them from inside your building so you will have the advantage of being able to see them in action, especially if you are discreet.

Even if you normally shy away from studying diagrams such as the ones in this chapter, we encourage you to take the time to look at our diagrams so that when you create your own, you will not leave out anything important. When you first start analyzing your buildings, it is easy to overlook key features, such as options surveillance might choose for a location from which to study you. However, once you understand the building review process, you will be able to very quickly perform on-the-spot reviews of unfamiliar buildings you are visiting and you will quickly notice both the security measures already in place and any gaps in security.

This review process is not rocket science. Unless you are in a high threat situation, you can take your time with it so that you feel comfortable and do not add stress to your already busy life. Even if route reviews and building reviews intimidate you, remember this is really just common sense. Give yourself permission to think like the bad guy; it may literally save your life one day! Plus, it is empowering to take control of your personal security by preparing yourself with this analysis work. Do remember to keep these maps in a secure location. If someone is really watching you, do not provide him with any helpful information which could be used against you.

Congratulations! You have completed the first and most difficult part of this book. You now have instruction on how to:

- Develop your situational awareness.
- Protect your privacy and identity.
- Create a risk/threat assessment.
- Establish a SUPNET.
- Conduct surveillance detection and develop an SD plan.
- Conduct route reviews for your routine travel.
- Conduct building reviews for your home and workplace.

In the second part of this book we explore how getting SASD and all of the other techniques you just learned apply to the specific threats women face in their daily lives. It is time to integrate all you have learned and put it to practical use to keep you and your children safe.

PART TWO

INTEGRATION: PREVENTING, DEFENDING, AND SURVIVING

CHAPTER EIGHT

DANGEROUS LIAISONS: DATING, RELATIONSHIPS, ABUSE, AND DOMESTIC VIOLENCE

*"Do you ever finally reach
a point of knowing
or do you just wake up one day
and say, I am going?"*

--Cowboy Junkies

Ming gasped: "You're kidding, right: Security for relationships? Relationships are complicated enough!" "How am I supposed to size up a guy after one date much less one year? Men are full of surprises and every relationship I have been in has not turned out like I expected."

Most of us can relate to Ming's exasperation; relationships often immerse us in complexities. Yet, since so much of our time and energy is invested in obtaining and maintaining romantic relationships, it makes sense that our personal security might be impacted at some point during the course of any courtship or relationship. Date rape and domestic violence statistics alone give us pause and compel us to realize that attraction and love do not always equal harmony and bliss.

Now that you have learned how to practice situational awareness and surveillance detection, we will explore how you can apply these skills to your romantic life, regardless if it is healthy and safe or has become soured by dysfunction and the potential for violence. Ironically, relationships present us with psychological challenges that impact our personal security. We all get drawn into a mythology about romance and love. Often this mythology separates us from our better judgment. It is difficult to maintain situational awareness when one's emotions are at the helm. Our emotions cloud our perceptions, causing us to ignore or overlook indicators of threat and danger.

Women must challenge themselves to embrace a more objective overview of their romantic endeavors. This does not mean we cannot enjoy all of the delights that accompany our romantic quests. It simply means that we need to develop the easy habit of taking a step back and realistically assessing early warning signals of potential danger. If you practice situational awareness in every aspect of your life, including your romantic life, you stand a much better chance of sensing danger from the get go and removing yourself from it. If you are well into a relationship that becomes dangerous, you can apply SA and SD techniques to keep yourself safe in the relationship and after the break up.

No matter what psychological complexities are embedded in your subconscious regarding your romantic liaisons, it is ultimately your responsibility to consciously protect yourself (unless you are a minor). Naturally you can elicit support from law enforcement and other groups, but this support does not always guarantee you will be kept safe. Ultimately you must be the one to first make the choice to be safe and to then follow through by being proactive with your own security (even if it means removing yourself from a relationship and enduring the pain and hardship of a break up or divorce).

Think about it this way: What if, on a first date, you both asked each other the question "Who are you at your worst?" We all have our worst moments and a side of our personality that emerges when we are unhappy or are under stress. In relationships, we often do not get to know one another well enough to expose that side of ourselves until months or years down the line. It would be a radical question to ask on a first date, but imagine if you got an honest answer (and you gave one). Suppose, for example, your date revealed something like: "I have a short, explosive temper and sometimes give the woman in my life the silent treatment if I am upset with her." Of course we never discuss such things on first dates because we are caught up in the attraction, the possibilities, and presenting ourselves in the most favorable light possible.

Imagine how efficient this line of questioning could be for both parties concerned. Perhaps each would learn about the other's darkest personality traits and the two would recognize instantly that they would be a bad match. They could save months, if not years of agony. At worst, each would reveal his/her distasteful traits and then both could choose to continue from a place of honesty about the possibilities for the match. In fact, perhaps the honesty itself would be a refreshing approach that both would deem a worthy component to a healthy relationship. Here is the rub: Even if you were to ask an abuser or a predator for the truth about who he really is deep down, you will not get it. His ugly truth will rear its head when you least expect it, so you *must pay attention to early warning signals.*

Part of our vision of the evolution of empowerment includes women taking charge of their own emotions so that they can maintain their personal security. This does not mean becoming an unfeeling robot who never abandons herself to love. Rather it means evolving to a place where you love *yourself* enough to prioritize your safety. Low self-esteem, loneliness, our need for love and connection, and our nurturing, trusting nature can all work against us if we do not consciously develop good, consistent habits regarding our personal security in the context of relationships. Love calls us to be vulnerable sometimes. We can accept ourselves as emotionally vulnerable and even fragile when it comes to love, but that vulnerability does not need to seep into the part of ourselves that governs personal security. We must evolve to a place where we establish boundaries in our romantic lives that are clear, true, and wholesome. Because love embraces the notion of forgiveness, many women forgive the violence perpetrated against them by loved ones. Forgiveness for instances of violence undermines the boundaries we have set and compromises our personal security if it means we brush off what happened and do not hold our partner accountable. Certainly, once you work with a professional to identify and resolve the issues associated with the violence, you may end up being able to forgive your aggressor someday, while at the same time insisting on keeping yourself safe. Just remember: you cannot forgive from the grave.

Testosterone levels alone separate women from men. We know men's physical make-up is different from ours. In some ways we totally cannot relate to their levels of aggression and violence. Living day to day with a man allows a woman to experience the ebb and flow of his particular disposition. So many factors can impact aggression and violence, including but not limited to: hormone levels; diet; lack of exercise; caffeine intake; use of alcohol or drugs; external circumstances and stress factors; emotional or mental problems; unhappiness in the relationship; and low self-esteem. Women often make the mistake of thinking they can control the level of aggression and violence in relationships. Women will work hard to appease, placate, and smooth over the instigators of this aggression and attempt to create that happy ending that is so indoctrinated and desired. Our nurturing nature backfires and we end up nurturing the aggression, allowing it to simmer slowly until it boils over into violence.

What we should be nurturing is our survival instinct. If we put our personal security first and refuse to tolerate any kind of abuse or violence, we will contribute to an evolving society. When women allow men to be abusive in relationships, they empower the aggression and violence against them by condoning it as acceptable attributes of love. In this chapter we hope to impact the evolution of empowerment by encouraging women to take a stand for their right to be safe in the context of relationships. In order to take this stand, we will provide you with the tools for doing so and instruct you in the application of prevention techniques. Please note: although we are focusing on male/female relationships, the same information and techniques certainly apply to same sex relationships. In addition, if you recognize that you are the one who is being abusive in your relationship and find yourself exhibiting cyclical patterns of abusive responses, you would be wise to seek professional help. As embarrassing or difficult as it may seem, admitting you are an abuser is the first step to transforming the behavior.

Dating

Let us begin at the beginning of a relationship. How can we know if the person we are interested in is a possible threat? It can be confusing because the early warning signals of predatory behavior are often very similar to the courting rituals of a suitor. Add to that the emotional soup-sandwich called desire that plays into the dynamics of a new relationship and you come out looking like a deer caught in the headlights. Your best asset when beginning a relationship is, once again, situational awareness. Pay attention to your intuition, your sensory responses, and any early warning signals that tell you something about this man is just not right. Do not sacrifice your security for the prospect of a meaningful relationship. Logically speaking, how meaningful can it be if the man is someone who might hurt you?

Women make enormous sacrifices all the time for love. Some sacrifice their self-esteem by overrating the men they love. Some sacrifice their personal security because they are so afraid of losing their partners. Do not project your desires about the relationship to the point that you overlook your safety. Even if you allow yourself to be motivated by your own fears and insecurities when you make decisions about dating, such as the fear of being alone or the fear of rejection, you must train yourself to prioritize your personal security. Perhaps your biological clock is ticking and you have high hopes of meeting Mr. Right so that you can have children. Romance is not the only reason we date. Most of us have ulterior motives where relationships are concerned. Still, you must avoid becoming so hypnotized by the prospect of love that you ignore the signals of danger.

It seems unthinkable to us to do any kind of background check on a man in whom we are interested. We could hire a private investigator to address our concerns, but what kind of relationship is based on such mistrust? Yet, often when we apply for employment we are screened by such things as applications, references, background checks, drug tests, and sometimes even security clearances. Conducting due diligence on a prospective mate is not necessarily an invasion of privacy. Rather it is a prudent option for both parties. If you identify early warning signals that cause you to wonder about the man you are dating, it is not expensive to do a simple background check on the internet (see Appendix E). No one has to know you are looking into his past for a possible criminal record. It is not, for example, difficult to go on the internet and do a search for sexual predators in your area. Any woman with children would be crazy not to, in this day and age. Why would the same logic not apply to dating?

Even if you are set up on a blind date, do some due diligence. Ask questions about the man and his background. How well do the people who are setting you up know him? For that matter, if you meet a man at a bar or in a café, you really can only do a certain amount of due diligence on him. For example, does he really work where he says he does? That is easy enough to check out for yourself by calling him at work or arranging to meet him there. Stay alert for discrepancies in his story about himself and his life. If he were wise, he would be on the lookout for the same from you. On the surface, he might appear to be the cat's meow, but do not assume you are in the clear until you take the time and effort to really get to know him.

Due to the spread of sexually transmitted diseases and H.I.V./A.I.D.S., women and men have become more cautious about their sexual practices, especially with partners they have not known for very long. This is one area where we have taken precautions to protect ourselves physically in a relationship. Why would we not extend our physical protection and consider our personal security as well? Similar trust issues arise. When we consider our partner's sexual history, some may want HIV test results, condoms, and screenings for STD's before hopping into bed together. It is not that we mistrust our prospective partner, per say; rather, we just want to be sure we are safe since his/her sexual history is out of our control. Likewise, we cannot control our partner's propensity towards violence, so why would we not do some due diligence in this area? Why would we not look into researching if this person has a criminal history, a drug problem, an alcohol problem, a gambling problem, or any history of mental illness?

We are not trying to be the 'Relationship Big Brother' here, but we are trying to get you to consider how much you dive into the unknown when first dating someone. It is a dive we all willingly take because life would be incomplete without love. We are simply proposing that you take that dive while maintaining situational awareness and conducting whatever due diligence you deem appropriate. The best way to accomplish this is to establish some dating ground rules for yourself and stick to them, no matter whom you meet. Communicate your ground rules clearly when necessary. These ground rules can apply to dating and can be modified once you are in a relationship. For example, one of your dating ground rules might be: I will always meet my first date rather than allowing him to drive and pick me up at my home. Obviously this rule will change once you have screened him and feel safe enough to be alone at your home with him.

Below is a list of sample ground rules for dating. Take what works for you and add more of your own.

Before the Date

1. Always limit the personal information you give out to someone until you have met with him at least once and feel comfortable. This applies to conversations in person, by telephone, via internet, or even personal ads in a newspaper. (For example, via the internet, your address can be gleaned from a phone number and your phone number can be found by using your full name).

2. Allow yourself time for your instincts to work and for evaluating whether or not your prospective date is being truthful before accepting an invitation for a date.

3. Listen to your intuition: Is it giving you any distinct signals that this man is somehow not right for you?

4. Know yourself. Are you emotionally vulnerable due to a recent break up? Are you feeling like your biological clock is ticking and you better meet Mr. Right soon? Is there any reason you might be feeling desperate to meet someone and would therefore overlook early warning signals of danger? Be honest with yourself. If you doubt in your ability to remain objective while dating, ask someone in your SUPNET to give you honest feedback about your level of vulnerability.

The First Few Dates

1. Arrange to meet in the daytime, at a busy, public location.

2. Have a "wing person" with pre-arranged signals for assistance such as a "coincidental" meeting or phone call or an emergency "get me out of here" plan. Keep your wing person informed of your date's name, phone number, vehicle description, and information about him, such as where he works. Schedule a phone call with this person, so that, if he/she does not hear from you or cannot reach you by a certain time he/she will know to come to your date location to check to see if you are okay.

3. During initial dates be alert for suspicious indicators such as: white lies, "eschew obfuscation" (purposefully confusing you), or an excess of information he offers to cloud the issue and change the subject.

4. During initial dates, do not: ride in his car; allow him to pick you up at your residence; go to his or one of his friend's residences; or invite him over to your residence.

5. During initial dates, be independent by: paying your own way; being involved in decisions; and not allowing yourself to be pressured.

Anytime Rules for Dating

1. Always trust your instincts. If you have a "funny feeling" that he is not being truthful, then he probably is not. Do not deny, rationalize, or talk yourself out of your intuitional nudge; just break contact at an appropriate time and in a way that will not antagonize him.

2. Always have a plan to break contact, cash, and a means to get home.

3. Always be specific about your boundaries and communicate them   clearly. "No means no" so do not joke about it or send him mixed messages.

4. Stay sober! Even if you meet at a nice restaurant and he orders a bottle of wine, you can graciously accept and sip but not drink too much.

5. Never get in a heated discussion with a man while he is driving. De-escalate the situation as soon as you see it heading in that direction   even if it means placating him by going along with what he says. You can always discuss the problem later. Do not get back in a car if your date has had an outburst and has stopped somewhere (once he has had one outburst he could easily have another since he is already upset by the argument).

6. Try to arrange break ups or cease the dating process over the phone or in a public place. Inform your SUPNET so that you can have someone nearby if you expect a negative response.

7. If you are on a date and are in a situation where the number of men surpasses the number of women, be on the lookout for any male peer pressure situations or territorial conflicts that may erupt into fights.

8. If you have an awkward or difficult end with the dating process with any man, be sure to conduct surveillance detection for awhile after you have broken off the connection with him. This includes paying attention while driving your routes and using SD when you are in and around your home and workplace. This will help you spot him early on if he stalks you.

Dating can and should be fun. If you practice situational awareness and use the above tips you will actually feel more at ease in this normally awkward realm. Likewise, if you end up forming a relationship with the person you are dating, you will have established yourself from the beginning as an empowered woman who takes her personal security seriously. Predators tend to shy away from women who demand to be taken seriously regarding their security.

Healthy Relationships

A healthy, romantic relationship that involves no verbal or physical abuse is an important part of life and most of us invest a lot of effort in finding one. When we are in healthy relationships we sometimes allow ourselves to ignore our situational awareness because we depend upon the men we are with to protect us. This is a bad habit because a man's perspective is totally different than a woman's and if we turn over our security to our partners, we may negatively impact our ability to respond to danger. Even if you feel confident in your partner's abilities and you trust that he understands what women face daily regarding the threats against them, you should never totally hand over your security to him.

If you pay attention to your partner's perspective, you will likely notice that, upon occasion, he will suggest doing things that were you alone, you would never consider doing. For example, he might ask if you know of any private places where the two of you could go swimming, such as a remote area near a lake or river. It would be normal for him to check out such places on his own because he does not feel the ever present threat of being raped. You, however, likely would not venture to such places alone because of the dangers such seclusion presents. Or, he might be more willing than you are to go to a rowdy party or a club that is located in a bad neighborhood. Men have more freedom to roam and explore the planet while feeling risk free than women do. This does not mean women cannot put themselves in isolated rural places or dangerous environments; it simply means that the threats they face when doing so are normally greater, in particular the threat of some type of sexually based attack. When you depend on the man you are with to protect you, he may make a choice (based on his desires or mental template) that actually puts you at risk, even though he does not intend to do so.

Keisha and her husband faced the consequences of this when their daughter ended up in a compromising situation one Sunday afternoon in the park. Keisha shared her story with us in hopes of helping other young girls to avoid making a similar mistake.

"It was a beautiful fall day and I was up to my ears with house work. My husband, Devon, and I decided to go grocery shopping. We were walking out the door when the phone rang. I remember having a sick feeling in my stomach that something was wrong. It was the police calling. Our fifteen year old daughter, Michelle, had been brought into the station with her seventeen year old boyfriend, Lamont. The police asked us to come down to the station immediately. They told us the kids were fine, but they were in some trouble.

When we got to the station, Michelle looked completely mortified. We could not imagine what she had done. She is a 'straight A' student, plays on the volleyball team, and volunteers at the local hospital. Lamont is a wonderful boy who never does drugs or runs with the wrong crowd. Devon and I felt blessed that Lamont and Michelle had had a steady relationship since Michelle was fourteen. Lamont was always very respectful towards our daughter and he never kept her out past her curfew, even though his curfew was later since he was older.

Officer Timmons asked us to come into a private office so he could speak with us before we talked to the kids. Lamont's parents arrived and we all went into the office. We were stunned to learn that Michelle and Lamont were caught by an off-duty officer in a small park having sex. To make matters worse, the officer detained a man who was in the park and who took photographs of the kids while in the act. Apparently Michelle was totally exposed while lying on top of Lamont.

My head was spinning. I was so shocked at Michelle. She was always such a careful girl who made mature decisions at an early age. How could she have been so reckless? Devon and I were devastated. We had assumed the kids had some degree of a sexual relationship, but all at once we learned that, not only were they fully sexually active, but also they were facing charges as a result and had been photographed by some pervert! I was beside myself.

Officer Timmons told us that the kids confessed that this was not the first time they used the park as a bedroom. He had concerns that the man with the camera may have photographed them on prior occasions if they had set any kind of pattern of this behavior. When we finally got to see Michelle, we felt relieved that she was okay. Devon gave me some time alone with her. I asked her why she did this, to which she replied: 'Lamont said it would be okay and that nobody would see us. I trust him, mom. I guess I just figured he'd protect me.'

The next few months were very difficult. It turned out that the man had taken other photos of the kids on prior occasions and had put some of them up on a website. Because of Michelle's age, he now faced child pornography charges. The media got wind of the story and Michelle's life became a living hell. Fortunately no criminal charges were filed against her, but we all paid for the choice she and Lamont made that day."

The point of Keisha's story is that her daughter abandoned her situational awareness and turned over her security to her boyfriend. Rather than protecting Michelle, Lamont actually put her in danger by encouraging her to have sex in the park. It is not our place to be the moral police regarding their choice to be sexually active, but we do feel compelled to offer a wake-up call to teenagers and their parents. This is a clear example of a potentially very dangerous situation. Predators are known to frequent parks looking for prey.

As a parent, you can use this example as a springboard for discussing with your daughter the importance of making wise choices regarding her personal security. You can also use this example to talk with your son about being responsible towards his girlfriend and considering her safety. Take a moment to consider what a nightmare this situation could have become for them. They were both lying down and were obviously completely distracted, leaving them physically vulnerable to an attack. Also, what if they had not been caught by the police officer and that creepy guy continued to photograph them and post the photos on the internet without being caught? Or worse, what if he raped, kidnapped, or murdered them?

Even healthy relationships can become a context for danger if the two people involved in the relationship lack situational awareness. Never hesitate to educate your partner on security issues. Remember that men do not face many of the same threats as women by virtue of the fact that they are, generally speaking, physically superior to women. Because women are 'the weaker sex' physically, it is our responsibility to educate the men in our lives if we are expecting protection from them. Even if you are in a healthy relationship with a man, a time may come when he makes some choice that impacts your personal security. Although he loves you, he may simply be unaware that this choice could have placed you in harm's way. Open his eyes to your perspective. Chances are he will immediately register that your point is valid and merits a kind of attention that is not part of his habitual practice. You might even create a code word or phrase to use when you think you are in danger. For example, you could use the phrase "no duff" (meaning, "for real" or "no kidding") to indicate that you detect an imminent threat. Empower yourself by educating him. Every little bit counts and creates a ripple of contribution towards the evolution of our personal security.

Abusive Relationships and Domestic Violence

Perhaps you have a secret. Many secrets are embarrassing and perhaps this one is no exception. Perhaps if you just said it aloud you could put some impetus behind it and gravitate towards change. You could privately whisper to the wind: "He hits me whenever he gets angry" or "He is so mean to me and I have become his prisoner" or "I have to protect my family so no one can ever know about this." Perhaps the secret is that he is a monster and you are afraid for your life. Then again, perhaps you have resigned yourself to keeping your secret and to quietly dying inside.

Abuse against women is a problem of epidemic proportions. Women of all ages, shapes, sizes, classes, and races are abused. Women who are strong, sweet, capable, confident, and loving are abused. Famous women, successful women, and happy home-makers are abused. Some statistics are alarming. For example, it is estimated that one in six pregnant women is physically abused during her pregnancy and that abuse is a more common pregnancy complication than diabetes. During the courtship period of a relationship you may not get any indicators that the man you have chosen is an abuser. However, after the honeymoon phase is over and you start to get serious about someone, the situation may change. As relationships unfold, so does the potential for dysfunction. Sometimes it can take years before any abuse or violence occurs, but the early warning signals are there and can be detected. In some cases the violent behavior may result as a reaction to something specific, such as marital problems, an impending divorce, a pregnancy, loss of employment, illness, alcohol or substance abuse, financial stress, or some traumatic experience. Still, early warning signals do develop.

Often women in abusive relationships wonder how it came to this. They reflect on the early parts of the courtship and find themselves years later stuck in a cycle and are too ashamed or embarrassed to admit they used such poor judgment in selecting a mate. They become isolated from their friends and family in that they present a façade rather than admitting what really goes on at home. (Note: If you are experiencing such shame and isolation, seek professional help, or at a minimum the support of friends and family). Since part of the abuse cycle involves remorse from the abuser, abused women succumb to believing it will all be okay and they just have to forgive and move on. They fall into a pattern of behavior wherein they continue to give their abusive partners the benefit of the doubt and will make endless excuses for the abusive behavior. When the abuse happens again they may swear up and down that this is the last time and they will break off the relationship. Then the complications surface (What about the children? How will I support myself and my kids without his help? What will people think? What about our commitment?), thus they opt to hang in there and convince themselves it will never get so bad that they might be seriously hurt or even die. This "head in the sand" approach can end up costing a woman her life.

One fascinating recurring theme we encountered during the course of many of our interviews for this book relates to women's misperception of the definition of abuse. Many women with whom we spoke had the perception that they had never been victims of violence even though they had been victims of abuse. The misperception resulted because they somehow categorized physical abuse from loved ones differently than physical abuse perpetrated by a total stranger. Lena's story captivated us because it is so precisely illustrative of this seriously dangerous misperception and emotional snare women often experience in any type of abusive relationship, whether it is romantic in nature or related to family life.

Lena's home is a work of art. She has a European sensibility and is at once creative and economical. Everything she touches becomes beautiful. She whips up an amazing vegetarian pasta dish as we sit in her kitchen for the interview. She is concentrating solely on our questions while magic appears on the stove.

Our intended focus in this interview was not abuse, but rather general fears women face every day regarding their personal security. We did not realize that this would become an interview that would contain such profound insights about abuse and domestic violence. Lena's answer to our question about her biggest fear was immediate.

"My biggest fear is that I would not be able to defend myself and that a man would be able to physically overcome me. Sometimes I think that, if I were raped, I would just go along with it so that I could live. I guess my fear is good because it makes me very aware of my surroundings. I use a lot of common sense and don't take any short cuts when it comes to my security. Fortunately, I've never really had anything awful happen to me."

The words Lena failed to add to the end of her last sentence were "by a stranger." Our conversation shifted to her years raising three small children after her divorce.

"Suddenly, I was alone and had these three kids to look out for. I remember the anxiety that would overcome me even taking them to a baseball game. I dreaded the thought that one of them could disappear. I used to nail my windows shut at night because I could not afford window locks. It was a difficult time."

As she delved into her past, Lena began to reveal incidents of abuse. She grew up with an angry, abusive father who used the belt on her and her brothers when they misbehaved. He pushed and shoved her mother during arguments and was verbally abusive to all of them. Lena married a man who abused her and made her fear for the safety of her children. On one occasion, Lena's then husband picked her up by the chin when she was six months pregnant and pressed her up against the wall in a rage. Another time he was drunk and picked up their three month old baby. She remembers feeling the imminent danger that he would be too rough with the child and having to talk him into letting her hold the baby. She bowed her head and lowered her voice before relaying the next incident.

"Once my brother, who at the time was suffering from mental illness, threw me on the ground and kicked the hell out of me. We are okay now and have worked through it all, but it was very terrifying. I knew he wouldn't kill me though, so that made it easier to endure. I guess these things are why now I set very clear boundaries in relationships. I told my boyfriend when we first met fifteen years ago that if he ever laid a hand on me, I would end the relationship immediately and would never take him back."

At this point in the interview it became clear to us that she was separating the real incidents of violence that had befallen her at the hands of her abusive father, husband, and brother and was categorizing them differently from the imaginary violent attacks by a stranger. Lena had been the victim of violence, but because it was perpetrated by people she knew and loved, it somehow did not equate with the idea of violence inflicted on her by a total stranger. She had an overwhelming fear of being attacked by a stranger and being unable to defend herself and yet she remained seemingly unscathed by the abuse she had suffered at the hands of those she loved. We asked her about this and she recognized the inconsistency in her thinking.

"Maybe it's why I have become so good at letting anger roll off of me. I had one incident in a parking lot where a man became very aggressive with me because he thought I stole the parking spot he had been waiting for. The truth was, I did not see him waiting, but nonetheless he was out of control and in my face about it. I just apologized and played dumb to placate him and then reported him to the store manager and had someone walk me to my car when I left. Another time, a guy who was painting my house became enraged when we disagreed about his lack of performance on the contract. Again, I acted like it was no big deal so that I could get him to leave my house. Once he left, I called the police. I definitely have a built-in fear of angry men so I will do whatever it takes to avoid their anger."

Lena became much more self-reflective as the conversation ensued. She, like many women, expressed the void that separates her emotional fears from her ability to take actions to prevent violence against her. True, she had learned to set boundaries in her relationships because of the abuse in her family life, yet she was still at a loss as to how to protect herself from a stranger.

"It's so abstract. I think about it all the time, yet I've never really done anything about it...I don't know what that's about! I mean, you can't drive a car without insurance but you can go through your whole life without learning some kind of self-defense. We take our daughters to ballet lessons and soccer practice, but very few people have their daughters go to martial arts or self-defense classes. I don't know what exactly I would want to do to make myself safer. I am afraid of the power of a gun, though I guess I could get training. My own denial keeps me from taking that extra step to invest the time in learning to protect myself."

Lena exhibits that human contradiction factor so many women display when it comes to their personal security. On the one hand they want to feel safe, yet they are unwilling to take precautionary measures. Or, even if they are very careful, their fears still elude them and make them feel inadequately prepared to defend themselves. We asked her if she resented having to even think about defending herself.

"Not really. I know from experience that I cannot stop an angry man from becoming violent. I can't do anything about him; I can only do something about me. And I don't know why I haven't been more proactive in being involved with myself in this area of my life. I guess on some level I assume I will be fine and nothing bad will happen to me. Maybe it's just easier to hold on to my denial."

We were appreciative of Lena's forthrightness. She was not judging herself, per se, but she was totally tuned in to her own incongruence. The black and white nature of abuse was actually in grey scale in her life; she could not equate the abuse she had experienced as being the same as violence against her inflicted by a stranger because her perspective was somewhat blurred by love for those who harmed her. On the other hand, because she learned how to handle abuse in a family and romantic setting, she was able to take some of those techniques and apply them to strangers, (letting the anger "roll off" her). By the same token, she had never mastered an ability to fight off abuse and was extremely fearful of a stranger who might become violent with her. She said that, because she could not be sure that a stranger would not kill her, she felt a total lack of control; whereas she knew in her heart that the abuse from loved ones would not be fatal.

What amazes us is that almost every woman we know or have met during the course of writing this book has a story, but she holds it deep. Violence against women has become integrated into this private place in our beings and we reveal it only with trust (trust that the person listening will not judge us or make us feel embarrassed). As women, we take on the blame, the shame, the embarrassment, and the guilt. We love so strongly that we forgive and endure abuse from those closest to us. We often opt to live with the dread and fear of future incidents of abuse rather than taking a stand to extract ourselves from the relationship. If you are in an abusive relationship, you may feel it is impossible to leave. Sometimes it truly is very difficult to remove yourself. Do not lose hope. Think creatively, seek out support, and commit to freeing yourself of the stress and burden of abuse. Regardless if you leave or stay in an abusive relationship, prevention of future incidents of abuse is possible. Getting SASD is the place to start. Be aware of the indicators that your partner is on his way to becoming abusive:

- Does he seem agitated, depressed, angry, defeated, or ready for an argument?
- Does he yell at you, call you names, or taunt you?
- Is he criticizing you or berating you?
- Is he becoming obsessive with you, overly jealous, or possessive?
- Is he monitoring your every move and trying to isolate you from friends and family?
- Is he ordering you around or refusing to participate in helping you around the house?
- Does he constantly complain that you are an unfit girlfriend, wife, or mother?
- Does he try to manipulate your emotions?
- Does he close in on your physical space in a way that makes you feel threatened?
- Does he threaten to use any weapons against you or to hurt you physically?

If you detect any indicators that lead you to believe he may become abusive, the best thing to do is to break contact with him immediately. Trying to placate him or talk him out of being violent may actually work against you. He may become enraged if you attempt to manipulate his mood. Your best chance to diffuse the situation is to remove yourself from it and give him time to calm himself.

You can also use a variation of surveillance detection to gain early notification that he is monitoring you. Pay attention to your personal belongings. Is he reading your mail, e-mails, or listening to your phone messages for ammunition to use against you? Does he show up at your workplace unannounced or at events with your kids when you had not planned to meet him there? Does he follow you when you are out running errands? Detect any unusual behavior on his part. Perhaps you will detect other strange things, such as unfamiliar calls on your phone bill or receipts that pinpoint his location at a time when you thought he was elsewhere. These are not necessarily indicators that he will become abusive, but they do imply that there are things about him that may leave you feeling mistrustful or afraid. Pay attention to your emotions, your intuition, and signals of potential danger of any kind.

If you are in an abusive relationship, it might help you to conduct a risk/threat assessment for the relationship. Obviously you will need to secure this document so that your abuser *never* finds it. This assessment may help you to think in a more objective way about your situation (one which is based on facts rather than emotions). It is also extremely important for you to develop your SUPNET. Even if you are too ashamed to discuss the abuse with your friends, family, and co-workers, you can still make a plan for contacting them for the various types of support you might need should the abuse escalate.

The Jekyll and Hyde Syndrome

Another dangerous pattern women experience in relationships is what we call the Jekyll and Hyde Syndrome. Some men are only abusive, either verbally or physically, when they are under the influence of either alcohol or drugs. These men experience a dramatic transformation when they are drunk or on drugs and engage in behavior that is totally foreign to their normal disposition. They may not be able to remember what they have said or done once they are sober.

If you are involved with a man who changes character so dramatically, you must consider some important points. First, if you have not done so already, let your partner know about any abusive behavior he exhibits when in an altered state. Next, if he continues to choose to drink or use drugs that put him in this altered state, knowing full well that he has the tendency to be abusive, suggest that he get appropriate professional help. Above all, take care of yourself. You are not in control of his problem or his addictions. You cannot force him to stop drinking or using drugs; he must make that choice on his own. You can, however, take care of yourself by breaking contact with him any time he is in a condition which may prompt him to become abusive. This may mean you refuse to go out to a party with him. It may mean you and your children go spend the night at a friend's or even a hotel to get away from him. You must take a stand against the abuse and refuse to be with him if he chooses to put you in a situation where you might become his victim. No matter how much you love him, his problem is *his* problem and you must not allow yourself to become the victim of his irresponsible choices.

Relationships are complex and both parties must work at keeping a relationship healthy so that it thrives. Your refusal to be anywhere near him when he drinks or uses drugs sends him a powerful message. It may be a message he chooses to ignore and, if that is the case, you may have to reassess your relationship. On the other hand, it may be a message that impacts his life profoundly in that he may face his problem and get the help he needs to transcend it. Regardless of which life path he chooses, your decision to protect yourself and remove yourself from any abusive behavior will empower you (even if it means you lose him). Any time women stand up and claim their right to deny abuse, the men on the other side of the equation are given the message that abuse (verbal, emotional, or physical) is intolerable and inexcusable. No matter how much he tries to rationalize his behavior ("But honey, I was drunk and didn't know what I was saying."), apologize for it, or act like it never happened (because he cannot remember it), the bottom line truth is that it is your responsibility to protect yourself from the behavior. You cannot rely on him to make that choice for you; you only have control over your response to the situation, not his.

Abuse Resulting from Mental Illness

Loving someone who suffers from mental illness can be extremely difficult and a heavy burden to bear. Certainly not all mentally ill men are abusive, but some are. Imagine if your soul mate or a beloved family member was bipolar or schizophrenic and experienced violent moods swings, during which he became verbally, emotionally, or physically abusive to you. How could you separate the love you have for this man and the impact of the abuse on your life, knowing that he really cannot control his behavior (even though he is on medication and is under medical and psychiatric supervision)?

If you are in such a situation and have committed to staying with a man who suffers from mental illness and is abusive as a result, you must still take precautions to protect yourself from the abuse. You must break contact with him whenever he is abusive and get as much outside professional support as possible to handle the abuse. Do not keep it a secret, especially from his doctors. Let your family and close friends know about the position you are in so they can support you. If the abuse is physical, be sure to follow the advice in this chapter for keeping yourself safe. The bottom line is that you cannot control another person's illness. Do not prioritize taking care of any man over protecting yourself. As difficult as it is to love someone who is mentally ill, you must love yourself enough to not allow his illness to destroy your life.

This chapter is not meant to be a psychological analysis of abusive relationships. Much exists on the subject and support networks and organizations can help you with the emotional aspects of being in an abusive relationship (see Appendix E). What we want to help you with is keeping yourself safe, should your boyfriend or spouse reach the point where he becomes abusive in any way. A woman in an abusive relationship often feels trapped and is unable to extricate herself from the relationship for a variety of reasons, including lack of financial independence and the complications of divorce and custody issues. If you are in such a situation, at the very least prepare yourself with every possible option should the abuse escalate. Establish a strong SUPNET and have emergency contact numbers ready, such as an abuse hotline number. Consider both the option of ending the relationship, staying in your home, and demanding that he moves out and the option of you escaping the situation and being the one to move. The former option requires you to get SASD so that you are warned in advance if he returns to seek revenge (see Chapter Nine for what to do he stalks you). The latter option requires you to prepare yourself by establishing an emergency evacuation plan. If you had to get out immediately, how would you do it? Your emergency evacuation plan should include the following preparation:

- Have a stash of emergency cash that you can access quickly (including both bills and coins).

- Keep your gas tank filled and have a spare set of car keys hidden with your cash stash.

- Always keep a spare house key on your person in case he steals your keys and locks you out of the house (this way, you can access your cash stash once you are certain he is out of the house).

- Identify safe locations you can drive to at any time of day or night, (these could include a police station, a hospital, a friend with whom you arrange a refuge plan, a battered women's shelter, etc.).

- Buy an emergency cell phone and/or calling card (if you do not already own a cell phone).

- Keep a list of important phone numbers in your purse and hidden in your car. Obviously you can call 911 in an emergency, but you might need other support, such as help from the administration at your children's school or from a neighbor.

- Join a support group if there is one in your area, (do *not* let him know that you are attending meetings with any group unless he is also willing to attend meetings and is actively working through his issues).

- Have your personal documents, such as your passport, social security card, credit cards, checkbook, and photo ID in a pouch, ready to take with you at any time.

- Pack a suitcase with spare clothing (including clothes for your children) and store it at a friend's house.
- Carry a small flashlight in your purse at all times (See Chapter Twelve)
- Consider buying a TASER device (See Chapter Twelve and be sure to research if you need a permit to own one in your state).
- Practice surveillance detection to determine if your abuser is following you or is planning to attack you along your routes or at your new location (if you are staying elsewhere).

Have a survival plan in the event that he attacks you in your home. First, do whatever it takes to diffuse the situation and calm him so that you can buy time to escape the situation. Do not add fuel to the fire by arguing or disagreeing with him. Try to distract him with something he likes (for example: "Honey, you relax and go watch the baseball game.").

Consider each room in the house and what you would do if he became violent with you there. The kitchen is obviously not a good room in which to have an argument if your spouse or significant other is prone to violent behavior. Remember that any object can be used as a weapon, either by him for the abuse or by you for self-defense. If he attacks you, one hard strike to his temple could buy you the time to get out of the house and run to a neighbor's for help (see Chapter Twelve). Your survival plan, in the event of an attack in your home, should include the following preparation regarding your home, family, and evidence collection:

- Always have access to a phone. If you own a cell phone, keep it on your person at all times.
- Determine which areas of your home can offer you safety in the event you cannot escape (e.g., a bathroom with a good lock on the door). Make sure you have access to a phone from this room (grab a portable or cell phone before entering the room or position a phone in the room).

- Instruct your children to hide in the home and not interfere in the situation. If your children are old enough, you may want to instruct them to call 911 or run to a neighbor's for help. Make sure they understand that they must do so only if they are certain the abuser will not be violent with them (for example, if your husband is beating you in the basement and they are upstairs and are able to call or get out for help without him knowing).

- Give your children phone numbers of family and friends they can call for help.

- If your potential attacker owns a gun, know where he hides it and if he keeps it loaded. Encourage him to keep it locked up (so that it takes him longer to access it in the event he is in a rage and tries to shoot you).

- Develop escape routes from your home. Determine which doors and windows you can use to get out of the house. Plan your escape route to safety, depending on which way you exit the home.

- Create a code word/phrase or a visual signal that you share with friends or neighbors which instructs them to call the police immediately.

- Be sure to have any third parties who witness any of the abuse fill out an incident report, noting the date, time, and what they saw.

- Have any evidence of the abuse that you collected (photos of bruises, incident reports, witness reports, police reports) stored in a separate location where your abuser cannot access them, such as a private safe deposit box or at the home of someone in your SUPNET.

To any woman reading this list of tips: If this rings true to your situation, please wake up! If you are in an abusive relationship, you are taking an enormous risk with your life. Your goal should be to extricate yourself from the relationship as soon as you can. This does not necessarily mean getting a divorce. You might separate until your husband gets the help he needs. If you are not married to your abuser, you can opt to break off the relationship until he agrees to get help. No matter how many times he apologizes and swears he will never hurt you again, do not believe him. He is fooling you and, more importantly, himself with these false promises. Until he gets professional help, you are at great risk. And even if he does seek help, you do not have a guarantee that it will cure him from his abusive behavior pattern. Be willing to lose him. Be willing to let go of your dependency on him. Be willing to face the complications and finality of a break up or divorce if there is no other way for you to be safe with this man. Do not overrate him. There are plenty of wonderful men in the world; love one who will never abuse you.

> *My fear of change*
> *renders me changeless*
> *even in death I will transform*
> *as my body decomposes*
> *it is time for me to change my fear*
> *and render myself living again*

Whether you go on a date with a man who turns out to be a threat or if you are in an abusive relationship, any dangerous liaison puts you at risk. Remember that practicing situational awareness will help you identify the early warning signals of impending danger or abuse. You can also implement some of the surveillance detection methods you have learned should you become afraid that the man you dated or the man with whom you are involved begins to follow you or even stalks you. In the next chapter we discuss what you can do to protect yourself if a dangerous man pursues you either after you have stopped dating him or have broken off an abusive relationship with him. At this point he becomes a stalker and you will need to take more drastic measures to protect yourself and your children.

CHAPTER NINE

STALKING

If I can make you mine
control your world
concentrate solely on you
If I can make you mine...

The most concise, accurate definition of stalking that we have seen states simply: "To pursue by tracking." Because all stalkers track their prey, situational awareness and surveillance detection are highly effective defenses. What better way for a stalker to "track his prey" than by conducting surveillance on his target? If you are being stalked, either by someone you know, (an abusive ex-husband, an employee you fired) or by someone you do not know, (a stranger who has developed an obsession with you) you can outsmart your stalker and avoid being attacked. The first point you must understand if you even suspect you have a stalker is that you must immediately go into "red alert mode," meaning you need to heighten your security straight away.

In an odd way, a stalker almost trains his/her victim in being SASD. If you have dealt with a stalker you probably learned to look ahead for that person before departing from or arriving at any location that you regularly frequented. You would also have been "trained" to heighten your situational awareness and to always be keeping an eye peeled for your stalker. You would naturally have limited the personal information the stalker could access. And reporting the stalker to the authorities probably became a habit since you were able to get a clear description of him because of the many encounters you had with him.

If you have never been stalked, it may interest you to know that, according to the Department of Justice, one in twelve women will be stalked in her lifetime. This is a startling statistic and one all women should register so that they understand how palpable this threat is. While conducting interviews for this book, almost every woman with whom we spoke knew of a woman who had been stalked, whether it was a friend, family member, co-worker, neighbor, or herself. Imagine if women took a stand around this statistic in the same way they have around the issue of breast cancer. There are countless support groups, fund-raising walks, media reports, and awareness programs that pertain to breast cancer because of the alarming statistics for this illness (one in eight women will develop breast cancer). If stalking received the same level of attention, perhaps more anti-stalking laws would be established and women everywhere would have a better handle on this threat.

Our objective in this chapter is to illustrate how the techniques we have discussed in previous chapters can apply to stalking. As a general rule, we recommend the following if you become the target of a stalker:

- Document all sightings or incidents related to your stalker. Log dates and times of sightings or incidents, and record any significant information (see Appendix D).
- Save any evidence (gifts, voice messages, photographs of vandalism, etc.).
- If possible, discreetly photograph or videotape your stalker. Do *not* overtly photograph your stalker or do anything confrontational because doing so may cause the danger to escalate.

- Do *not* confront your stalker directly. Ignoring him by refusing to interact with him is the better course of action, though it will in no way guarantee a cease-fire.

- Consider the possible consequences before deciding to take legal action against your stalker. Court protection orders (restraining orders) against stalkers can sometimes backfire by aggravating the situation.

- Inform everyone in your SUPNET about your stalker so that you can begin to seek support and avoid isolating yourself.

- Immediately implement a surveillance detection plan, including using SD along your routes and at key locations in which you spend time.

When an Abuser or Someone You Know Becomes a Stalker

Many women end up being stalked by someone they know. Sometimes the stalker is an abusive spouse, lover, or ex-husband/boyfriend. Sometimes the stalker is a co-worker, a casual acquaintance, or a suitor who becomes obsessed. In Molly's case, her stalker was a man she dated for a few months.

Molly is a licensed social worker, a painter, a poet, a mother, a daughter and the survivor of one man's vendetta against her. Not long after the attacks of September eleventh, Molly was in a place in her life where she was very vulnerable. All of her friends were paired up with someone they loved and Molly was newly divorced and very lonely.

"I was so vulnerable back then. I so wanted to find someone special and to begin a new relationship. When I met Omar I was ready for love. I never ever would have imagined how things would turn out."

Molly met Omar at a bar when her friend, Julie, introduced them. She thought her friend knew Omar, but found out much later that Julie had also just been introduced to him that night. Omar was Iranian and pulled on Molly's sympathy strings telling her he had been discriminated against after 9/11 and had even received death threats. Molly, accustomed to comforting patients in need, listened and consoled him.

"When Omar approached me at the bar I was immediately taken by how well dressed, educated, and interesting he was. He was worldly, or seemingly so, and I found him very attractive and intelligent. Later I learned that much of what he told me about himself that night was untrue, but I fell for it all, hook, line and sinker. We dated for three months. He showered me with attention, bought me nice things, cooked fabulous meals for me, and even brought me breakfast in bed. I was in heaven. For years I had felt invisible in my marriage, so this kind of adoration was just what I craved. We were together constantly."

Molly explained how, even though everything changed almost overnight, she remained in a state of disbelief at his actions and could not perceive the early warning signals objectively.

"Omar became very mistrustful of me. He was obsessed with knowing my every move. If I went to visit my friend Julie, he would call her house literally seven times in less than an hour. He told me he did not trust anyone. The signs were there and looking back on it I realize how foolish I was not to catch on sooner that he was a sick man. I tried to break it off with him three times. He would respond with panic attacks, pleading for me to stay with him and apologizing for being overbearing. I fell for it and took him back. I feel stupid even now telling the story. How could I have been so blind? I am a well-educated clinical social worker, for heaven's sake!"

Had Molly informed her SUPNET about Omar's desperate pleas, they probably would have warned her to get him out of her life. We explained to Molly that Omar's panic attacks and desperate pleas were early warning signals because his behavior was obviously so over the top. Molly understood and felt embarrassed but was eager to continue, if for no other reason than to understand her own actions and make some sense out of her story.

"I felt really sorry for him and even located an Iranian male therapist he could work with, but he refused to go. The last straw came when I attended a three hour seminar for my job. It was a licensing workshop that was mandatory. I worked one-on-one with a man. Later, when I excitedly relayed what I had learned to Omar, he freaked out. He called me a whore, accused me of having sex

with my co-worker, and became enraged. He pounded on my son's bedroom door, shouting obscenities and degrading me. He even called me a 'filthy Jew.' I broke it off with Omar immediately. I finally set my boundary with him, but it was too late."

The situation escalated. Molly received over one hundred phone calls from Omar in just two days. She ignored the calls but saved the angry messages he left on her voice mail, including a death threat. A few weeks went by and things quieted down with Omar. Molly moved on and met Robert. When Robert called and left Molly a message about going out on a date, Omar resurfaced and more trouble ensued. Omar had the access code to Molly's voice mail and Molly had forgotten to change it, (Molly had given the code to him once when she was out of town and needed him to check her messages for her). He had been monitoring her voice mail and Robert's call sent him over the edge. Omar also had a key to Molly's apartment building. He broke into her apartment while she was home and attacked her, backing her into a closet. She pleaded her way out of the situation, begging for her life. He did not harm her but she was terrified.

Molly filed a court protection order against Omar. Shortly thereafter her boss received a letter from Omar in which he accused Molly of having an affair with a co-worker. The day the letter arrived, the office received an anonymous bomb threat. At this point, Molly called the F.B.I. hoping for added support. She hired a bodyguard, a private investigator, and had three police departments involved in the case. Finally her landlord agreed to change the locks on her apartment building. Molly felt judged and even hated by other tenants who were inconvenienced by the change and intimated that her bad judgment was the cause.

"Even some of my friends judged me. People acted like it was my fault somehow because I made a bad choice in getting involved with Omar in the first place. But how could I have predicted this behavior until I got to know him? Sure, I did some foolish things, like not breaking it off with him right away, but I never asked him to stalk me!"

Omar continued to follow Molly. On one occasion she took an impromptu trip to the east coast. On her return she had to change her flight at the last minute. When she arrived at the airport in her home city, Omar was at the airport. Molly *had no idea if he actually followed her to the east coast for the duration of her trip. All she knew was that the airport sighting made her skin crawl.*

Fed up with the entire situation, Molly became desperate. She worked with her private investigator and the police to set up Omar. Her private investigator had coached her to keep her access code to her messages unchanged so that they could use this in a sting operation. She purposely set up a fake date with a male friend, via her voice mail, and had her private investigator and the police show up to apprehend Omar if he entered the bar. Sure enough, Omar did show up and was arrested for violating the court order. Fortunately the judge was strict and sentenced Omar to six months in jail. Molly had to appear in court twice. She wishes she had also brought a civil suit against Omar because her expenses were so high.

"It is so sad to me that only women of means can afford to protect themselves. This cost me thousands of dollars and I wish I had taken action to get the money back. I'm glad it's over but it took a great toll on me. I had a serious bout with PTSD {Post Traumatic Stress Disorder}. Fortunately I found a great therapist who helped me by using EMDR therapy {Eye Movement Desensitization and Reprocessing: See Notes section}. But there again, I was able to afford the help, even though I am angry as hell that I had to spend my money to survive and prevail. What about all the women out there who are stalked who cannot afford the specialized help? I wish I could have read your book before I ever met him."

Certainly we wish that every woman we interviewed could have read our book before experiencing her story. In fact, several months after we interviewed Molly, her stalker resurfaced. It had been over two years since he had been released from jail so Molly thought she was in the clear until one day his phone number showed up on her caller ID. Molly reported the incident to the police immediately and they contacted him and warned him to stay away from her. Molly called us for some surveillance detection training. We took her out along her routes and in the area of her home, instructing her where, when and how to look for Omar. She told us: "What you did was huge in terms of helping me realize how much control I have over my own safety. I had no idea how much I can participate in protecting myself instead of always just relying on others."

We can learn important lessons from Molly's story, especially if we look at how she could have applied the techniques in this book to her situation. First, if she had been practicing situational awareness and had established better communication with her friend (Julie) the night she met Omar, she would have realized that he was a total stranger to both of them. Knowing this, she could have then been more careful and have applied some of our rules for initial dates. Even if she did not detect any early warning signals during the first few dates, she still might have been more careful about releasing her private information (voice mail access code, apartment building key) to Omar so early on in the relationship.

As the relationship progressed and Omar exhibited his irrational behavior (showering her with adoration; tracking her while at her friend Julie's; pleading with her not to break things off with him), she would have been able to establish firm boundaries with him and begin the process of protecting herself using a surveillance detection plan, which would include both route and building reviews. Using SD, she would have been able to determine if he actually followed her on her trip back east. She likely would have detected him in many of the places she habitually frequents.

She would also have involved her SUPNET to a greater degree, informing everyone she knew about Omar and his stalker-like actions. In her situation, she would want to air her 'dirty laundry' as a way to involve as many people as possible to help protect her. By notifying the tenants in her building to report Omar to the police if they saw him in or around the building, for example, she might have avoided the attack inside her apartment. The point is, because she was being stalked, she had to immediately get as much support as possible.

Finally, if Molly had had access to a more affordable prevention approach (such as this book) she may have been able to take more control over her situation early on, thereby reducing the costs she incurred as a result of her lack of timely action. However, stalkers are loose cannons so we do advise you get all the help you can afford and be sure to take care of the problem legally. We are in no way trying to talk you out of hiring a private investigator, lawyer, or bodyguard. On the contrary, if you need a "threat management team" comprised of professionals in your corner (and can afford one), we say go for it. Likewise, if you cannot afford to hire a threat management team, do not lose hope. You can do a lot on your own and with the help of your support network. In addition, you have community resources available, such as women's organizations and local law enforcement (see Appendix E).

Molly's story only scratches the surface regarding the plight of women who are stalked by people they know. Regardless if your stalker is a boyfriend, spouse, co-worker or friend, consider the options for defending yourself against an abusive person who is stalking you. Depending on how serious the threat is, you may need to take some drastic measures, like moving in to a shelter for battered women. However, we understand that in the majority of cases, women who face being threatened from a former abusive partner do not have the option to freeze their lives and hide away from harm indefinitely. You must become much more proactive to protect yourself.

Once you get SASD and become proactive about prevention, what you will realize is that, rather than restricting your freedom, you will actually gain more freedom from fear and you will become more relaxed. There is no need for you to be overcome emotionally with fear, to feel inconvenienced, or even defiant about being stalked. In fact, if you take on a defiant attitude against your stalker ("To hell with him; I'm living my life!") you may put yourself in greater danger. The idea is to outsmart him, not to make him angry.

The techniques presented in the first seven chapters of this book apply to your situation, so we suggest you implement them immediately if you have a stalker. Use your situational awareness. Protect your privacy and identity. Conduct a risk/threat assessment for this particular threat. Establish your SUPNET. Create and implement a surveillance detection plan and conduct route and building reviews.

In addition we have a list of tips that can also help you secure yourself and your environment, especially if the situation escalates.

Responding to Being Stalked by Someone You Know

- Consider filing a temporary restraining order/court protection order, if you have not already done so. Be warned that this is not a guarantee that you will be protected by law enforcement since they will not be able to be with you 24/7. Also, your stalker may be further agitated by this move, so use your judgment given your particular situation before deciding to go ahead with this action. If you do get a court protective order, keep it on your person at all times.

- Visit the police stations in the areas where you are experiencing the stalking. Actually meet face to face with an officer (preferably one who specializes in stalking cases) and establish a connection. If possible, get his/her cell phone number in addition to the direct number of the station.

- Conduct a risk/threat assessment for the stalking threat, identifying all of the possible threats you face as a result of the stalking.

- Have an emergency contact plan with all the necessary phone numbers of your SUPNET.

- Conduct a building review for your home, workplace, and any other location you regularly frequent. Consider it a very real possibility that your stalker will try to attack you in or around any of these locations. Once you have identified your vulnerable areas, make all necessary adjustments to reduce your risk of being attacked in these locations. Conduct routine building sweeps in which you look for anything suspicious (anything that has been moved, such as yard tools or anything out of place). Do these sweeps twice a day or as needed.

- Secure your residence. Change the locks immediately and install deadbolts and an alarm system if you can afford one (or get a dog). Make sure all entrances, (windows and doors) are secured at all times. Exterior motion lights will help alert you if anyone is lurking around your home.

- Identify what you can use as defensive tools in and around your home and workplace, as well as inside your vehicle (see Chapter Twelve).

- Consider installing a surveillance camera to capture your stalker on film. Be sure to use the date/time settings. Position the camera to cover the most likely areas your stalker would use to watch you. Instruct the company that provides the camera to use an unmarked vehicle when working at your home. If possible, schedule a time for them to install the camera/s when you know your stalker will not be in the area.

- Develop a surveillance detection plan which includes SD along your routes and near the buildings in which you spend time.

- Always have a working phone on your person. A cell phone is the best option in case he cuts your phone lines.

- Make a flyer with your stalker's photograph and vehicle description information to distribute to neighbors, co-workers, family, friends, and teachers at your children's schools.

- Ask your employer, co-workers, and neighbors to call the police immediately if they see him in the vicinity.

- Talk with the administrators and teachers at your children's school and advise them to notify you if your stalker is seen anywhere on or around school property. (However, if you have a custody issue and he has visitation rights then this may alter your ability to keep him away from your children).

- Change your phone number to an unlisted number. Get "Caller ID" so that you can screen all phone calls. Allow your voice mail to pick up the messages and save them as evidence. Instruct co-workers to send his calls to your voice mail as well. Listening to the messages will likely be upsetting, but we feel it is important to do so. If you can afford to hire a Threat Management Team, let them listen to the messages. The point is he may say something that gives you an indicator of what his next action will be.

- Conduct route reviews for all of your routine travel. Incorporate surveillance detection in key locations along your routes. At a minimum, conduct SD yourself from inside your vehicle while driving your routes each day.

- Break your routines. Vary your schedule and the routes you travel often and randomly. Do not establish any kind of pattern your stalker can study and use to predict your whereabouts.

- Carry a personal alarm or air horn in your vehicle and on your person at all times (see Chapter Twelve).

- Avoid being alone, both at home and in public, if possible. At a minimum, have someone walk you to your car or front doorstep and go in the house with you to be sure you have no intruders.

- If you are forced to relocate and go into hiding, be sure to keep your address and phone number secured. Do not give specific information as to your whereabouts to anyone you leave behind. Allow people to contact your cell phone only.

- Use surveillance detection techniques to *discreetly* acquire photographs of your stalker. Attach a printed copy of the photograph to your hard copy "Stalking Incident Log" so that you build a record of the evidence against him. Document every stalking incident. You can photocopy the blank form we provide in Appendix D.

- Create an emergency evacuation plan so that you are ready to evacuate at a moment's notice. Inform your children of the plan and have them rehearse it with you. Inform your SUPNET of your plan and give them any specific instructions if they are to support you in any aspect of the plan.

When You are Stalked by Someone You Do Not Know

Surveillance detection is a powerful tool for determining if you are being stalked by someone you do not know and for preventing being harmed by a stalker. The disadvantage of being stalked by an unknown predator is that it may take you longer to realize you are being tracked. However, if you practice SD on a regular basis, you can quickly and easily identify a stalker. Think about it: your predator will have to come out into the open to collect information on you because he probably does not know one or more of the following:

- Your address and phone numbers (home, work, and cell).
- Your schedule (what time you leave for work in the morning; what time you get off work; what scheduled weekly events you attend; what time you turn out the lights and go to sleep at night, etc.).
- Where you work, how you go in and out of the building, and what security measures and procedures exist at your workplace.
- What routes you travel and if you travel alone.

- Where you park your car; if you keep it locked while you are driving and while it is parked; if your car has an alarm system.
- Where you hang out during your free time, including any routine activities you attend such as church, working out at a health club, hair and manicure appointments, regular social engagements, and any routines you establish with your children.
- Information about your friends, family, co-workers, or neighbors.
- Your level of situational awareness (if you pay attention to your surroundings or if you are often distracted and unaware of who and what is around you).
- Your personality or disposition (if you are an approachable, kind person who does not easily reject advances from strangers or if you are a guarded person who does not easily warm up to strangers).
- What security you have around your residence (motion lights; locked gates and doors; if you close your curtains at night; if you have a dog; if you have a placard or sticker on your door indicating that you have a home alarm system; if there are any entry points he can exploit, such as a basement window that is easy to open). Although your stalker can only study your home security from the outside (unless he breaks in for reconnaissance purposes), he can still learn a lot from what is visible to him while he is parked in a car on the street watching your home.

As you can see, your stalker will be interested in collecting various types of information about you and your life. If he plans to be successful in attacking you, he will need this information. Even if he is stalking you in an overt manner, he will still be collecting the details which help him sort out the logistics of his endeavors, meaning both his stalking activities and his attack planning. If you tap in to his mindset and his tactics, you can learn a lot about how to defend yourself against him. *You must study yourself the same way he will study you.* Completing the personal security profile (Appendix B), conducting a risk/threat assessment (Chapter Three), reviewing your routes, and analyzing your residence and workplace (Chapters Six and Seven) will keep you steps ahead of him. Remember: If you even suspect you are being stalked by a stranger, you must use great discretion when completing all of this work. Do not let him know that you are aware of him.

After you have completed the same type of analysis of yourself that he will conduct on you, you will then use this information to detect him, identify him, and report him to the authorities with solid proof of his activities. You will also be able to use the information as a shield to protect yourself from his attacks. Since you will have analyzed where and when he is likely to attack you, you will be able to implement the necessary measures to protect yourself from harm. Although this may sound like a lot of work, it is worth your time and effort. For some women, it will take you just a few hours to complete. For others, it could take a few days to complete. However long it takes, this ground work will empower you to be proactive in defending yourself, without having to become a fighting machine in order to do so. Certainly, if you are physically capable, taking any kind of self-defense class will also help you feel empowered and will increase your situational awareness. In addition, since no prevention method works one hundred percent of the time, learning any physical self-defense tactics might come in handy (see Chapter Twelve). The work we are putting before you is focused on prevention, not deterrence. We are encouraging you to step way back and tap in to your stalker's early planning stage of his efforts against you.

Something magical happens when you study yourself as a target. Your eyes are opened to your vulnerabilities. You will see yourself in ways that you never considered before. It is similar to talking with a therapist; parts of your "security personality" will unravel before your eyes and you will likely realize how remiss you have been against the very real threats that most women confront every day. You will also likely see how competent you are in certain aspects of your personal security. Analyzing yourself as a target is similar to taking medical tests to analyze your risk of illness. For example, if you just consider your dietary habits and your exercise routines, you do not get a full picture of the real threat you may face with the condition of your heart. However, if you get a heart scan or other cardiac tests, you can get a totally realistic picture of the true health risks you face. Once you have analyzed yourself as a target, you then get to decide how often you will allow your stalker to see you. This does not mean hiding out in your home and avoiding all public places. Rather this means you can now orchestrate situations where you can be sure he will show up and you can attempt to have law enforcement there waiting for him every time. Or, at a minimum, you can record the incident and build your evidence against him. You get to set your own patterns. He is studying these patterns so make yourself available to him only in locations where you know you are safe because you have support.

Imagine that your stalker has learned where you live and what car you drive. You can now fabricate a pattern to draw him in and expose him. You may start by eliciting help from a friend who positions her/himself in a surveillance detection location to watch the location where you will lead your stalker. Let your friend record the information and, if possible, discreetly obtain a photograph of the stalker in action. Once you have safely and legally accumulated evidence against this person, you can then proceed with any actions you plan to take against your stalker, such as filing a court protection order.

The following is a list of tips you can use to: reduce your risk of being stalked; determine if you have a stalker; respond to your stalker's actions; and control your own safety if the situation escalates. (Note: you will notice overlaps in the tips listed in various parts of this chapter. We want to be sure that readers who skip right to the parts that apply to their situations do not miss critical tips that may have already been mentioned in previous sections).

Reduce your Risk of Being Stalked by Someone You Do Not Know

- Listen to, trust in, and act on your intuition!
- Identify the early warning signals and respond by heightening your situational awareness.
- Conduct basic surveillance detection to help you determine early on if you have a stalker.

- Notice any unwanted attention given to you by a stranger.

- Extract yourself from interactions with strangers who appear to be trying to lock you into their sphere.

- Instruct people you know to keep your personal information private (phone numbers, addresses, hobbies, family history).

- Tell your family and co-workers to alert you to any hang-up calls that persist. If possible, try to obtain the phone number (off caller ID or from the operator).

- Set clear boundaries with all those you encounter so that people take you seriously and do not attempt to infringe on your good nature (you can still be polite, kind, charitable, and gracious, but be so with the intention of always protecting yourself against any aberrant person on the receiving end of your goodness).

- Use a mailbox that locks. If you suspect any mail tampering, report it immediately to the post office and the police.

- Request that your address is kept private through the DMV, the telephone book, and voter's registration.

- If possible, have an unlisted phone number.

How to Determine if You Have a Stalker

Pay attention to the following behaviors, indicators, and incidents:

- Anyone who calls you excessively, especially after you have asked him/her not to.

- Any threatening, harassing, or menacing messages on your voice mail or answering machine (often the stalker will use obscenities or threats).

- Anyone appearing frequently in the area of your residence or workplace or any other location you frequent (using basic SD on a regular basis will help you to notice these "coincidences").

- Anyone who tries to intimidate you.
- Receiving unwanted letters, cards, gifts, attention.
- Being followed, watched, photographed or filmed (again, you will determine this by using basic SD). If you suspect you are being followed, do not drive home. Your stalker may not have collected information on your home address yet and perhaps he is following you in order to do so. Go somewhere safe, such as a police station, hospital, or crowded public place. Be careful not to tip off your stalker that you know he is following you. Do not make a series of turns that are illogical; he will know you are onto him. Make sure to discreetly write down his license plate number and vehicle description.
- Anyone who contacts, threatens, or harasses your family, friends, neighbors, co-workers or boss as a way to get your attention and evoke a response from you.
- Anyone who uses a third party to make contact with you directly or indirectly.
- Anyone trespassing or vandalizing your property, including your vehicle. Look for graffiti, mail tampering, vehicle tampering, or any signs of destruction of property.
- Any hostile or aggressive action taken towards your pets (wounding, abducting, poisoning, etc.).
- Anyone using threats to manipulate a response out of you, such as promising to commit suicide if you do not return his phone calls.
- Anyone who defames you publicly and thereby becomes enraged against you (he might claim you are having an affair or are embezzling money from your employer).
- Anyone who objectifies you by belittling you so that he can vent his anger and make you the object of his rage (for example, if you are an IRS employee he may rationalize the injustice of tax collection methods as a way of justifying his anger so that he can take it out on you).

How to Respond if You are Stalked

- Accept the fact that your life is now in danger. Never underestimate the threat against you. Stalking is a crime and can result in physical violence, rape, abduction, or murder. Commit to resolving the situation without being harmed.

- Give your stalker a firm "No" and do not engage in any further contact with him, no matter how many attempts he makes (you do not want to convey the message to him that his actions will continue to elicit a response from you, because that is precisely his objective). Do not try to negotiate with him (unless it is a temporary ruse), reason with him, or have someone (other than the police or experts) intervene on your behalf; just break contact.

- Consider all threats to be serious, even if they appear ambiguous or are nonspecific in nature. Stalkers, especially those who are strangers, are emotionally unstable and are therefore unpredictable to a certain degree. Do not take risks by assuming that your stalker will respond in a rational, logical manner.

- Make sure your residence number is visible and easy to find so that emergency responders will not be delayed. (In some counties you can use reflective paint to mark your house number on the street for good visibility after dark).

- Ask the police to drive by your home whenever possible. Visit the police station and make contact with an officer so that you put a face to your name. Ask if anyone at the station specializes in stalking cases.

- If you can afford to, hire a threat management team, including a lawyer, private investigator, and anti-stalking experts.

- Consider having your lawyer send a registered letter to the stalker telling him to stop.

- Record and report all incidences to the police (and to your Threat Management Team if you have one). Log all incidents using the form in Appendix D.

- Obtain a photograph of your stalker (discreetly) and any information, such as his vehicle license plate number.

- Increase your home security (install deadbolts, an alarm system, and motion lights; get a dog; keep all doors and windows locked at all times).

- Increase your vehicle security (install a car alarm; always keep doors locked and windows up; park in well lit, visible places; do not allow your gas tank to go below the half way marker).

- Implement a surveillance detection plan, including conducting route and building reviews.

- Vary your schedule, including departure and arrival times to locations you frequent habitually, such as work.

- Do not walk or jog alone in remote areas.

- Always carry a cell phone. If he has your current cell phone number, keep that phone but do not answer any unfamiliar calls. Keep all evidence, including phone bill records of incoming calls and any voice mail messages he leaves.

- Do not attempt to respond to or return any correspondences or gifts. Save all letters, cards, notes, gifts, and messages as evidence. Handle items as little as possible. Store them in sealed, dated, plastic bags. Keep all of the packaging materials in which the items were delivered. Photocopy and photograph all evidence before turning it over to the police, using rulers positioned at right angles in the photographs to indicate measurements of objects.

- Inform everyone you know and trust about your stalker, including your neighbors, apartment manager, doorman, valet, co-workers, employers, friends, family, and school administrators. Give them a flyer with his picture and any descriptive information about him and his vehicle. Ask them to help you by being on the lookout for him and reporting him to you or the police (photocopy some incident forms from Appendix D for them to use). Tell them not to release information about you to your stalker, should he try to elicit any from them.

- Always carry a SureFire flashlight, a TASER device, or pepper spray (See Chapter Twelve. We advise you receive training in using them for self-defense purposes).
- If you can afford to, get SD, evasive driving, and self-defense training (See Appendixes A and E).
- Inform anyone who could become a collateral target (such as your boyfriend, close friends, co-workers, or family).

Control Your Safety if the Situation Escalates

- Consider obtaining a court protection order. Research the local laws and find out what the implications are if your stalker violates the court order. Your goal is to get him in front of a judge. Keep in mind that a court order may backfire and further antagonize him.
- Consider filing a civil suit against him for damages. If you have incurred serious expenses while protecting yourself from him, you might want to try to get reimbursed. Keep in mind this may aggravate the stalking. It could also work as a tool to get him to stop. Use your judgment and seek advice from professionals in order to make the best decision.
- Work with a Threat Management Team if at all possible, including law enforcement, an attorney, a private investigator, crisis management services, and professionals who specialize in stalking cases. Do *not* allow friends, family, co-workers, and neighbors or anyone who could be considered a collateral target to intervene on your behalf.
- Inspect your vehicle each morning. Look for any evidence of tampering or damage to: tires, hubcaps, lug nuts, gas cap, leaking

brake fluid, or anything suspicious under the hood or attached to the under-carriage of the vehicle. If you find anything, realize it is evidence and do not touch it. Call the police and report it.

- If you have children, use all the necessary precautionary measures in the event that your stalker turns his attention towards them as a way to get to you. Notify their schools of the situation and do not allow anyone to pick up your children after school except a family member. Have them escorted in and out of school.

- Be especially careful during transition times (for example, when leaving the house in the morning, when arriving to work, etc.).

- Break your routines. Vary your schedule and the routes you travel often and randomly. Do not establish any kind of pattern your stalker can study and use to predict your whereabouts.

- Carry a personal alarm or air horn in your vehicle and on your person at all times.

- Avoid being alone, both at home and in public, if possible. At a minimum, have someone walk you to your car or front doorstep and go in the house with you to be sure you have no intruders.

- Have an emergency contact plan with all the necessary phone numbers of your SUPNET.

- Identify what you can use as defensive tools in and around your home and workplace, as well as inside your vehicle (see Chapter Twelve).

- If you are forced to move as a result of the stalking, do not leave a paper trail. Limit the information you release regarding the whereabouts of your new residence.

- Keep your fuse box, telephone box, gas cap, vehicle, and home secured at all times.

- In extreme cases, remove your name from all properties and put them in the name of a trusted family member. Seek advice from a lawyer before doing so.

In order to illustrate how our prevention process works for handling being stalked by someone you do not know, let us return to our high threat character, Kate, and complete her story. Although Kate determined late in the game that she was being stalked by a stranger, she was able to prevent being attacked.

Kate's suspicions that she had a stalker were warranted; she did. Her first inkling came one day when she was eating lunch at the plaza in front of the office building where she works. She noticed a man sitting across the plaza and she felt like he was watching her. Uncomfortable, she took her lunch and went back inside to her desk. Two days later, the same thing happened. Kate assumed the man worked in her building and just happened to take his lunch break at the same time she did. A week later, when on her coffee break in the building cafeteria, he was standing behind her in line and started to chat with her about the weather. Now Kate became very uneasy. It was just a feeling, but she decided to pay attention to it.

Kate had heard about us from a friend and called us that afternoon. She had the usual trepidation in her voice: "I'm probably over-reacting, but something just doesn't feel right." We reassured her that she was not over-reacting and, since the odds are so high that she will be stalked in her lifetime, why not conduct the prevention process anyway. In other words, we encouraged her to study herself as a target so that she is ahead of the game even if it turns out that she has no real immediate threat.

After completing her personal security survey and risk/threat assessment, Kate had a much more objective view of her own patterns. Kate rated herself as having average situational awareness when she completed her personal security profile. She gasped with a mixture of horror and amusement: "I can't believe how predictable I am!" We then took her through the route review process so that she could study herself as a moving target (see Chapter Six). Sure enough, she spotted her suspected stalker in one of the key surveillance locations she identified on her route map from her home to work. There he was, walking his dog in the park up the street from her home. Kate became understandably alarmed and spiraled into that powerless place where any woman would go when she realizes she is being tracked by a predator. She tried to shake it off as a coincidence: "Maybe he just lives near here," she whimpered with the slightest bit of hope.

Now that Kate had four incidents of seeing this man, all of which she documented and reported to the police, she eagerly continued studying herself as a target. She now considered what information her stalker would need to collect if he were to attack her as a static target, meaning if he were to come after her at any of the locations she frequents regularly, beginning with her home and workplace. Once she completed her route review maps and building review maps, we positioned surveillance detection support specialists in several of the surveillance detection locations that Kate identified and indicated on her route and building maps (see Chapters Six and Seven). Since Kate's threat was imminent, she completed this process hastily, regretting out loud: "If I had only done this before I ever noticed this guy, I probably would have been on to him a lot sooner. Who knows how long he's been out there watching me. If he has already figured out what street I live on, then that probably means he has figured out other things about me too."

Kate was correct; one of our surveillance detection support staff saw the man parked in the lot at the strip mall where Kate does her grocery shopping every Sunday afternoon. Since that was a pattern Kate could easily change, she avoided going to the grocery store that Sunday, but our people were there for her. At this point, Kate now had new information about her predator, namely a vehicle description and license plate number. The police were able to match the vehicle to his driver's license. Kate could now potentially learn more about her stalker. The police discovered he had no record, for stalking or any other crime. Kate felt completely helpless all over again. She had high hopes that he was violating his parole and would be arrested immediately for his actions against her. She agonized: "By the time the police will be able to help me, he may have already succeeded in attacking me. How am I supposed to defend myself against this guy? Who is he and why is he after me?"

We coached Kate to make herself as inaccessible to him as possible. She brought in her lunch and coffee thermos to work and only took breaks in her company's secured employee lounge. She notified everyone at her office about the situation, including the parking garage security staff, and gave them a photo and description of the man and his vehicle information. Kate agreed to have an escort walk her to her car. She never entered or remained in an elevator alone. She totally avoided using the stairs. She even had a female co-worker accompany her to the ladies' room. She instructed that no unidentified packages or deliveries should be accepted on her behalf. Somehow her stalker obtained her home phone number and called her to ask her out on a date. She gave him a firm response ("No and never call me again.") and logged the date, time, and content of the call. He then began leaving threatening messages on her voice mail, saying "I am sure we are meant to be together. Please just have coffee with me. I'll never stop calling you until you say yes." She saved all of the messages and turned them over to the police.

Over the course of several weeks, Kate practiced surveillance detection along her routes and at her home and workplace. She radically changed her routines, including her departure schedule to and from work. She tightened her security in and around her home and informed all her neighbors about her stalker. She enlisted surveillance detection support from us and from her friends. She took back her power and put herself in charge of the situation.

Initially Kate opted to forego getting a court protection order against her stalker because, since he was a total stranger to her, she felt he must be seriously mentally disturbed to be fixating on her. This element of unpredictability made her wary of taking any aggressive action towards him. Instead she focused her energies on doing everything possible to deny him access to her. Using her surveillance detection plan, Kate was able to detect her stalker on several occasions hiding in the woods behind her home. She was able to photograph him discreetly from inside her home. Since the woods were part of her property, she reported him to the police for trespassing but did not press charges against him. At this point she felt compelled to get a court protection order. He violated the order and returned to the woods behind her home. She photographed him and logged the incident and then called the police and had him picked up for both trespassing and violating the court order.

Although she felt frightened by his irrational behavior, Kate also told us that she felt much more secure because she knew, based on her route and building reviews, *where and when to look for him. She said she felt much more control over her situation because she knew it would be hard for him to sneak up on her by surprise. A month went by and things were quiet. Her stalker was never sent to jail or fined. Kate ruminated, "The silence is eerie. I know he's still out there and I'm not convinced he is over me." Once again, she was correct.*

On the day her stalker attempted his attack, Kate was steps ahead of him. She had not abandoned her surveillance detection practice simply because things had quieted down. Instead, she intensified it and her efforts paid off when it counted most. She was driving to work an hour early one morning. As she approached the intersection where she had identified one of her predictable travel locations on her route review map, she spotted him in one of the surveillance locations she had identified. He was in his car and began following her vehicle. Kate discreetly dialed 911 on her cell phone and reported him. She proceeded to follow her normal route and was ready to use one of her safe locations if the police did not get there in time. She stayed on the phone with the operator and provided the necessary information about her safe location so that the police would know where to intercept her stalker. As she pulled into the parking lot of her safe location, the police arrived. Her stalker was arrested and, because he had an illegal firearm in his possession, spent time in jail.

Kate learned how to make herself a "hard target" (meaning difficult to access). Even though she had to catch up on implementing her prevention process rather late in game, she was still able to utilize the techniques to keep herself safe.

Regardless if you know your stalker or he is a stranger, you should assume that he will try to hurt or kill you and then work hard analyzing where, when, and how he could be successful doing so. Once you have this information, do whatever it takes to deny him the opportunity to get near you. In extreme situations, this may mean relocating and going into hiding. In most situations, if you make it impossible for him to get close to you (both physically and verbally) your ability to protect yourself will outweigh his ability to harm you. "The best defense is a good offense."

Cyber Stalking

With the increasing popularity of the internet and e-mailing, stalking has taken on a new face. A cyber stalker can be someone you know or a total stranger. Essentially, when a woman becomes the victim of cyber stalking it means that she is monitored and harassed via the internet and/or through e-mails. A cyber stalker might write a malicious e-mail about you and spread it around using the internet. He might harass people who visit your website and write in their comments (thereby providing their e-mail addresses for him to exploit). He might use a blog or website to spread lies or rumors about you. He could send you menacing e-mails and threaten you. The options are only as limited as his creativity and computer expertise. If you become the victim of cyber stalking, it is important for you to realize that you should take it very seriously. Cyber stalking can escalate into regular stalking if your stalker is able to obtain the necessary information about where you live and work. In addition, cyber stalking could put you at risk of having your identity stolen.

Reduce the Risk of Cyber Stalking

- Use a gender neutral e-mail address so that you cannot be identified as being female.
- Only open e-mails from originators with whom you are familiar.
- Keep your computer virus protection and spyware updated.
- Turn off the headers in your e-mail so that your name is not released every time you send an e-mail.
- Guard the information you release to profiles or online directories.
- If you visit chat rooms, internet dating services, newsgroups, or have a blog, limit the personal information you release to strangers.
- If you have a website for a business, use a P.O. Box rather than your home address. Limit any personal details that can be used against you.
- If your children use the internet, install a software program to track their use. If they are using one of the free blog sites or are "instant

messaging," find out what information they are releasing about themselves which a predator could exploit. Make sure they know they should *never* arrange a meeting with anyone they communicate with on-line, even if that person encourages them to meet in a busy public place.

What to Do if You are Cyber Stalked

- Seek professional help from an information technology (IT) specialist.
- Document all evidence of the stalking. Save all original documents and correspondences. Use a back-up drive to save additional copies. Print out a hard copy for your records as well.
- Do not respond to the stalker or initiate any contact with him.
- Research the laws on cyber stalking in your state.
- Report your stalker to the authorities.

What to Do if the Cyber Stalking Escalates

- Form a team for support, including community resources, law enforcement, and an IT specialist.
- Proceed with great caution and follow the above tips in this chapter for handling a stalking situation that has escalated.
- Assume your cyber stalker knows where you live and work. Even if he does not, you cannot afford to risk believing you are safe because you think he is only stalking you from a distance.
- Inform all of your loved ones, neighbors, and co-workers about the stalking so that, if he does begin stalking you physically, others will be apprised of the threat and may notice someone who is out of place or is fixating on you or your home.

In some ways we feel this is the most important chapter in this book. The odds are so high that many of our readers will be stalked. Not only does the U.S. Justice Department find that your chances of being stalked are one in twelve, they also found that almost fifty percent of stalking victims never report the problem to law enforcement. To us this says that probably more than one in twelve women is stalked because all of those women who never reported it are unaccounted for in the one in twelve statistic.

Imagine if we declared an anti-stalking day and on that day every woman who has been stalked or is being stalked right now wore an adapted version of a "Scarlet Letter" (a large red letter "S" pinned to her shirt). It is a feminist twist to the idea behind the book by Nathaniel Hawthorne, published in 1850, wherein the main character, Hester Prynne, was shamed and publicly vilified by being forced to wear the letter "A" on her clothing to expose her adulterous actions. We could turn around this concept and make it work *for* us. If women took it upon themselves to expose this oppressive crime, perhaps we could bring more attention to this horrible plight we face and gain more support from those in our communities. Rather than embarrassing or shaming us, this bold action would empower us to take a public stand and announce this problem to the world. It is a radical idea but stalking is a very real threat and it is not going away any time soon. Certainly, were women to implement such an idea, we would have to take into consideration the possible security issues involved. Because the idea is somewhat confrontational in nature, women who have stalkers would want to be careful not to provoke a reaction. On the other hand, when women unify against violence they send predators a powerful message.

The salient point is: If you have a stalker, report him. You are playing with fire if you try to go it alone. You are not required to take legal action against him, but if you let him get away with stalking and threatening you, you may put yourself or your family at greater risk. In addition, if he is never reported to the authorities, other women will likely become his future victims. The idea behind becoming empowered is that you take charge and refuse to be a victim.

CHAPTER TEN

SEXUAL SEDUCTION:
THE BIG CREEPY

But he was such a nice man
and he seemed like a normal person.
I never would have imagined...

Each state in our country establishes what is known as an "age of consent." This is the age at which an individual is considered competent to give consent to having sexual relations. Regardless of the state in which you live, consider that there is exactly one day between the time an individual is classified as a minor and then as an adult in terms of her/his ability to consent to sex. This is significant to this topic because having consensual sex with an individual who is not of the age of consent may be classified as statutory rape, while having consensual sex with an individual who has reached the age of consent is legal. Murky waters churn at the bottom of the river.

In this chapter we will explore the disturbing similarities between the techniques that pedophiles are using illegally on minors and some sexual seducers are implementing legally on adult, unsuspecting women. We will also look at other sexually deviant behaviors that threaten women. Be prepared for a rude awakening, but know also that your best defense against these types of sexually deviant behaviors and crimes is information. You cannot prevent becoming a victim of something about which you know nothing.

Sexual Seduction

One of the most disturbing threats, yet also one of the most overlooked, is something called sexual seduction. Oprah Winfrey has brought much needed attention to this subject, as seen in her efforts to expose pedophiles who target children. Kudos to Oprah because this technique is a silent danger about which many women and parents are unaware. If you are a single woman out in the dating world, a high school or college girl, or a mother of either daughters or sons, you need to read this. The most disturbing part of this subject is that, although techniques of sexual seduction are not illegal to use on adult women, it is not a far leap for the sexual seducer to use them illegally on a minor. In addition, the techniques are so psychologically manipulative that when they are used as a pick-up strategy on an adult woman, they are akin to the worst kind of trickery. Stated another way, some men are using very similar techniques to the ones that pedophiles use to get you to have sex with them. How creepy is that?!

Sexual seduction of an adult woman consists of a series of manipulative techniques which are used, unbeknownst to the woman, in order to convince her to have sex with the seducer. Sexual seduction of a minor is a manipulative, calculated process a molester uses in order to "groom" his victim to become receptive to inappropriate sexual advances. What both targets (the adult woman and the minor) have in common is:

- They are secretly being manipulated and often isolated from others who could warn them about the seduction process.
- They often enjoy some aspect of the seduction process.

- They develop some degree of a relationship with the seducer.
- They experience shame at having been a participant in the seduction process.

The important distinction is that even if the minor becomes a willing participant, the seduction process and molestation are crimes because the minor is too young to protect her/himself. The adult woman, even if she is tricked and manipulated because she is ignorant of the tactics her seducer is using, is old enough to be capable of refusing sex from her seducer. Your best defenses against these unsolicited advances are, once again, situational awareness and surveillance detection.

Sexual Seduction of Adult Women

Subliminal Conquest Techniques

At this point in history, if you have a particular problem to research, all you have to do is use the internet to conduct a keyword search on the topic and almost instantly an answer will be provided. So, for example, a man who is desperate to learn how to get women to have sex with him is just keystrokes away from a solution to his problem. For whatever reason, some men have difficulty meeting women who will have sex with them. Perhaps these men are unattractive, lack confidence, or have no social skills. Perhaps they are simply too lazy to court women and wait patiently until they feel ready for sexual intimacy. What all men now have access to is training in sexual seduction techniques. Some men are actually paying good money to learn how to lure women into bed using subliminal conquest techniques. They are practicing these techniques and claiming to be successful.

Sexual seduction techniques are based on using neuro-linguistic programming against a target (a woman to have sex with). Basically men can receive training in these techniques via seminars and video tapes/DVD's. The training focuses on the use of subliminal verbal patterns, including key words and phrases, which prompt sexual responses in their unsuspecting victims (oops—these guys do not like the word 'victim' because they do not consider themselves to be predators). It works like this:

Jennifer and Stephanie, both twenty-one years old, are at a local bar that is popular with college students from a nearby campus. They are out with the intention of meeting interesting men, possibly men they would like to date in the future. The bar is not crowded and the two women are deep in conversation about dating and relationships.

Mike is sitting nearby. He is thirty-five and a frequent customer of college bars because he likes to pick up college girls, especially ones who are open to having sex with an older man. Mike is, unbeknownst to the women, eavesdropping on their conversation because that is the first technique he always uses. He will surreptitiously collect information on his target to enable him to develop a more effective strategy. Mike overhears Jennifer saying: "I just want to meet a guy I feel comfortable enough with to hang out in my pajamas and watch DVD's on a Saturday night. I'm so sick of this dating scene and all the jerks out there. I'm so tired of guys who are just interested in having sex. Don't get me wrong; sex is an important part of a relationship. I just want it to mean something to both of us."

Tom, Mike's friend and 'wingman' is sitting at the other end of the bar. Mike discreetly points to Jennifer, basically calling dibs on her and giving Tom the cue to work on Stephanie. Mike and Tom's objective is to isolate the women from each other so that the two men can tag-team off of each other's seduction strategy. Mike and Tom both attended a course on sexual seduction and learned to exploit women's potential competitive nature with each other where sexual experience is concerned. In other words, if Mike can get Jennifer to assume that Tom and Stephanie are hitting it off, then Jennifer might be more apt to succumb to Mike's advances. Also, if the girls are separated from each other, they may be more receptive to being seduced and touched since no one is there to witness it or question it. Since each woman will be removed from the influence of the verbal or nonverbal cues of her friend, she will also be removed from negative judgments that may influence whether or not she is willing to become physical or sexual with her suitor.

Mike approaches the bar and stands next to Jennifer to order his drink. He tells the bartender: "I guess I'll have one more but then I'm off to chill in bed with my DVD player. I rented some great movies." He turns to Jennifer: "I don't know why I even bothered coming out to a smoky bar in the first place. Hi, I'm Mike." They shake hands and Jennifer introduces herself and Stephanie. Mike continues talking directly to Jennifer, (after all, he knows Tom will be moving in on Stephanie soon enough and she will be more apt to talk to Tom if she is being ignored by Mike).

"My intuition tells me you are not that into this bar scene either." Jennifer lights up because she thinks she is about to make a real connection with Mike, not the usual bar pick-up charade. They continue to chat about movies. He inquires about her favorites and affirms some of them are his too. He mentions a romantic movie and then adds emphasis to strengthen his position. "What I love about the two characters is how deeply they connect right on the spot, as though they were destined to be together." He uses a hand gesture and points back and forth between himself and Jennifer to emphasize the idea.

Meanwhile, Tom has approached Stephanie, who is happy to be receiving some attention now, since Jennifer is otherwise distracted. Tom uses light-hearted conversation and makes Stephanie laugh. Mike moves in closer to Jennifer and asks: "Looks like your friend has met someone she likes. Maybe we should give them some space. Want to go over and sit at a table? I have to confess, I am enjoying having someone I can really talk to." Jennifer agrees.

When they sit at the table Mike opens the discussion with a variation on one of the conversation patterns he learned at his sexual seduction training. He will use subtle suggestions to bring Jennifer closer to the subject of sex, without ever directly mentioning the word sex.

"I was watching this show the other night on public television about attraction. They said that the ideal attraction has three components. First, when you experience it you feel a high state of arousal. Second, it makes your heart beat really fast and your breathing accelerates as you feel an enormous rush all over your body and third, it fascinates you and enthralls you. It's kind of like an amazing ride at a carnival; as soon as you get off, you want to get back on, over and over again." He then introduces another pattern he learned which he hopes

will help him reinforce the idea of a meaningful connection: "Actually, for me attraction has to do much more with feeling comfortable with the other person. You know, like you were meant to be together and like your perfect match is sitting right next to you." He points to himself coyly and gazes into her eyes.

Mike takes time to let Jennifer talk about herself, as he listens intently. He has scripted his techniques and has practiced them so often that he knows exactly when to insert each one into the conversation in order to guide Jennifer's thoughts in his chosen direction (towards sex). When Mike feels Jennifer is ripe for manipulation, he begins to integrate some patterns into the conversation to more assertively program the idea of a sexual encounter into Jennifer's mind. His objective is to arouse Jennifer and make her experience sexual thoughts without explicitly bringing up the subject of sex. That way, Jennifer might feel as though the thoughts were her own and she was not pushed into them but arrived at them all by herself, thereby giving her the false perception of being in control of her part in the seduction process. At this stage, Mike begins with a technique wherein he will make statements that are seemingly normal but, because he will alter his pronunciation and slur some words together, he adds a subliminal sexual overtone to the conversation. Because Jennifer believes that Mike might be that real love she is waiting for, her mind is open to experiences she desires, such as lovemaking that is deeply satisfying because she has a potential partner who truly cares for her.

"You know, Jennifer, I used to think I was being selfish trying to attain happiness {pronounced 'ha-penis'} through a relationship. You know, like it was below me {pronounced 'blow me'} to let love play such a big role in my life and penetrate my existence so thoroughly that I would ignore doing other things with my life. But now I'm starting to believe...{a long pause to create anticipation}... that I should surrender and allow love to come deep inside me. At my age, I am thinking more and more about getting serious with the right person." At this point he shifts to joining words together so that they come out sounding like a command. "Have you ever felt like you just want to say: 'Go for it and just do it'? With me, it's like that sometimes." {He binds together the words "just do it with me"}.

Next Mike shifts gears to his carefully crafted technique for subliminally influencing Jennifer in the direction of oral sex. "I'm really craving something sweet right now. Have you ever had a chocolate covered strawberry? I went to a wedding last week and they served chocolate covered strawberries with champagne. It's like an explosion of pleasure in your mouth. I'd love to have one right now. They should serve them here. Who cares about drinking beer; I'll take chocolate and champagne any day over beer!"

Stephanie interrupts and tells Jennifer that she and Tom are leaving together. Jennifer can tell that her friend is very excited about Tom. Once they have departed Mike states sarcastically "Nothing going on there, huh!" He then offers to walk Jennifer back to her apartment. "Don't worry; I won't try to invite myself inside." He leans in, rests his hand on her knee, and whispers sweetly, "Unless of course you insist I do."

Certainly men and women have played courtship and seduction games since day one of human history. Jennifer is not necessarily a victim if she chooses to have sex with Mike. She may end up disappointed if all Mike is really interested in is sex and does not have any interest in her as a person. Likewise, Mike might be fooling himself with his seduction techniques. Perhaps he is the one who will be duped when he ends up falling in love with a woman he only had intentions of seducing. What we find alarming about sexual seducers is that they are walking such a fine line in terms of predatory behavior. The fact that they are using a calculated process of deception and manipulation is what gives us pause. Surely, if a woman were repulsed by a man who approached her using these techniques, they would not work. However, if she is neutral to or attracted to the seducer, she might succumb, especially if she is in any altered emotional state (for example if she has had too much to drink or she is in a celebratory mood).

The question remains: Is a woman in danger if a sexual seducer targets her? Not necessarily, but if a man is willing to use calculated techniques in an effort to manipulate her, would she feel safe trusting him enough to bring him into her life? If a man is routinely using seduction techniques so that he can have a trophy collection of sexual experiences perhaps he will also take the next step and capture those experiences on film or discuss them in detail with his friends who capitalize on the same techniques. A woman who encounters such a man should wonder how far he is willing to go to have sex with her. If he is willing and even proud of having manipulated her verbally and emotionally by dominating and steering the conversation, would he take other manipulative actions towards her, including dangerous ones?

If you encounter this type of situation and feel you are being verbally manipulated take a moment and break contact with the seducer. Go to the ladies' room and regroup. If you are with a friend, make her go with you and explain to her what you think is happening. Even if you decide he is a man you would like to have sex with, breaking contact temporarily will give you time to identify if he may be a serious threat. You can collect yourself and take the time to notice if he, for example, is working with a wingman. If you step back from the seduction process, you deflate its emotional power over you and you can then decide if you are being duped. Breaking contact will give you a clearer perspective as to whether or not your seducer could be a predator with hostile intentions. When you return from the ladies' room, you can take control over the conversation and discover if there is really anything more to him than a desperate man in search of sex. Heighten your situational awareness and practice surveillance detection when you depart the location to be sure he (or his wingman) does not follow you.

Our emphasis is on helping women stay safe. We surmise that the more women become aware of this deceptive seduction process, the more capable they will be of protecting themselves from an experience that might eventually place them in harm's way. In addition, as women we must band together and help each other against potential predators. Imagine if you, now that you are informed about this subject, were sitting at the bar watching Mike and Tom in action. Probably your instinct would cause you to find some opportunity to warn the women they are targeting about what is happening. Or, if you are a mother and your daughter is about to leave home for college, would you not want her to be aware of this strategy that might be used against her without her knowledge? And, if you are a single woman out in the dating scene, even if you do go out with the intention of meeting someone with whom you can have sex, are you willing to be the target of any man's deceptive scheme? More important, would you not want to do everything in your power to avoid potential predators? Women have the right to expect men to be on the level with them, even if women's desires are in alignment with men's.

Sexual Seduction of Minors

If we return for a moment to Mike and Jennifer from the scenario discussed above, imagine that Mike is still thirty-five but that Jennifer is thirteen. She and her friend Stephanie are now sitting in a coffee shop instead of a bar. Mike uses eavesdropping to collect information on his target. He finds out that Jennifer wishes she had a boyfriend who likes movies and will go shopping at the mall with her. Mike moves in to talk to Jennifer when Stephanie is standing in line to buy a coffee. Jennifer is isolated from her source of protection so Mike takes advantage of the moment. He quickly gains her trust by discussing subjects that he now knows are important to her (such as meeting someone with whom she can watch movies). He tells Jennifer he is a college student and asks to meet her again at the coffee shop, telling her he would rather be alone with her so that he could get to know her better. Jennifer agrees and meets him again. Over time, Mike uses conversation patterns to dominate Jennifer's emotions. He develops a level of intimacy and trust before attempting to isolate her further at his apartment. They make trips to the mall together and he buys her nice things. He takes her to "R" rated movies and treats her like an adult. He tells her to keep their friendship a secret because her parents and friends will probably not approve of her dating a college student. Jennifer is thrilled to keep their secret because it is exciting and she feels special. Over time Mike introduces the subject of sex and uses visual images to lead her into thinking about sex. He only introduces 'safe' touching after he has established trust and a 'meaningful' connection with Jennifer.

We refer to the sexual seduction of minors as 'The Big Creepy' because it is one of the most disturbing threats both girls and boys (even ones who are teenagers) face in terms of child endangerment. We are including this segment because we want as many women as possible to become more aware of this threat. Many of you are mothers, teachers, child-care workers, older sisters, aunts, friends, and neighbors of minors who may need you to be the one to notice when something is amiss. Our female, intuitive maternal instincts are powerful when it comes to protecting children. Our radar for detecting predators who target children is instinctively honed and we should trust it.

Sexual seduction of a minor is a threat because it normally will result in some type of violent or criminal behavior against the child. Many cases of sexual seduction result in molestation, sexual abuse, or rape. Kidnapping and murder are other possible outcomes of a case that may begin with the sexual seduction process and then lead to something far worse. Child pornography is another common crime that results from the sexual seduction process.

The process of sexually seducing a minor with the objective of sexually abusing the child is a slow, deliberate, calculated manipulation. Often the predator is someone the child and her/his family knows, such as a neighbor, friend, coach, teacher, employee at a store where the family shops, or even the parent of a friend of the child's. The predator begins by establishing a friendly relationship with the child. He will show interest in the child and will work to establish trust with the parents so that he can gain access to his victim. He might offer some type of help, like tutoring or babysitting. He may approach single mothers whose children need a father figure in the picture. Once he has unrestricted access to his target, he will work hard at "grooming" the child so that he can form a bond of trust and friendship. The grooming process will include activities like special games just the two of them will play together. This gives the child the message that she/he is important, unique, and fun to be around. Building the child's self-confidence is all part of the larger plan.

The sexual abuser who is willing to invest the time and energy in the grooming process is a patient predator. He will craft an entire seduction process so that, by the time he introduces the sexual abuse, he has a context of collusion with the victim within which he can safely maintain and perpetuate the abuse. He makes his victim a "willing" party to the seduction process. The molester will often use the special game he has devised to first isolate the child and then to develop an oath of secrecy. He might use a tactic such as convincing the child that, "If your parents knew we played our game, they might make us stop. They won't understand how fun it is. Why don't we make it our secret game?"

The molester will extract information from the child that he can exploit. For example, if the minor were a thirteen year old girl the molester might try to learn any potentially useful information about her relationship with her parents. Perhaps her parents will not buy her clothes or phone cards for her cell phone. The molester will exploit this information and use it as an opportunity to build an alliance with his victim against those who are most invested in her protection. He might buy her clothes and phone cards, telling her, "You deserve to be treated like a princess; don't your parents understand how special you are?" He will take his time and infiltrate her psyche with these types of devious manipulations.

He will nurture the relationship over time, perhaps as long as months or even years. He will be the constant provider of affection, gifts, self-esteem, attention, and trust. By the time the molester is ready to introduce sexual contact with his target, the victim is well groomed and likely has developed a strong emotional attachment to the abuser. At this stage, the abuser will begin using what is sometimes referred to as "the collection" to lure his target towards sexual contact. He will introduce something that evokes the subject of sex, such as a pornographic photograph or an explicit sex scene in a popular movie. At this point, depending on the age of his target, he may be opening a dialogue about sex with a young child or using items from the collection to arouse the adolescent. He may also attempt to use the guise of providing "appropriate" sex education to the child by offering: "If you want to learn more about sex, we can discuss it. I think you are old enough and smart enough to hear about it and it might help you to know more about what sex is really like." Again, he is adding adhesive to the bond of collusion he is developing with his target. Now, even if the child is uncomfortable, the predator can refer to the time when the child asked him about sex and begin to blame the child with statements like: "Well, you asked me about it so I thought you were grown up enough to talk about it." In this way the predator sets the stage for the victim to feel responsibility for the abuse that is to come.

Once items from the collection have been introduced and this Pandora's Box of abusive entanglement has been opened, the victim is now being escorted through the dark hallways of her/his complex emotions. On the one hand, the victim's inhibitions are lowered regarding the subject of sex. On the other hand, the child may feel fear or, at a minimum, uneasy talking about the subject. Yet she/he may also feel secretly thrilled at this type of attention or flattered that the predator finds her/him to be so mature. The victim may also feel guilty for doubting him, like she/he caused a conflict and should patch up things so as not to lose this trusted friend. The predator is gleeful about his manipulations and will waste no time moving to the next stage.

The molester is now ready to introduce touching as his catalyst to sex. At first the touching may be interpreted by the victim as innocuous. He may tickle, tease or wrestle with his target, slowly and methodically introducing inappropriate touching that may at first seem to be accidental (for example, he may brush against a girl's breast or a boy's penis while tackling her/him to the floor as though they were playing football). Eventually he may use items of erotica or even child pornography from his "collection" to convince his target that it is normal for adults and minors to have sex with each other. This sends the signal to the victim that it is acceptable for the adult to now initiate more direct inappropriate touching. The predator will keep it light-hearted and will incorporate promises of fun and rewards into the abusive activity. The predator may also resort to using alcohol or even drugs to help relax his target and make her/him more receptive or even helpless.

If the victim tries to resist, the blackmailing process is already in place. The molester has already assigned the blame to the victim for being willing to talk about sex and look at 'dirty' pictures. A common technique that has become popular among molesters involves photographing the victim in compromising situations and threatening to post the photos on the internet. The photos also become a part of the molester's collection (this is important because he will likely keep them and laws against child pornography will apply in an investigation that turns up this type of evidence). Since the secret game that the molester and his victim play now includes sexual abuse, the molester will blackmail any victim who threatens to expose him. He may have an emotional hold on the victim by threatening to tell her/his parents about the alcohol/drugs, the photos, and the abuse itself. He may say things like: "You never said you didn't want to play our game" or "You asked me to tell you what intercourse is like." He also may convince his victim that "It would ruin your family if you tell them the truth." Often years will go by before the victim can disclose what really happened, if ever.

Defenses against Sexual Seduction of Minors

Parents please pay attention to the behavior of any adult who has a relationship with your child. We understand that it is difficult to live with suspicions and we are not suggesting you make any premature accusations. What we are saying is, the signs will be present, but you have to look. If you are practicing situational awareness, you will be looking as a habit and you will notice early warning signals of trouble. You must also educate your child about inappropriate interactions with adults. You have to be the one to ask your child the right questions in order to determine if any threats exist with any adults in your child's life. You also may have to be the one to educate your husband about this issue if he is unfamiliar with it.

None of us wants to imagine that our best friend, our brother, our co-worker, the scout leader, or the coach would ever harm our child in such an abhorrent way. It happens! Parents would be crazy not to accept the reality that this malfunction of humankind exists. Do whatever you can to avoid allowing your child to have isolated time with any adult on any regular basis. If your child spends a lot of time at a friend's house, make a surprise visit. If you notice your child is on the computer chatting or instant messaging, look into it and see what you can learn about the person with whom your child is communicating (see the section on cyber stalking in Chapter Nine). If necessary, contact your internet service provider or install parental controls on your computer.

You can also practice surveillance detection in order to pick up any indicators that an adult is fixating on your child. Do any adults try to elicit information about your child's activities and schedule? Pay attention at any activities your child attends. Is anyone there spending a lot of time with your child or photographing your child? Watch any adults who seem to be captivated by the children and barely interact with other adults. Trust your instincts! Be on the lookout for inappropriate verbal contact or even the smallest gesture that might indicate an inappropriate intimacy between your child and the adult in question. If an adult is transporting your child, watch from your window during pick up and drop off times. Often these moments of greeting or saying goodbye between the victim and predator are telling signs that there is some inappropriate relationship that has developed or is in the process of developing.

Most of all, talk to your child about the "secret game" strategy. Let your child know that she/he can trust you and that if any adult tries to make a game for her/him to play that you want to be notified. Stress to the child that she/he will not be in trouble and you will not punish her/him or embarrass her/him. Make it emotionally safe for your child to confide in you. In addition, teach your child, especially if she/he is young, to *never* allow her/himself to be photographed in private by any adult even if it is a 'trusted' person.

In addition to paying attention to the behavior of adults, watch your child closely for indicators of sexual abuse. Some of the common signs of a child who is being sexually abused include:

- Loss of appetite.
- Inability to sleep or nightmares.
- Withdrawn, introverted behavior or excessive clinging.
- Changes in your child's disposition.

- Changes in your child's behavior towards adults, such as aggressive, fearful, shy, or nervous behaviors when in the presence of adults.
- Explicit sexual behavior, abnormal fixation on genitalia, or an advanced degree of knowledge about sex that seems inappropriate given your child's age.
- Inflicting harm on her/himself or engaging in self-destructive activities such as drug or alcohol abuse.
- A sudden drop in grades or changes in performance at school.
- Any onset of emotional changes such as the development of fears, excessive crying or depression, or regressive behaviors such as thumb sucking or bed-wetting.

This list is only a partial look at the indicators. Multiple resources exist to help you with the issue of sexual seduction and abuse (see Appendix E). Certainly the above indicators could also result from other traumas in a child's life. Before you panic and assume your child is being sexually abused, you may want to seek professional help for your child in order to determine the cause of the changes in behavior.

If your child is a post pubescent adolescent, you should be informed about two types of predatory behavior used against post pubescent minors (mostly boys). The first is ephebophilia, a sexually deviant condition wherein an adult is primarily or exclusively attracted to post pubescent adolescents and may become obsessed with and attempt to engage in sexual relations with an adolescent. The other type of pedophilia is called pederasty, wherein an adult male will form a bond or relationship with an adolescent boy, including a sexual relationship. Since adolescents generally have more opportunities for unsupervised contact with adults, pay attention to any adults who make concerted efforts to spend time with your teenager. Do not assume that, because your adolescent is growing up, he or she cannot be targeted by sexual predators.

It is easy to see the similarities between the tactics of child molesters and sexual seducers of adult women. Now that you have more information on the topic of sexual seduction and how it applies to both adult women and to minors, you are well on your way to being able to heighten your situational awareness and detect the early warning signals. Sexual seduction is not a pleasant subject. The incidence of abductions and murders of children by sexual predators is on the rise in our country, while in other countries children have long been victimized by the sex industry. This aberrant aspect of human nature is both sickening and profoundly disturbing. As women, we have more power now to take a stand against pedophiles and to defend ourselves and our children against sexual abuse. Our voices are stronger and we must continue to refuse to tolerate the most base and ugly behavior from those in our lives who are deviant. None of us wants to be put in the position to be forced to confront this issue, and yet it looms as a menacing, silent enemy against the purity of our children and our own sexual integrity.

Other Creepy and Potentially Threatening Sexually Deviant Behaviors

Unfortunately the creepiness does not end with pedophiles and sexual seducers. Women should be aware of the potential threat posed by men who engage in sexually deviant behaviors known as "paraphilias." Paraphilias are impulse control behavioral disorders that manifest themselves in the form of inappropriate (and often criminal) sexual behaviors, such as uncontrollable urges, fantasies, and socially inappropriate sexual displays. Pedophilia is classified as a paraphilia. Other paraphilias that are criminal in nature include:

- **Exhibitionism (Flashing):** An exhibitionist will expose his genitals to an unsuspecting victim and will sometimes masturbate in public. Normally an exhibitionist will not physically attack his victim, as his objective is to shock her with his blatant behavior.
- **Voyeurism (Peeping Tom):** This predator seeks sexual gratification by watching women (without their consent) who are either undressing,

using the toilet, or are engaging in sexual activity. Again, this predator will normally not seek physical contact with his victims, but he may obtain photographs or film footage and post them on the internet. A recent trend includes activities called "down-blousing" and "up-skirting." These voyeurs take photographs using cell phone cameras or hidden surveillance cameras to obtain photographs of women's body parts. Websites exist with posted photos taken without consent of unsuspecting women.

- **Frotteurism:** This predator will seek physical contact and attempt to touch a woman without her consent or rub his genitalia against the body of his victim. He may press up against a woman on a crowded subway car, for example, in order to achieve sexual gratification.
- **Sexual Masochism/Sadism:** Although these are normally not criminal acts, both sexual masochism and sadism can become criminal acts if the dominant party engages in violent behavior towards his victim. One example of a fantasy based practice that can become a crime is called "autoerotic partial asphyxiation." Here the dominant partner will attempt to induce a temporary state of asphyxiation in his submissive partner during orgasm. Obviously this can result in death. In addition, sadistic sexual behaviors become criminal if they result in rape, torture, or murder.

Paraphilias are much more common in men than women. In order to defend yourself against these deviant behaviors, you must first become better informed about them so that you can detect these behaviors and not be taken by surprise. You must also be aware that these deviants often do not realize they are committing a crime. Many of them believe their behavior is benign and that no one is victimized by their actions. Even the ones who realize they are doing something wrong cannot control their impulses. They attempt to elicit reactions from their victims and are motivated by the thrill of the forbidden nature of the experience (which for them is sexually gratifying). It is important that you understand these aspects of their psychology because their behaviors will seem bizarre to you. If you apply logical thinking, it is difficult to fathom that these men either do not realize their actions are inappropriate (much less criminal), or they simply cannot control themselves. In order to defend yourself, stay SASD and pay attention to any early warning signals of these behaviors:

Exhibitionism: If you see a man who is fondling himself or is attempting to unbutton his pants, you are getting early warning signals that he is probably an exhibitionist. However, many exhibitionists will not give you early warning signals because they obtain their thrill by totally surprising and shocking you. If you are taken by surprise by an exhibitionist and others are nearby, make noise and call for help. If you have a cell phone with you, call the police and report him. If you are alone and isolated, break contact immediately and go to a safe location. Sometimes an exhibitionist will follow a woman for a short time before exposing himself. Use basic surveillance detection to notice anyone who is following you, especially if you are entering an isolated area.

One woman we interviewed had witnessed four incidents of public masturbation in her life. With each incident, she did not see the man until he was already engaged in the act; there were no early warning signals. Exhibitionism of any kind is such a shocking thing to witness and it can be very difficult to respond appropriately. She never reported any of the events (which she told us she regrets to this day) mostly because she was young, uninformed, and thought no one would believe her. She also did not know if these men would attack her so she simply removed herself from their presence. In all four cases she was in a public location with many other people near the area, thus the behavior seemed totally insane to her. In three of the incidents she was with others who also witnessed the behavior. Only once was she alone, though others were very close by and could have easily walked into the area.

Voyeurism: Because a voyeur will attempt to remain concealed, you must pay attention when you are in any location where you are undressing, bathing, using the toilet, or are being intimate with partners. Gyms, fitness centers, changing rooms, public bathrooms, and new or temporary residences are key locations that voyeurs use. If you use a women's locker room at your gym or move into a new apartment take note of any areas/rooms/utility closets that border the bathrooms and bedrooms but to which you are denied access. Note any activity or suspicious sounds that come from those areas that correlate to your use of these rooms and your activities in them. Inspect likely areas where clandestine camera lenses could be emplaced, bearing in mind what body parts/activities predators would want to be filming. In other words, could a predator film anything in line of sight of that camera lens, such as your bathtub or bed? Focus on anything that sticks out as odd or anything that looks like a camera lens. Pay attention to cracks, gaps, and holes in walls. Look for any location or appliance that has a small dark circle the size of a dime or less, or an object/surface with an opaque or clear glass covering. Notice any newly repaired or temporarily repaired (jury-rigged) items. Many varieties of "nanny cams" are available that come camouflaged in ordinary looking household objects such as smoke detectors, clocks, and fans.

When out in public pay attention to anyone using cell phone cameras to take photos of your body parts. If you are wearing revealing clothing, such as low-cut shirts, bathing suits, or mini skirts, you may be at greater risk. First, check a man's hands for objects, such as cameras. Then, look at his accessories. Is he wearing glasses or sunglasses? If so, notice if you can see a tiny lens in the third eye position in the center of the forehead. Wireless video cameras hidden in glasses are available off the internet. (Our research revealed that one man has a pornography site on which he shows videos he made of girls he picked up and had oral sex with while filming them, without their consent, using these glasses). Also check the shoes for a tiny hidden camera with which the predator may be attempting to film up your skirt. If you work at any kind of a drive-thru or tollbooth, look for evidence that a predator may be taking a photo or filming you as you lean over towards his window, possibly exposing your cleavage.

Voyeurs who are attempting to film women will often choose busy public locations or activities where excessive partying is going on (such as nightclubs, wild college parties, or beaches at spring break). The large amount of distraction works to their advantage. Listen to your intuition when in crowds. Pay attention to any man who is closing the physical distance between you and him. If he wants to film up your skirt using a camera that is lodged in his shoe, he has to get the lens in the correct position. Pay attention to any men who appear to be working together as voyeurs. Perhaps one man will distract you with conversation while the other gets in range in order to film you. Use surveillance detection to make sure you are not followed.

Frotteurism: Pay particular attention if any man rubs himself against your body. Even though he may make it seem accidental, such behavior could be sexually deviant. Anytime you are crowded into a space and a man is standing behind you, use your situational awareness and define your boundaries. If he persists, break contact and firmly announce the violation if others are in earshot so that he cannot continue without being witnessed (for example, "Stop rubbing up against me."). If possible, report the incident to the police. Use surveillance detection to make sure he does not follow you as you exit the area.

Sexual Masochism/Sadism: Your sexual practices are up to you. If you decide to engage in such behaviors willingly, be sure that your partner is clear that you have boundaries and are not willing to be victimized in any way. Remember that the person you are trusting may be secretly filming you. Since he will likely not allow you to "sweep" his home for hidden cameras, ask yourself if the experience is worth the risk to you. Realize also that if you consent to being handcuffed or bound in any way, you put yourself at great risk of being unable to defend yourself in the event your sexual partner becomes violent.

For all of the above paraphilias, know that you must break contact immediately should any men engage in the above listed behaviors as a means of victimizing you. Often women will be either too shocked or embarrassed to respond appropriately. Many women will not report such behaviors, even if they are certain that someone is attempting to victimize them. Our methodology involves having a plan for what you would do in the event you were victimized in a variety of ways. Consider your 'what if' plan for such behaviors. If you were in public and a man victimized you by pulling down his pants and exposing himself, would you be able to respond by breaking contact and immediately reporting him to the police? In order to prevent being victimized, you must learn to take away the element of surprise from your predator. When women are caught in an awkward moment, a moment they have never considered, they often make the wrong choices based on their reactions to what is happening to them. Being SASD means staying ahead of this element of surprise by eliminating it as a possibility.

If you identify or even suspect any of the above deviant behaviors we recommend that you remain as calm as possible. Be discreet; do not alert the predator that you are on to him unless others are close by and can assist you. If it is possible for you to document the incident do so, but only if you can remain at a safe distance from the predator. If you can discreetly photograph him in the act, do so. Record other key information, such as the date, time, location, and a description of the incident. Report the incident to law enforcement as soon as possible. Immediately practice surveillance detection to ensure he does not follow you. *Never* attempt to detain or pursue a predator.

Finally, be aware that men who are "curb-crawlers" will drive around in bad neighborhoods and harass women verbally. Normally they operate in areas of town where prostitutes work. In addition, realize that the common behaviors of catcalling and wolf-whistling must on some level reward men who engage in these types of harassing behaviors. Your concern with any level of harassment should be escalation. If you walk by a construction site every day on your way to work and men harass you by catcalling or wolf-whistling, consider reporting them to the owner of the project site. The more proactive women become about reporting all of these behaviors, the better chance we stand of eliminating them as threats to our security.

Prosecuting these predators is becoming easier because legislation is being passed all over the world to close loopholes and deficiencies in existing privacy laws (such as the "in public view" right that paparazzi and up-skirters/down-blousers have used to evade prosecution in the past). Radical measures are taking place to protect women from these predators. In Japan, for example, they have women-only train cars because of the increase in public voyeuristic practices such as up-skirting and down-blousing.

The Dark Side of Cyber Space

We feel compelled in this chapter to take a strong look at how the internet and the World Wide Web have impacted the victimization of women and children, especially where sexually deviant behaviors are concerned. Sexually explicit material, be it pornography or other less graphic sexual content, is on its way to becoming a cyber genre of epic proportions. Many women are willingly playing a big role in this as models or actresses on porn sites. Even young high school and college girls post soft porn pictures of themselves on their blogs. Although some women may be enjoying this new freedom of sexual expression and exploration, they may also be elevating their risk of becoming victimized. Likewise, more and more men are visiting pornographic websites as a routine part of their lives. Naturally, this widespread interest impacts the porn industry, as supply and demand remain at the helm of any business venture. The fact that pornography is a twelve *billion* dollar industry in the United States alone speaks for itself. Capitalism and our first amendment rights merge in cyberspace and a new realm of sexual impetus, opportunity, and access has emerged.

One wonders if men who are addicted to viewing pornography on the web eventually begin to perceive it as the norm for human existence. If so, when they are out in the real world among women, will they begin to approach women believing that pornography is the norm and that all women are willing to partake of their fantasies? In a recent case a man was caught videotaping cheerleaders at high school sporting events. Unbeknownst to anyone, he was filming close-ups of their private parts when they were performing the splits, bending over, or jumping and causing their skirts rise. He then posted the close-up photos on the internet. Every day it seems there is a new story about the exploitation of women as a result of the internet. Will violence against women increase as a result of this exploitation and the permeation of pornography in our society? Certainly the crime of child pornography is on the rise. As society evolves, the balance between good and evil is always in question.

We interviewed one woman in her seventies who told us that she witnessed an incident of public masturbation when she was a college student in the 1950's. She also remembered that the nuns at her grade school used to warn the girls against wearing shiny patent leather shoes so that the boys could not use the reflection to look up their skirts. The point is, sexually deviant behaviors are not unique to the men of today's world; predators have been out there for centuries. The difference is that, due to the internet and World Wide Web, predators have exponentially increased their access to sexually motivating material which they can use as their impetus to target women and children.

The supposed anonymity the internet appears to provide makes people feel safe enough to venture out into uncharted sexual territory. However, every new- found freedom has its price. The dark side of all of this technology is its potential impact on the victimization of women and children. Remember that male predators have the advantage of knowing that, generally speaking, women will not resort to sexual predatory behavior as a means to victimize men. Therefore, the only retribution male predators have to fear is being caught by law enforcement or other authorities. We do *not* encourage or advise women to use any predatory behaviors as a means of defending themselves against becoming victims of violence. We do, however, want women to use prevention methods such as getting SASD as a means of reducing their victimization.

How Women Participate in Elevating the Risk

We also feel compelled to address women who are participating in perpetuating the marginalization of women by engaging in promiscuous and high risk behaviors. In our highly sexualized society there appears to be a tug of war between some women's desire to have power and be treated equally and other women's willingness to marginalize themselves in order to obtain this power. For example, some women are embracing their sexuality by indulging in the freedom of sexual expression the internet provides. On the one hand, this freedom can be positive because women are no longer sexually repressed by society's limitations and harsh judgments of their sexual activities. On the other hand, some women willingly continue to be marginalized by men who exploit them for money. Certain trends of this exploitation have emerged. One popular trend among young women includes the spring break wet t-shirt contests and videos of women flashing their breasts. It is primarily men (not women) who are making money from these contests and videos. When a predator encounters a woman who is willing to exploit herself, he may wonder what else she is willing to do. In his twisted mind, she may appear to be an accommodating victim. He may even try to blackmail her by threatening to tell her family or boss about her indiscriminate behavior. At the very least a woman who willingly participates in exploitive activities increases her risk by drawing attention to herself from the wrong men, namely predators.

In addition, any woman working in the sex industry must understand that she faces unique challenges concerning her risk of being victimized as a result of her chosen profession. The statistics of violence against women who work as strippers, for example, are startlingly high. If you choose to be sexually permissive at work, you are essentially sending the message that you will accept a certain degree of what some might perceive as a willingness to be exploited (for payment). It is not a far leap for a predator to believe you will also accept being victimized. He may capitalize on your involvement in any illicit activities as a way to manipulate you. For example, if he learned about an outstanding warrant for your arrest he might deduce that he can rape you and you will not report him.

Another example of exploitation that encourages violence against women is evident in the music video industry. Certain genres of music are using images of women and language about women to advocate violence against women. Again, women are participating in this industry by purchasing and listening to this music and by performing in these videos, thereby contributing to endorsing the message that violence against women is acceptable. Know that if you decide to participate in self-exploiting activities, you are increasing your own risk level and are potentially increasing the risk level of other women. If even one woman sends the message that violence against women is acceptable, all women suffer the potential consequences of that message.

Women must participate in squelching the messages of violence that permeate our culture and put us all at greater risk. We spoke with one woman during the course of writing this book who gave us a unique insight into the subtle ways in which women participate in promulgating the message that violence against women is acceptable. This woman (we will call her Myra) had recently undergone cosmetic surgery, having a partial face-lift. Myra, like many women who have had cosmetic surgery, did not want anyone to know she had "work" done on her face. Myra told us that she went to the grocery store shortly after her surgery, her face still bruised and swollen. She said that she could tell that the checkout girl: *"...felt sorry for me because she thought I had been beaten."* Myra confessed she struggled with the notion that, on some level, she actually preferred that the checkout girl thought she had been beaten rather than knowing that she had undergone cosmetic surgery. Myra's perception caused us to ponder the opposite scenario: Would a woman who was beaten prefer a stranger to think she had recently undergone a face-lift? It is fascinating to consider how a woman's issues with her own self-image can become a contributing factor to spreading the message that violence against women is acceptable.

Conclusion

Part of our vision for the evolution of women's empowerment includes teaching women to apply proactive prevention methods against sexual predators. Women are slowly evolving out of a place where they have taken a survival approach to violence against them and their children and they are beginning to develop what we like to refer to as a "refusal approach." This means that, rather than accepting violence against us as a given and accommodating it by saying "Okay, it's going to happen so let's set up shelters and create hotlines and support groups," women are gradually moving into a state of refusal by saying "Let's *refuse* to tolerate this anymore and work to change the laws and make the consequences severe so that pedophiles and rapists will not be able to do this anymore."

Oprah Winfrey has taken a refusal stance against pedophiles by displaying their photographs on her T.V. show and website so that she can assist the F.B.I. in their nation-wide search for these criminals. Eve Ensler (author of *The Vagina Monologues*) has started a global movement called V-Day to educate people about violence against girls and women. In an interview with the St. Louis Post Dispatch she said: "There's a completely different mentality between treating it [the violence] as though you want to end it and treating it as though it will happen again."

In order to refuse to tolerate the violence against us and our children, we must evolve to a place where we are willing to literally prevent it from happening, rather than focusing all of our energies on accommodating it when it does. Since we cannot control the deviant behavior of others, it would be naive to think that the violent behavior against us will not happen again. It will. This does not mean, however, that we should simply accept this fact and continue to accommodate it. Nor should we shut down our shelters and hotlines. Rather, it means as women we must take ownership of prevention and our role in it as a means towards evolving to a place where we can eventually successfully refuse to tolerate the violence against us. We can take ownership of prevention and work to evolve to a place where we can refuse to be victims by getting SASD, by implementing all the prevention techniques discussed in this book, by working to change laws, and by educating ourselves and our communities. It is an ongoing process. Our desire with this book is to enhance women's evolution by providing women with tangible methods they can put into practice in their daily lives to prevent the violence against them. Philosophy and action must merge if we expect real change to occur.

CHAPTER ELEVEN

PREVENTING THE WORST: ABDUCTION, RAPE, AND MURDER

When the out of nowhere comes
and the you that was
slips out the back door
and the you that remains
is an empty house
dusty rooms that echo ruined laughter
and your morning cup of coffee
will never taste the same

As we complete the final editing of this chapter another story appears in the newspaper. This time the girl happens to be from a neighboring suburb, very close to home. She, like the many victims who seem to pop up in the news more frequently every year, was a good girl with a bright future who came from a loving family. She was twenty, in college, and then she was strangled to death. For her and her family, the out of nowhere has come.

The impact of the crimes of abduction, rape, and murder oppresses us with tremendous gravity, mostly resulting from our false perception that these crimes come from that 'out of nowhere' realm. We confuse the impact they have on us with the occurrence of them. We come unhinged. Our lives are suddenly and permanently altered as a result of these crimes because they shock us into new realities of hardship and loss. But at the crux of this book is the truth about the nature of violence against women: *these crimes do not come out of nowhere.* We can study and increase our knowledge base about how predators operate; we do receive early warning signals; and we have prevention techniques and defenses we can use to avoid becoming victims.

It makes no sense for women to do nothing proactive to prevent these crimes except to sit back and hope we are never victimized, just like it makes no sense to drive a car without wearing a seatbelt and to then be stunned by resulting fatalities from a serious accident. Taking responsibility to prevent these crimes is our duty to ourselves. We cannot control the sickness of predators and we cannot count on our criminal justice system or law enforcement to protect us all of the time. We can only do our best to keep the seemingly 'out of nowhere' realm at bay by accepting our own responsibility where survival is concerned. If we want to survive at the hands of sick and violent predators, we have to learn how they operate and outsmart them.

We would like to use the promise of empowerment as our motivator to get you to read this chapter. Although reading it may be upsetting to you, "knowledge is power." The more you know about how predators operate and what motivates them (especially the worst ones) the better armed you will be to prevent becoming one of their victims. These crimes are the really scary stuff we all would rather avoid in hopes that our lives are never damaged by them. However, egregious acts of violence against us will never stop until we take more control over our own security and work to make it impossible for predators to victimize us. In this chapter we will look at how the techniques you have learned in this book apply to preventing becoming a victim of abduction, rape, and murder. (Note: We use the term "abduction" for women and "kidnapping" for children, though their meaning is interchangeable).

We would like to share our expertise in security, prevention, surveillance detection, and military precepts and then translate this into teaching you to detect the early warning signals of these crimes so that you can prevent becoming a victim. Abductors, rapists, and murderers use common techniques, which we will discuss at length later in this chapter. Some abductions, rapes, and murders are seemingly random crimes of opportunity. This means the predator is out and happens upon an easy target, snatches her and either abducts her, rapes her, kills her or all of the above. Random crimes do involve some planning, even though they seemingly come out of nowhere. Many abductions, rapes, and murders involve extensive planning. What is critical for you to understand is that both random and planned acts of violence against women involve some degree of surveillance of the target (even if the surveillance only occurs over a very short time period). These predators will be interested in the habits and routines of their targets. They will collect information on their targets' routes, on the times their targets move, and on the security around their targets' domiciles and workplaces.

All of the techniques you have learned in this book will assist you in preventing becoming a victim of these three heinous crimes. Situational awareness is your best ally in preventing these crimes because you must be able to tune in to and recognize behaviors that are threatening. Protecting your identity and privacy on a regular basis will help you set up a barrier against these predators. Knowing how to conduct a risk/threat assessment, even on the spot if you find yourself in a dangerous neighborhood or situation will help you make appropriate decisions as a threat unfolds. Creating a support network will allow you to quickly respond should you feel threatened by any of these types of predators. Practicing surveillance detection as a habit, even to the smallest degree, will allow you to notice if such a predator is studying you. Conducting route and building reviews will allow you to determine if any predator is exploiting your vulnerabilities or planning to attack you along your routes or near your home or workplace. Learning about defensive tactics and tools (Chapter Twelve) will empower you to find a comfortable defensive posturing for all threats. Learning how to respond if you are ever under attack will increase your chances of survival (see Chapter Thirteen). Learning to travel, date, work, socialize, and live life with greater security will keep you steps ahead of becoming the victim of a heinous crime.

Security is a lot like insurance; you hope you never need it but when you do, you need it one hundred percent. This is especially true for the crimes discussed below, so allow yourself to feel your most primal fears and stare death in the face for a few moments. Let yourself think like these predators and consider how they might approach you. Allow yourself to be empowered with prevention. Realize that, even if you are trained in self-defense or have some defensive tool or weapon with you, you must still heighten your situational awareness and ability to respond according to what the situation dictates. What works in one woman's story may not work in another's.

You must also know yourself, both physically and emotionally. Ask yourself right now: "In this very moment, if I were about to be raped would I fight even if it meant I might die? Would I acquiesce to my rapist's demands in order to survive? Would I physically be able to fight or would I have limitations that would require me to come up with an alternate solution to escape and survive?" You have to think ahead and create a 'what if' plan that matches your physical, moral, ethical, and spiritual limitations and boundaries. Knowing yourself and thinking ahead as to your stance on defending yourself will actually help you to be better prepared to respond if you are ever attacked by an abductor, rapist, or murderer. Some women are so non-violent in their nature that they would rather be raped than physically harm another human being. Some women read this last sentence and cringe, thinking to themselves: "I would fight like hell and kill him if I had to." What type of woman are you? If you decide that you could not accept being abducted or raped or murdered and that you would fight your way out of it, we strongly suggest you take a self-defense class, at least once in your life, if you are physically able to do so.

The Worst Crimes: An Overview

Before delving into the common techniques abductors, rapists, and murderers use for attacking their victims and enacting their crimes, let us examine each of these crimes separately.

Abduction

Abduction is the illegal capturing or detaining of an individual against her/his will. We tend to have the impression that abduction/kidnapping only pertains to people of importance who have money for ransom. Perhaps many readers will skip this portion thinking the odds that they might be abducted are slim. If you are a reader in Latin America this portion will be of great interest to you because kidnapping for ransom has become a business. The kidnappers even take their victims to "Kidnap Hotels" where they hold them until the ransom is paid. This problem runs rampant in many countries, yet in the United States we tend to perceive abduction/kidnapping as a more unusual crime, one about which we do not have to be very concerned unless we have children.

The growing number of missing children has startled us into paying more attention to kidnapping. Still, grown women do not seem to worry about being abducted as much as they do about being raped, battered, and abused. What is important to realize is that abduction is a possible consequence of any attack. If an attacker is unsuccessful or makes mistakes, he may opt to abduct and even murder his victim. Adult women do go missing. Just because the odds of it happening to you may be relatively slim, it is worth your time and effort to learn how to prevent becoming the victim of such a crime. None of us is impervious to danger. In addition, abduction can be the end result of an abusive relationship or domestic violence incident. Women are abducted at the hands of both men they know and by strangers.

Types of Abductions

Abductors who take women for purposes other than ransom are motivated by a variety of factors. Sometimes rape or sexually based crimes drive them to abduct. Sometimes abductions occur as the direct result of some stressor, incident, or precipitating event that has nothing to do with the target. For example, the predator may have just been dumped by his girlfriend and he becomes rattled enough to abduct a woman and release his rage about his girlfriend against an innocent woman. Some abductors are sadists or serial killers. Women can also be abducted by someone who is seeking ransom or is trying to make a political statement. Other women are abducted as the result of some other crime, such as a car jacking. We have all heard the horror stories of women who are held captive and tortured by maniacal killers or who are sold into slavery as part of the sex industry. Abduction is one crime where you should assume that you may be up against more than one predator. Abductors often work in teams. However, an abductor can also work alone, thus you should not discount this possibility. A woman can be the victim of abduction due to a relationship gone sour, if she is a target of opportunity, because she is in the wrong place at the wrong time, or because she is unaware and attracts a predator by being too friendly and approachable.

People at high risk of abduction include: international aid workers; ex-patriots; people serving in the military (especially in war zones); executives and their families (especially those living in high risk countries); and people who have some type of celebrity status. If you live in a high risk area or are at high risk of becoming the target of abductors, consult a professional kidnap and ransom company (see Appendix E). Your insurance company will likely have some arrangement or clause for this problem. Having a surveillance detection plan which includes route reviews and building reviews is critical for you. You might be surprised, if you have bodyguards, to learn that they will very likely have never come into contact with some of the surveillance detection concepts and techniques in this book. For a more comprehensive study on surveillance detection, read our book on it and have your security staff read it as well (see Appendix A).

Rape

The word originates from the Latin verb *rapere*, which means "to seize." For any woman, the idea of being seized in a violent sexual manner is terrifying.

Rape is a profound violation and an ever present threat for all women. The idea of being over-powered and controlled by a man who is performing violent sexual acts upon one's body is such an awful prospect that most women prefer to put the subject at bay and hope it never happens to them or to any woman they know. What makes the threat of rape even worse is that it can happen at the hands of a man whom a woman knows. Women are sometimes raped by men they trust and even love.

Rapists come in all shapes and sizes, races and socioeconomic classes. Some rapists are motivated by their desires to degrade women or humiliate them. Some are sadistic and wish to torture women. Others seek power over women because they suffer from low self-esteem or are driven by some severe emotional insecurity. Rape can also happen as a result of some environmental influence on the rapist, such as some stress factor or a significant incident (perhaps he was recently fired from his job). A rapist may be driven by his desire to act out a fantasy. A rapist may suffer from feelings of sexual inadequacy. He may in some way be repressed or he may have a degree of sexually indiscriminate behavior (such as an indulgence in pornography). He may be influenced by some type of peer pressure situation that makes him prone to committing rape (such as being teased by his peers for being a virgin).

For most women, the prospect of being raped is our most primal fear. The many cases of women who were victimized by total strangers have made us all ill at ease with men we do not know. When we hear of women who have been abducted, raped, or murdered, we take pause. Could it happen to us, to our mothers, sisters, daughters? The answer (yes) makes us feel out of control and terrified. Denial is an easier place in which to reside. Even if we are cautious, that unknown threat looms in our subconscious. We empathize with rape victims and their families. We get involved in organizations and marches, donate and raise money for awareness, and support women who have become victims. But our fear, our lack of control continues to plague us and creates a low level of constant stress in our daily lives. This stress is the end result of feeling disempowered about preventing becoming a rape victim.

Our primal fear of being raped should lead us back home to our forgotten instinct (our situational awareness), not further away from it.

Rape instills the most primal fear in a woman because of its violent nature and the emotionally, socially, and sexually charged repercussions associated with it. We wonder how we could ever feel clean again in our bodies were we to be overtaken and brutally raped. We question if we will ever be able to have normal sexual relationships if we are victimized by rape. And we fear we will never again know the peace and security we felt in our lives before the rape occurred. We struggle because the men in our lives who love us cannot really relate to this constant, undercurrent of vulnerability we experience. The reality is that, unless a man is about to be sent off to prison, rape is not normally a viable threat in his life. Even if it were, most men would stand a much better chance of physically protecting themselves against a rapist than women would, due to our physical inferiority regarding brute strength.

Types of Rapes

Rape is a crime that is about control, not sex. Rape is motivated by a variety of factors, thus women face the threat of various types of rape. Rape can happen as the result of another crime or as a random act of violence. For example, a woman might be at home when a burglar enters and decides to rape her before leaving the home. Or a rapist may select a target who is in an opportune location. Women are raped by men they know (from work, a friend, and sometimes their own husbands) and men they do not know. Some women fall prey to a serial rapist. Gang rape is a more drastic threat, yet women worldwide continue to experience it. Rape may also be used as a means of victimizing a woman in order to prepare her to enter into the sex industry, either for sex trafficking or for pornography.

Date rape is another type of rape for which there is a growing concern among women, in particular young college students. Some date rapes are truly crimes of passion, meaning the rapist did not begin with the intention of raping, but the situation unraveled in such a way that he lost control. The example of this would be the date that goes bad when the woman says "No" to the man's sexual advances and he, in the heat of the moment, refuses to accept her "No." His reasons could be related to peer pressure, embarrassment, the influence of drugs or alcohol, or because he is socially inexperienced and dysfunctional. Maybe he thought she was playing mind games. No matter the reason, her "No means no" and if he ignores it, he is committing rape. Other date rapes are premeditated and date rape drugs are used to gain control over the victims.

Murder

The worst of the worst is murder. People tend to avoid the subject of murder because it is so unpalatable. However, it would make no sense for us to exclude it from this book, as it is the ultimate threat women face because it is almost always a possible consequence of any other crime or act of violence committed against a woman. Women who are carjacked, raped, assaulted, burglarized in their homes, abducted, stalked, abused, and molested are sometimes murdered as a result of these attacks. This alone should motivate you to read more about preventing being murdered.

Murder involves what is known in legalese as "malice aforethought," or a depraved indifference to human life. Some murders are planned and involve premeditation and some happen in the moment, without premeditation. What all women must realize is that preventing a murder does not require you to understand or differentiate the various degrees of the crime of murder. Your only concern if you are ever faced with the prospect of being killed by another human being is *survival.* Unfortunately many victims of murder are completely unprepared to survive being in the presence of another human being who literally has no regard for human life.

A murderer may be motivated by a variety of factors, some psychological and others environmental. Your best chance of survival is if you accept that you are at the mercy of a monster. This means that you must grab hold of the reality that your predator may be getting a thrill just by having the power to decide if you live or die. Perhaps his need to control and dominate you or to punish you is what is driving him. He might be so sick as to enjoy the idea of torturing and killing you. Maybe because you are a woman he holds great hatred and rage against you and therefore wants to annihilate you. Perhaps he is totally delusional and thinks he is acting in God's best interest by taking your life. Or it could be that some incident or stress factor has caused him to cross over and release his rage. You must, in the moment, realize that he is not operating under normal standards of human compassion and accountability and embrace the fact that he intends to kill you.

Types of Murders

Some murders are well planned and the target is studied over a period of time so that the predator ensures a successful attack. Other murders appear to be more random in that they are crimes of opportunity. Usually these murders happen because the predator has made the decision to take a life and will wait for a convenient target of opportunity. Other murders are the result of another crime, such as a robbery, rape, or car jacking. Incidents of domestic violence can also result in murder. Some murders are crimes of passion, such as a love triangle situation that escalates into a violent incident, or an incident of workplace violence from a disgruntled employee, or a courtroom shooting.

Serial killings are the extreme, but every woman should educate herself about the basics of these types of murders. Often when a serial killer is caught, neighbors and associates will report that they never would have expected this person to be a madman (incidentally we say 'man' because serial killers are almost exclusively male). Early warning signals of a man's propensity to become a serial killer do exist. Serial killers often come from broken or dysfunctional homes, have very low self-esteem, and will blame the world for their problems. They exhibit three identifiable behaviors: bed-wetting well into adulthood; lighting fires/pyromania; and exhibiting cruelty to animals. They are also quite adept at manipulating people. In addition, virtually all serial murders are sexually-based crimes and serial killers normally have low self-esteem regarding their sexuality.

Techniques Used by Abductors, Rapists, and Murderers

Our goal is to broaden your perspective about how abductors, rapists, and murderers enact their crimes, what early warning signals you should look for, and what defenses you have against them. You will also see that the most heinous of crimes are addressed here, such as serial killing and murder that involves torture. We apologize in advance for the graphic nature of this section; if it saves your life or the life of a woman you know we have done our job.

One important rule applies to all women. If you are living in an area where a serial rapist or murderer is operating, learn what his "modus operendi" is, meaning his method of attack. For example, the serial rapist may always break into homes during the day and wait for his victim to arrive. Or the serial killer may always abduct a woman whose car has broken down on the shoulder of the freeway. In addition, if you fit the description of his preferred type of target, take extra precautions to heighten your situational awareness and to vigilantly practice surveillance detection. Obtain as much information as possible about his attack techniques from the police.

The following are common techniques used by abductors, rapists, and murderers. We also include lists of early warning signals and defenses against these techniques. You will notice some overlapping information, as predators sometimes combine certain aspects of different techniques.

Ambush/Location

When a predator ambushes his target, he is relying heavily on the element of surprise. He will lie in wait, usually from a concealed position, with the intention of designing a trap for his victim. Ambushes are always location driven because the lay of the ground is what dictates the success of this type of attack. In other words, a predator cannot surprise and entrap his victim if the location does not provide him with the ability to be concealed and lie in wait to surprise his victim. The predator will design his attack around a specific site so that he is able to control his victim and avoid getting caught in the act.

Ambush locations are almost exclusively dictated by terrain. A predator will pick an ambush site that channels, restricts, slows down, or pins the target. He may use turns, corners, stop signs, dark areas, bushes, or may even hide inside a vehicle. He will be out of line of sight, at least momentarily, so that he can surprise the target. He will choose places that offer the opportunity for concealment, such as dark areas, vegetation, hiding in a car, van, behind a door, or around a corner. The predator will look for an easy way in and out of the ambush location, for example by using dead ground (areas not used for normal foot traffic), waiting in a vehicle or isolated area, or hiding in a room inside a building. He may also use high ground for watching the target because he knows that most people never look up when they are walking or driving in a vehicle.

If his intended victim is traveling in a vehicle, the predator will lie in wait until she arrives at a designated location (one he chose from studying her routes when he put her under surveillance). When her vehicle arrives, the ambush occurs. There are multiple possible scenarios. Perhaps he will pull out his vehicle in front of hers and stop while his partner pulls up directly behind her, trapping her. If the target is moving on foot the predator may hide in bushes or around a blind corner and snatch her and throw her in the back of his pre-positioned vehicle. The predator's primary objectives are to act quickly and discreetly and not attract any attention or witnesses to the attack. He may lurk in a grocery store parking lot, watch her go inside, wait near her vehicle until she returns, grab her as she is loading her groceries into her car and drag her into his car (or throw her into her trunk and steal her car).

A predator intent on killing a woman may choose a specific ambush location or type of location from where he can attract an appropriate target. For example, a serial killer often choose to look for their victims on freeways or in areas of cities that provide him with the type of target he prefers (if he wants to kill prostitutes, he will cruise areas where they work). If a man is intent upon killing a woman and he uses an ambush as his technique for catching her and then isolating her, his ambush could only be the beginning of his violent act. He may try to knock her out, tie her up, or even use a knife or gun to force her to go to an isolated location with him.

Some predators will use the technique of taking the target by storm or ambushing the target with some type of blitz attack. For example, the predator/s will take the target by storm by invading a facility, such as a home or workplace. In such a case, the predators are using the facility as the venue of isolation so that they can contain and control the target inside before transporting her elsewhere. They may gag and bind the victim or put her inside some type of container and then remove her from the location.

Another type of ambush involves outnumbering the target. For example, the most serious threat of rape happens when a woman is outnumbered by men who have the intention of gang raping her. These men will isolate the target, possibly by abducting her or channeling her into a remote location where she is removed from others who could help her. Anytime you are in a situation where you are closed in by more than one man who is threatening you the possibility exists that you may be gang raped.

Common Ambush Locations:

- Parking lots or garages (grocery stores/health clubs/shopping malls, convenience stores, etc.).
- Rest stops (avoid if you are alone, elderly, or frail).
- Public restrooms.
- Predator's vehicle (He can use vehicle as a location to conceal himself until target arrives or he can park next to target's vehicle to gain proximity).

- Real estate listings (a growing number of female real estate agents are targeted by predators who lie in wait near homes that are being shown, especially at night).
- Dark or overgrown areas (near home/on jogging trails).
- Isolated corners or underneath staircases.
- Long corridors and staircases in buildings.
- Alleys or restricted streets, especially ones lined with dumpsters.
- Any location where there are women who might be weakened or compromised due to any emotional or physical state (such as an alcoholics' recovery meeting, a church support group meeting, a counseling center, an abortion clinic, etc.).
- Any location where the consumption of alcohol is normal (outside bars, nightclubs, parties, or other social/public events).
- Freeways (predators out looking for targets can cover more distance faster and easier. Freeways have fewer police and offer isolation and remote areas. Often no cars pass for some time, or if they do the traffic flow is fast and it is therefore difficult for people to witness the ambush. When on freeways be wary of someone flagging you down, especially at night and during inclement weather).

Early Warning Signals of an Ambush:

- Being in the vicinity of any location that provides isolated areas or opportunities for a predator to remain hidden.
- Men loitering in or near any location conducive to an ambush (see list above).
- Any information you collect using situational awareness and surveillance detection that leads you to suspect you are in danger of being ambushed. Pay special attention to your intuition, noticing if someone or someplace feels threatening. Respect your nudges and act on the cumulative early warning signals.

- Indicators of surveillance. (To plan a successful ambush the predator will often put the target under surveillance, study her routes and the locations she frequents, and determine the best ambush location, bearing in mind his need to be discreet and have no witnesses to the attack).

- Any man who seems to be lurking around with no purpose and who is fixating on women or is following women.

- Any man near or in a women's public restroom. If a man is lurking outside of the ladies room he may just be waiting for his wife or girlfriend to come out. Delay going in until after you see him depart or choose another restroom.

- Any man who is obviously positioning himself in relation to you (he crosses the street to get closer to you or he pulls his vehicle in front of yours and tries to control yours).

- Any vehicle or person trying to control your vehicle or your body.

- Any man who is fixating on you and then signals to another person as he closes the distance between you and himself.

- Any unsolicited approach by any unknown man or men (or potentially a man who is with a woman) that occurs in a potential ambush location.

- Any man who seems to be out of his normal environment (normally indicated by his clothing and/or behavior) and is seeking some type of assistance or attention.

- Any vehicle breakdowns, accidents, bumps or interactions with any man who threatens to control you in any way.

- Any man cruising in a vehicle who makes multiple passes, pulls over near you, or correlates with your movements. Be ready for him to park and approach you on foot.

- Any service trucks or vans parked in your neighborhood or near your workplace that are suspicious (meaning you never see the service men working or dismounting the vehicle).

- Any sudden appearance of someone at your door, especially if it is more than one person.
- Being in a location where men are grouping together and are fixating their attention on you and are signaling to each other. For example, you could be at a party and two or more men might target you, use a date rape drug, take you to an isolated location, and take turns raping you. Or, you could be in a bad neighborhood and happen upon a group of men who target you. Sometimes groups of men will travel together looking to ambush a woman, abduct her, and gang rape her.
- Locations frequented by dominant or dysfunctional/anti-social males. Engaging in social activities or partying with men from this social spectrum whom you do not know (or know casually but do not trust) puts you at risk of being ambushed.
- Conspiratorial communication between men who then position themselves so as to herd females into a restricted area or room or to block access to exits.
- Sudden changes in the social atmosphere or any rise in hostility or aggression among the men.

Defenses Against an Ambush:

- Situational Awareness and Surveillance Detection (SASD).
- Risk assessment. Analyze your patterns to see if you regularly put yourself in any locations where you might be ambushed.
- Acknowledge the early warning signals of an ambush. Slow down and tune in.
- Varying your routes and conducting route reviews (the attack locations you label on your route reviews will include any ambush sites).
- Conduct building reviews for your home and workplace (again, any attack locations you label on these reviews will include ambush sites). Conducting building reviews and identifying the vulnerable areas for

break-ins will also help you strengthen the security at your residence or work place.

- Install surveillance cameras to monitor any ambush locations near your home (and advise your employer to install them at your workplace).
- Never open the door to strangers.
- Place defensive tools in strategic locations in your home and workplace (if you are trained and ready to use them).
- If you are a high profile target for abduction for ransom, be sure to consult with your insurance company and have a kidnap and ransom specialist lined up in the event you are abducted.
- Carry a cell phone that has an activated GPS device in it. If you have a GPS device in your vehicle, consider using the service so that authorities have a way to track you if you go missing.
- Be alert to any pity plays or any attempts to evoke your sympathy or win rapport from any unknown man.
- Use the buddy system, even with a woman who is a stranger at the scene if you feel you are at risk of being ambushed. Keep others informed of potential danger by giving a heads-up warning to any women in the area.
- Have a 'what if' plan for breaking contact with any man who poses a threat. Rehearse a mantra or cadence you can say to yourself silently to coach yourself out of the situation, such as "Time to go; no delay." Imagine an ambush situation and rehearse using your mantra as you visualize extracting yourself safely from the imaginary threat.
- Report any suspicious men to security or to store managers.
- If you are wary of any man in a parking lot, go back into the store and notify security and have someone escort you to your vehicle.
- Check in public restrooms to see if stalls are occupied by looking at the shoes of women in the other stalls. If you suspect a man is hiding in one of the stalls, exit immediately and report him to security.

- If you do not feel the threat is imminent, discreetly take a photo of a potential predator with your cell phone camera and send it to someone in your SUPNET or call someone in your SUPNET and apprise them of the potentially threatening situation. That way if the situation escalates you can tell a predator "I just called my friend and gave him your description (sent him your picture)." If the threat level is imminent, call the police or dial 911 immediately.

- When walking near or in a potential ambush location, dial 911 and be ready to press the "send" or "enter" button to connect the call. Carry a personal alarm and be ready to sound it.

- Identify safe locations and have a plan for transitions so that you have a policy to follow if a threatening event occurs.

- Maintain 360 degree awareness, meaning you are paying attention to what is in front of you, at your sides, behind you, above you, and below you. If you sense an imminent ambush, run to a safe location, make noise to attract attention to yourself, present any defensive tools you have with you, and immediately attempt to escape the situation.

- When traveling on foot or jogging, vary your pattern, routes, times, clothing, and appearance.

- Keep your distance when any unknown man approaches you. Move to a safe location. Attract attention to yourself. Pay attention to any signals that this man is out of place.

- Look for areas where an unknown man may be planning to force you to go, such as hidden areas or his vehicle.

- Avoid allowing an unknown man to isolate you in any way.

- Never turn your back on any unknown man. Watch his hands for weapons.

- Break contact if you are in a location where you notice a group of men fixating on you.

- Do not under any circumstances isolate yourself with any group of men if you feel a threat.

- Stay away from neighborhoods that you suspect could be dangerous.

Ruses and Lures

Ruse: An attempt to confuse or mislead.

Another favorite technique for predators is creating some type of ruse. The objective is to coax the target close in so that the predator can control her. Serial killer, Ted Bundy, used a fake cast on his arm to draw women close to his vehicle or to an isolated location. He would drop something and ask for help, using his supposedly broken arm as a means of playing on a woman's sympathy and then hit her over the head with his cast and either force her into his car or drag her to an isolated area.

The predator may use a ruse to move the woman to an isolated location or to get within arm's reach of her so that he can control her. For example, he may pretend his car is broken down and ask her if she has a pair of jumper cables. At an opportune moment he may force her into one of the vehicles and rape her at gunpoint. Or he could come to your home or apartment using the guise of being a solicitor or having a petition that he wants you to sign. He will then force his way into your home. If a predator is using a ruse, his main purpose is to create a distraction or a story. His hope is to trick a woman into participating in his charade or to distract and confuse her enough that she ignores the early warning signals of his attack. Serial killers and rapists often use ruses, so if one is active in your area of town, be sure to study his tactics and learn everything you can about how he operates.

Lure: An attempt to entice, tempt, or attract with the promise of gaining a reward (potentially by using a decoy as bait to catch a target).

One of the most blatant examples of a successful lure is often used by predators targeting children. The predator may use a puppy or even just a dog's leash as a decoy to lure a child into conversation with him ("Do you want to pet my puppy?" or "Can you help me find my lost dog?"). If the opportunity arises, he will snatch the child. Luring an adult can be more complicated, thus a predator must carefully craft a lure in order to attract a woman. In one case a serial killer used the recording of a baby crying to lure women out of their homes at night. A predator intent upon securing a target may use immense charm and deceptiveness to lure his victim into his trap. He may design a complex scenario, one that he has planned for a long time. By watching and studying his target, he will tailor-make a plan which will incorporate elements to which he is certain his target will respond. For example, an internet predator who is targeting a woman with whom he has initiated contact may use the information he has read about her in her personal profile to tempt her to meet him. She may, for example, mention a particular musician she likes and he may entice her with the promise of concert tickets. Perhaps the predator is someone the woman knows, such as a man in her economics class at the university. Perhaps he will put her under surveillance and observe that she swims at the pool everyday from five to six in the evening. He may arrange to "coincidentally" show up one day to swim at the same time and then offer her a ride back to her dorm.

If a predator has not selected a specific target, he may craft a scenario to lure a target he happens upon in the moment. For example, he might notice a woman who is struggling to fix a flat tire. Again, he will be very charming and appealing and will not necessarily put off the vibe of being at all dangerous. He might suggest she sit in his air conditioned car while he finishes changing her tire. He may then explain that she is missing a lug nut and that there is a hardware store close by where they can get one. He may then get in the car with her, point a gun at her, and demand that she cooperate.

Early Warning Signals of Ruses/Lures:

- Any unsolicited contact from a stranger or unknown man should prompt you to heighten your situational awareness, especially if he is attempting to get you to go somewhere with him, if he is turning on the charm, or if he is asking you to assist him with some problem.

- Any unsolicited contact from an unknown man who is behaving in a theatrical, dramatic manner.
- Any unsolicited contact from any unknown man who has a sense of urgency and requests your assistance.
- Any unsolicited contact from an unknown man who is providing an excess of trivial information, maintaining irrelevant conversation, or attempting to confuse you.
- Any man who refuses to take your "No" seriously and attempts to talk you into his agenda.
- Any man who is attempting to con you in any way.
- Any man who attempts to bond with you and make you indebted to him because he offered you assistance.
- Any man who gives you verbal commands or tries to order you to help him.

Defenses Against Ruses/Lures:

- Heighten your situational awareness any time you receive any unsolicited approach from any unknown man. Listen to what he says so that you can distinguish if he may be attempting to use a ruse or lure against you. If you receive any of the early warning signals above, know that you may be required to break contact immediately and move to a safe location. Be alert and do not immediately assume that this is a harmless encounter.
- Maintain a safe physical distance between yourself and any unknown man who is approaching you.
- If any man is clearly using a ruse, break contact immediately and move to a safe location where people are present to witness him in action. Warn other women in the vicinity if you suspect he may target one of them.
- If you are in your car, keep the doors locked and drive away from him to a safe location. Do not become verbally confrontational with

him. Ignore him and refuse to engage in conversation with him. If necessary, use clear hand signals to communicate to him that you want him to stay away from you.

- Look to see if unknown man who approaches you is working with a partner, male or female.
- Use surveillance detection and create a detour or reverse direction to determine if he is following you.
- Create obstacles between you and him so that you can break contact and get help.
- If the situation escalates and you feel imminent danger (or if he attacks you), stun and run (see Chapter Twelve).

Targets of Opportunity

A completely random abduction, rape, or murder, one that is not precipitated by lengthy surveillance, is a possibility. However, the word 'random' is misleading. It is inaccurate to believe that a predator has a sudden onset of desire to attack a woman. Actually the opposite is true; the predator has a simmering intention and the only aspect that ends up being truly random is that a satisfactory target appears in an appropriate location and the predator is then able to gratify his need to attack. This type of seemingly random target is called a target of opportunity. This means the predator's intention to find a victim is realized only when the opportunity arises for him to attack a target who meets his needs. Because his chance encounter with an appealing target may happen quickly, the predator may be unable to conduct lengthy surveillance on the target. He may be required to quickly arrange an attack so his desired target does not slip from his grasp.

Even if you become a predator's target of opportunity, there are early warning signals that you can detect using your situational awareness and by practicing surveillance detection. Many women who end up becoming a predator's target of opportunity are attacked while in transition or while in a location that offers the predator the elements he requires to conduct a successful attack. These so-called random crimes are usually situation and area dependent, thus there are still ways to avoid placing yourself in the danger zone of the dark alley or remote wilderness. Predators will sometimes use a specific location in order to find a vulnerable target. Parking lots and public restrooms are two locations that they use frequently because they have access to many women and are able to isolate their targets in these locations. The predator visits these locations with the intention of attacking a woman and waits for the opportunity to do so. Use common sense, situational awareness, surveillance detection, and avoid dangerous places when alone. Pay extra attention when you are in transition and are walking from your car into your home or work place and vice versa.

Even if an attack is premeditated, that does not necessarily mean the target has already been selected. A predator may have the intention to rape or kill but will wait until the opportunity arises for him to select a target that meets his needs. Often law enforcement will uncover a murderer's intentions after the fact once they have collected the evidence from his home and computer. They then realize that he had been planning to kill, was researching some aspect of his crime, had purchased special equipment to use in the murder, but waited until the perfect target arrived. In other cases, a killer who did not necessarily plan a murder may encounter a target of opportunity and a situation may unfold in which he is driven to take her life. For example, a date rape could escalate and result in murder.

Predators intuitively identify the weaknesses of their targets. They learn by trial and error and through spending time observing their potential prey. If a predator finds a target of opportunity he will look for an angle he can exploit or manipulate. Perhaps he notices the woman is somehow: needy; vulnerable; insecure; lost; lonely; upset; not grounded; isolated; or approachable. Perhaps she is: shy; starved for attention; easily flattered; or is simply sheltered, young and inexperienced. When selecting a target, the predator may prefer a particular type of woman, such as a college student or a nurse. Or, he may base his target selection solely on a location, such as a shopping mall parking lot. His location will be terrain driven, meaning that he will choose a location that offers him a variety of potential targets and the elements he requires for his type of attack. If he plans to ambush the target, he will need a location that gives him opportunity to do so (see list of ambush locations above).

Since the majority of predators are recidivists, it is safe to assume they learn from both their successes and failures. Many predators will use their past successes as the basis for their future target selection. For example, if a rapist has been successful in getting away with raping women who jog alone at night, his past experience may lead him to select his future target from this same pool of women. His past successes give him the confidence to attack again and he improves his techniques each time he succeeds. (If you are a jogger/walker, make it a habit to take a "snap shot" look behind you every ten steps).

It is important for you to realize that, even if you are selected as a predator's target of opportunity because of your location or activity or because you are his preferred type, there will be early warning signals and he will be required to study you even if only for a few moments before the attack. His surveillance of you may only include a small amount of reconnaissance on his part. This is why practicing basic situational awareness and surveillance detection as a habit increases your chances of preventing becoming a target of opportunity.

Often a predator will go out trolling for a target, meaning he will drive around town, often slowly, with the intention of identifying a woman who is, for some reason, a target who meets his needs. The predator may use his vehicle to drive around unfamiliar areas looking for a victim or he may troll for a target every day on his way to work or as he is driving home. His vehicle may actually serve as the bait, in that he may offer a woman a ride. It also provides him with a safe way to keep his distance while studying an area for potential targets. Perhaps the predator will spot his preferred type of target, or he might spot a target who is easy to ambush in that moment at that location. In the beginning of this chapter we mentioned the college girl who was tragically murdered by being strangled to death. Upon detaining the accused attacker the authorities reported: "It is our information he was driving around in the (victim's) neighborhood and saw her and he liked her looks." As the investigation unfolds, more information about how the attacker proceeded from seeing her while out trolling to ending up in her apartment will likely be revealed. Until then we wonder: How long did he study her before determining where she lived? Once he determined where she lived, did he watch her come and go from her apartment? Did he follow her for any length of time before the attack? These critical details are often never revealed until the predator is on trial. Yet these are the details that are most pertinent because they teach us how the predator operates and what we can do to prevent becoming his victim.

We were hesitant to include this story because this young woman's family is surely suffering beyond comprehension. Yet, her story may save a life one day. Another college girl may be influenced by her tragedy and act on it by using the techniques in this book to notice a predator who is watching her and prevent becoming his victim. As women, we share a collective bond through victimization. Our stories have value. Sadly, this young woman's death was the direct result of a judicial system that is not only failing women but is also actively endangering us by placing us at greater risk of being attacked. This particular predator was released from prison early and, although he was a registered sex offender, he was not under close supervision by the authorities. Thus, he was able to drive every day to neighboring states trolling for targets. He was not monitored by any GPS device nor was his movement in any way restricted. The end result was he was free to realize his intention to attack a woman and when his preferred target crossed his path he was able to enact his vicious plan. His release from prison and lack of supervision, in addition to the abysmal lack of affordable and available training for women in prevention against violence resulted in the tragic loss of life of this promising member of society.

Early Warning Signals That You Are at Risk of Becoming a Target of Opportunity:

- Being in any location that makes you vulnerable to becoming a target of opportunity (parking lots, public restrooms, jogging trails, etc.).

- Indicators that you are under surveillance, even if this occurs suddenly and for a very short time (for example, you may notice a man whom you have never seen before parked in a car in front of your apartment building, fixating his attention on you).

- Any sudden fixation on you, unsolicited approach, or obvious attempt to engage you in conversation or in any activity.

- Any man in a vehicle who appears to be trolling or lying in wait and is fixating his attention on women.

- Any man approaching a woman by driving up to and stopping beside her while engaging her in conversation.

- Indicators of the attack methods discussed above (ambush, ruse or lure).

- Any reckless or direct assault. Even if you are taken by surprise, there is time to respond and you must act immediately (see Chapters Twelve and Thirteen).

Defenses Against Becoming a Target of Opportunity:

- Read the expressions of any man who shows a sudden interest in you. If his face is lighting up or he is approaching you abruptly, seemingly out of the blue, take heed and prepare for the worst. Notice if he is fixating on anything in particular. For example, he may be using his eyes to negotiate the amount of space between you and a secluded staircase. He may be observing who might witness any attempt he makes to grab you. Or he may be fabricating a story to use as a means of moving you in a particular direction of his choice. Check his hands for a weapon and look for anything nearby you can use as a weapon to defend yourself.

- Realize his attack may be bold, decisive and he will act quickly.

- Accept that his nerve and confidence may be boosted by being under the influence of drugs or alcohol. He may be strongly influenced by anger, excitement, or be experiencing a manic episode.

- Use situational awareness to pay attention to a man who approaches you in a vehicle or on foot. Use surveillance detection to notice if he follows you or reappears in various locations you frequent over a short period of time.

- Any unsolicited contact and any closing the distance between you and any man should cause you to take a defensive action such as crossing the street, moving to a safe location, or making noise to attract attention and help.

- Record the license plate number of any vehicle with a male driver who appears to be trolling and report the information to the police.

- If you are carrying any defensive tools, have them out and ready for use. Carry a personal alarm when in transition or in any likely attack location.

- Realize that because *any* woman can become a target of opportunity, *every* woman must learn to get SASD and use the most basic security measures (for example, locking doors and not being out alone after dark).

How to Recognize a Predator Who Uses a Social Setting to Select a Target of Opportunity:

Some predators will use a social setting as the location for selecting their targets. This means the predator will go out to a bar or party or some type of social gathering and strike up a conversation with a woman in order to set the groundwork for his attack. He might use some type of ruse or lure, or he might simply present himself as a man looking to meet an attractive single woman. Regardless of the context, early warnings of his anti-social disposition and behavior will surface. Pay attention for the following signals:

- Limits revealing information about himself.
- Refuses to have conversations about the past.

- Redirects or reverses questions or changes the subject to avoid talking about himself.
- Any discussion or indicators of drug use, including prescription, over the counter, illegal drugs, steroids, or any mix of drugs. Any attempts to get you to use drugs with him or any offers of selling drugs.
- Any indication of an alcohol related problem.
- Any indication that he is hormonally imbalanced or adrift (perhaps due to youth).
- Any mention of a significant day or event that obviously distresses or upsets him.
- Any obsessive talk about his dysfunctional history, home life, or family.
- Indicators that he is socially inexperienced or somehow intolerant in a social setting (such as overt aggression towards strangers or bullying the waitress, etc.).
- Indicators that he has an anger management problem.
- Indicators of inappropriate jealousy.
- Any mention of being influenced by any current crisis or negative family situation.
- Significant age or socioeconomic class differences between you and him.
- Discrepancy or noticeable disparity in attractiveness between the two of you. Sometimes an unattractive predator will target a very attractive woman because she is his preferred type or a very attractive predator might target a woman who is less attractive because he is counting on her being weakened by receiving attention from such an attractive man.
- Any bold invitations to get you to leave the location with him or any attempts to isolate you.

Defenses Against Anti-Social Predators:

- Use the social setting as your means of protecting yourself. Plenty of people are around, so do not leave and isolate yourself.

- Break contact politely and unobtrusively. You might enlist the help of another woman or man or someone working at the event. Try not to make a scene or embarrass him. Excuse yourself to go to the ladies room but be careful he does not follow you.

- Once you break contact, notice if he targets other women and report him to someone working at the event. If you can do so discreetly, warn the woman whom he is targeting.

- Call someone in your SUPNET to report the incident and provide a description of him.

- When leaving the event, have someone escort you to your vehicle. Be alert and practice surveillance detection to make sure he does not follow you home.

- If you feel a threat is imminent, stay at the event and call the police to report him.

Drugging

The widespread use of date rape drugs has become a serious threat about which women of all ages should be aware. Date rape will likely continue as a growing threat as more of these drugs are developed. At present some date rape drugs are being used in conjunction with other drugs as recreational substances that are circulating in communities as party drugs. One example is something called "Special K" which is a combination of GHB (a date rape drug) and a horse tranquilizer.

When a woman is given a date rape drug, the consequences can include abduction, rape, murder or all of the above. The availability and use of date rape drugs has created an evolving threat for women, especially since most of these drugs render a woman helpless and leave her with no memory of the attack. This newfound method of overpowering a woman has given predators an edge because they can get away with rape since it is difficult to prosecute a predator if the victim has no memory of the incident and no witnesses can support her story.

Because date rape has become more prevalent, women who are being courted by men should consider the possibility that some level of courtship may be used as a ruse for getting close enough to the woman to slip her the drug and rape her. A predator may attempt to contextualize the attack with some degree of a relationship with his victim. This relationship might afford him an alibi in that he can always say she willingly took the drug to party with him and consented to the sex. He will argue that it was not rape but rather consensual sex (she went to his home willingly; she called him; they had a developing relationship, etc.).

Early Warning Signals of Drugging:

- Experiencing the symptoms of a sudden onset of a drug. Realization of slurred speech and blurred vision. Loss of fine motor skills. Others may be the ones to first notice and make you aware of your symptoms.

- If you suddenly and inexplicably become emotional, paranoid or overly affectionate and indiscriminately social.

- Being in an area or location where these drugs have been used before (college parties, bars, raves, nightclubs).

- Any man encouraging you to drink a beverage he brings to you.

- Any man who is exhibiting controlling behavior and is trying to get you to go to a second location with him, even if you have already refused.

- If you notice a man reaching into his pocket and using his hands to manipulate some small object anywhere near your drink.

- Any man who is behaving in a cagey, aggressive, domineering manner who is attempting to have a drink with you or get close to your drink.

- Clandestine or non-verbal communication between men who are exhibiting suspicious behavior or who are fixating on a particular woman or group of women. Consider the potential that they will create some type of wingman scenario to use as a distraction so that a drug can be slipped into your drink.

- Any man attempting to get your attention by using inappropriate nonverbal communication such as overtly staring at you, making obscene gestures, leering at you, or any indication that he is becoming sexually aroused.

- Any man attempting to control your behavior by channeling you into an isolated area or manipulating you and trying to "cut you from the herd" (separate you from your friends and witnesses).

- Any inappropriate talk about sex (like he is doing you a favor by offering to be intimate with you). Any crude expressions ("I bet you like it hot and nasty"), mannerisms or sexual references.

- If he goes from treating you with respect, turning on the charm, and showering you with attention to suddenly controlling you and becoming domineering.

- If he shifts and starts dehumanizing or objectifying you and exalts in sexualizing you.

- If his physical advances towards you make you feel uncomfortable because he is overly pushy, aggressive, or domineering.

- If he becomes antagonistic or aggressive if you refuse physical contact. He may try to use a guilt trip on you or make threatening comments such as "You shouldn't be such a tease because you're asking for it."

- Any attempts to lure you into buying or taking drugs.

- For an ongoing courtship, consider the following questions: Does he display any overt jealously, moodiness, and/or controlling behaviors? Does he instruct you to be discreet about your time together? Does he make attempts to isolate you from friends and family? Does he make multiple sexual innuendos or ask you to discuss sexual matters early on in the courtship (fantasies, sexual practices, etc.)? Are you involved in any kind of a love triangle and is he displaying jealousy or rage as a result? (Realize that he may use the context of the courtship as a way of creating his opportunity to drug you).

Defenses Against Drugging:

- Procure your own drinks at parties, bars, clubs, and social events.
- Do not leave your drink unattended, even if it means taking it with you when you visit the ladies' room.
- Cover your drink with a napkin or use your thumb to cover a beer bottle or can.
- Have a plan. If you intend to go to a location that is high risk because of past incidences of the use of date rape drugs, prepare yourself and be extra cautious with your drinks. Use the buddy system to protect yourself and your friends. Just like having a designated driver, designate one person to assist with watching the drinks.
- Drink before you go to the location or bring your own bottled water and keep the cap closed unless you are taking a sip.
- Only drink out of sealed bottles or cans that you open yourself and over which you maintain control.
- Remember you do not have to be rude and refuse to accept a drink but you can discreetly dispose of it without ever taking a sip.
- Use a date rape drug test kit to determine if your drink has been drugged (the kit allows you to place a drop of your drink onto a card which will change color if the drink has been drugged).
- Arrange an emergency signal with one of your friends so that you can effectively communicate if you think you are in trouble or if one of you notices suspicious behaviors and indicators of possible drugging.
- If you realize the threat has escalated, stay calm and maintain your friendly demeanor while you calculate your options for safely breaking contact from this man. Use all of your assets, including your SUPNET, intuition, feminine wiles, and rational mind to craft a safe

exit. Do *not* take a sip of your drink, even if you think it has not yet been drugged.

- Enlist help from security staff or female strangers if you are alone.
- Use stall tactics and remove yourself from the situation if any man tries to take you somewhere isolated.
- If a man has managed to isolate you and is aggressively forcing you to take a drink, look for the right opportunity to deliver a direct assault (see Chapter Twelve).
- Break out of any encirclement by any group of men. You may need to do so using a sudden and swift movement in the direction of your best escape route. You might first fool them by appearing to be oblivious about the danger or by tricking them into thinking you accept that they are in control until you find the opportunity to make your move to escape.
- Report any man whom you suspect is using date rape drugs to the owners of the establishment and the police.
- For an ongoing courtship: Breaking contact is your best defense against any man who makes you feel uncomfortable. If you are using situational awareness and are protecting yourself by using the dating tips in Chapter Eight, you should be able to limit his access to you and break contact with him safely by ending the courtship if you feel at risk of being drugged by any man you are dating. If he refuses to allow you to stop dating him you will need to consider him to be dangerous. You should now view him as a likely stalker and respond accordingly (see Chapter Nine).

Blackmail/Coercion

Some rapists will blackmail their victims by using some type of threat as a means of coercing the woman into having sexual relations. This is not to be confused with sexual harassment. In other words, the casting couch example, where the movie director or producer tries to trade sex for a role in the film, is a clear example of sexual harassment. Blackmailing a woman into having sex involves a threat. Perhaps the rapist will threaten to harm a child if the woman does not have sex with him. Perhaps he threatens to frame her for some type of crime. Blackmail is usually used against women who are for some reason in a weakened position or are frail. Examples of women who are at high risk of being blackmailed include: illegal immigrants facing the threat of deportation; elderly women; mentally impaired women; women who are in the porn industry; and women who suffer from emotional abuse and are easy to blackmail as a result.

Early Warning Signals of Blackmail/Coercion:

- In most cases, if a man were to blackmail a woman into having sex with him, he would require some type of leverage. If a man you know positions himself in such a way as to create a source of leverage, be wary. For example, he might be privy to a secret about you which he could use against you.
- Men who are friends or even relatives who spend isolated time with women who are at high risk of being blackmailed.
- Men who team up and have conspiratorial talks when interacting with women who are at high risk of becoming victims.
- Men who take advantage of fear and manipulate stressful situations faced by women who are at high risk of being blackmailed.
- Physical or verbal bullying from men towards women at high risk of being blackmailed.
- Men who do too many favors for women who are at high risk of becoming victims, thereby putting them in the position to feel obligated to pay them back with sex.

Defenses Against Blackmail/Coercion:

- Avoid giving any man leverage against you. Just say no to any blackmail attempts. Do not play his game.
- If a man attempts to blackmail you for sex, report him to your friends, family, and to the police.
- If the threat is immediate, look for an opportunity to stall him by arranging an encounter at a specific location and time and then call the police and have them show up at the meeting. He will likely deny that he threatened you, but at least the authorities will be onto him.
- Keep an eye on relatives, friends, and neighbors when they are near frail or high risk women. This means keeping careful watch over them as often as necessary or as dictated by situation, area, and threat. Accompany these women to any appointments.
- Keep in daily contact with neighbors and caregivers if you are in a high risk category due to a weakened position.
- Be prepared for violence if any man begins to verbally blackmail or coerce you.
- Gather evidence of his blackmail attempts using a nanny cam or audio recorder and report him to the police.

The Role of Force and Your Response to It

If ever attacked, you must be psychologically prepared to endure crude and vulgar language, meanness and brutality, overpowering strength, and potentially sadistic and insane behavior from your attacker. These are all methods your attacker might use to increase his control over you. You will be required to adapt in a moment to any sudden, dramatic change in his behavior. His objective is to put you into a realm which is clearly uncomfortable, anti-social, and far beyond your normal reality. He may use force against you in order to debilitate your will and resolve and to shock you into submission. Often when an attacker threatens a woman and uses some type of force against her it is an indicator that he needs to overpower his victim because he is not yet in total control of her. His use of any kind of force is a message to you that he is not yet confident that he has total control over you. Listen to his words and actions for this hidden message and look for openings so that you can prevent him from gaining total control over you.

In other cases, the use of force is his sick way of gaining gratification and the pleasure he is seeking from the attack. This, of course, will terrify you. How can a woman not be horrified when in the presence of someone who is so sick that he is actually enjoying hurting her? By contemplating this type of scenario now, you can instruct yourself to respond by not allowing yourself to be mentally caught off-guard by the evil of another human being. Rather than wasting your time and energy trying to catch up to his insane reality, you can instruct yourself right now, that if you are ever confronted by such a monster, you will not be surprised or distracted by his terrifying antics. Instead, you will identify the severity of the threat and fight with everything you have to survive and escape. Have a plan for how you would handle having force used against you and rehearse it in your mind. Your internal monologue in such a situation should not be bogged down with thoughts such as: "How can he be doing this to me?" Rather you should be giving yourself short, powerful verbal commands such as "Survive" or "Escape" so that you can function and respond rather than wasting your energy trying to understand or rationalize the actions of someone who is clearly insane and sadistic. Rehearse your survival commands and visualize yourself escaping.

When preparing yourself to handle force, you must also understand that a predator might deliver a sudden, direct attack as a means of gaining control over you. This means that the attacker will waste no time with a lure or ruse, he will rather deliver a powerful, direct attack and allow his crime to progress from there. He will begin the sequence of events with power and force and the threat of serious, imminent harm. He could use a gun or he could strike you, but be certain he will waste no time in overpowering you. He may push or pull you, grab your arm or hair, or even lock his arm around your neck.

In other situations, a predator might enact a sudden, violent reversal. This means that he is likely mentally disturbed, thus his behavior may change in an instant. He may surprise you by some sudden, violent reversal, either in his manner of speaking, acting, or in his facial expressions and appearance. He may begin his interaction with you by being charming or engaging. He may use a ruse or try to solicit some type of help from you. He may be the man you just started dating and suddenly during one of your conversations he becomes instantly aggressive or controlling. Or he may be a boyfriend or spouse who is suffering from some type of mental illness and suddenly he snaps. In the event he makes any kind of sudden, violent reversal, you will have very limited time to respond so you must take measures to escape immediately.

You may or may not receive early warning signals that your attacker will use force. If he is closing the physical distance between you or aggressively moving towards you, or handling you in a rough manner, you may have a moment to respond by moving away from him and attempting to escape. He may give you a verbal early warning signal by changing the tone of his voice and becoming more threatening. Or you may notice a drastic change in his mood or demeanor (trembling, nervousness, frantic pacing) that signals you to be wary that he is about to become violent. All of this will happen in a split second, thus you must trust your intuition and act immediately.

Your defenses against the use of force include:

- Do not allow any man to close the physical distance or remove obstacles that separate you and him if you feel threatened.
- Break contact and move to a safe location.
- Create a distraction, make noise, and draw attention to yourself.
- Negotiate your way out of the threat if possible.
- Use self-defense techniques and available tools to protect yourself (see Chapter Twelve).

- Accept the reality of the danger so that you do not go into a state of shock wherein you lose your ability to respond (see Chapter Thirteen).

- Use a verbal command (preferably one you have already rehearsed) to anchor yourself while enduring the violence to increase your chances of survival.

- Do not give up! You can survive having force used against you. Keep defending yourself and looking for ways to escape.

One preventative technique you can rehearse now is to anchor yourself with some type of verbal command. The command "SURVIVE!" is a powerful choice. Say it over and over and over in the thick of the situation so that your brain is doing everything it can to send the proper signals to your body to aid you in your survival. Plan your word and anchor it with a powerful memory or feeling. Imagine yourself under attack and in the heat of a survival situation. The word "SURVIVE" should be both a mental and verbal command to yourself. It is a strong motivator.

Another technique for motivating yourself to survive a life threatening situation is to create some type of very short cadence. Military cadences are used to motivate and focus the mind. You can create your own cadence for surviving in a high threat situation by taking a line from a song you find inspiring or singing a verbal command to a tune you find energizing. For example: the *Green Day* song "*Warning*" begins: "*Warning, live without warning.*" You can change that to: "Warning live with early warning" to keep yourself SASD and ready for anything.

In the U.S. Army Special Forces the word "SURVIVAL" is an acronym:

*S*ize up the situation.
*U*se all your senses.
*R*emember where you are.
*V*anquish fear and panic.
*I*mprovise.
*V*alue living.
*A*ct like the natives.
*L*ive by your wits

Your best chance for surviving having force inflicted upon you is having a plan which includes mental preparation and acceptance of the fact that it is possible you could become a victim of violence. It is natural that we would all rather not have to think about this truth, but denial is what keeps us downtrodden and victimized. Preparation, prevention, and acceptance of the truth about the threats against us empower us to defend ourselves.

If prevention measures fail and you find yourself under attack, you still have many techniques at your disposal for surviving. In Chapters Twelve and Thirteen we elaborate on specific tactics and general responses to all attacks. Below, we examine possible responses to the three types of attacks discussed in this chapter.

Responding if Abducted

If you examine case histories of abductions of politicians, diplomats, executives and other high profile individuals, what you will learn is that the attackers are successful because they bypass the visible security protecting the target. This means that they will study the target to determine the obstacles they must overcome. For example, does the target travel with bodyguards or in an armored vehicle? Once they determine the obstacles, they can then craft an attack plan which will ensure their ability to overcome these obstacles. For example, the hijackers for the attacks of September eleven determined that the cockpit doors were unsecured on U.S. aircraft. They also learned that it was possible to pass box cutters through security checks at airports. Using this information, they were able to execute successful attacks. Any visible security methods are at risk of being bypassed by watchful attackers.

The reason surveillance detection is so effective in preventing abductions is that, if conducted correctly the abductors will never realize they are being detected in their planning. Surveillance detection is a covert security measure, one which attackers will have great difficulty defeating. By implementing a surveillance detection plan you can expose attackers in the very early planning stage of their efforts to abduct you. You will likely have to hire some surveillance detection operators if you are under credible threat of being abducted, as the abductors will recognize your security staff. You must place people in positions where they can watch the abductors and their associates plan the attack. You and your security support have to outsmart the abductors rather than waiting for them to overpower you.

Imagine the amount of planning required for abductors to be successful. They must study the target carefully so they know exactly where and when to snatch her/him without getting caught. If you are targeted by abductors, you will have plenty of opportunities to see them out there while they are in the surveillance phase of their attack planning. A woman who is SASD stands a very good chance of preventing being abducted because she will notice early on that she is under surveillance and can then take the appropriate actions to protect herself and involve the proper authorities.

Regardless if you face a very real threat of being abducted or if you are an ordinary person who is not under high threat of being abducted, we have some basic advice for surviving abduction in the event that you are unable to prevent it from occurring. First, do your best to get attention during the initial attack. If you carry a personal alarm, sound it. Scream, shout, and yell for help. Expose your abductors to the scrutiny of others. *Do everything possible to avoid being taken to a second location.* If they do manage to control you and get you into a vehicle unnoticed, you will likely have to become compliant until an opportunity arises for you to either escape or foil their plan. Fighting them when you are totally under their control and out of sight of others could get you killed. Wait, stay aware, and maintain your resolve to survive. Assess your available options. If they are driving you in a car, can you discreetly signal to another driver that you are in trouble? Look for any opportunity that might make them ineffective in abducting you.

If they take you to a second location, do your best to study the route and pay attention to turns and directions and to any special odors or sounds that may help you identify where you are. Always look for escape routes and be aware of as many of the entrances and exits as possible in any building where they hold you. If you are held for any length of time, study the sun so that you have some basic sense of direction. That way, if you escape, you will have a better chance of knowing which way to run. Do your best to keep them calm so that they do not escalate their violence against you. Remember that your survival is all that matters. You can get therapy and medical treatment to overcome the trauma, but your life is irreplaceable. Try to develop some rapport with your abductors so that it is easier for you to convince them not to harm you. If you can get on a first name basis with them you will personalize the situation and stand a better chance of them not harming you. You may assess that the strategy of 'divide and conquer' will be effective. For example, you may befriend one of them and get him to betray the others. The possibilities are endless. You must retain your situational awareness and be in the present moment, always using your every skill and looking for opportunities to remove yourself from the situation and survive.

If you are in a high risk category of being abducted then you should know your ransom will be negotiated by your employer, insurance company, or by a professional kidnap/ransom company. Follow the professional advice of those who are protecting you. Prepare yourself for the real possibility that you may be abducted for ransom and know what to do and how to proceed with your abductors so that you mitigate your chances of being harmed or killed as a result of negotiations going wrong. Be patient. The longer you are held captive, the better your chances are of being released.

If you are abducted by someone who intends to kill you, the abduction is all part of the larger plan and is only a means to an end. A murderer will not necessarily inform his victim of his plans. This is why it is so important to do anything you can to avoid being taken to a second location. He could have a hideout where he plans to hold you, rape you, torture you, and eventually kill you. Perhaps you are not his first victim. If a murderer abducts you, he will likely have planned his crime so that he has a place to take you. If he has not prearranged a location, he will seek a deserted spot. Once you are held captive, he will have the control he seeks and will enact the murder in his own time unless you do something to provoke him to kill you or some random element changes the situation and he is forced to kill you sooner than he intended. Having control over his victim is part of his depraved desire. You must identify any depraved behaviors or tendencies of your abductor and muster your resolve to find an opening to escape or defend your life. (Again, Chapters Twelve and Thirteen contain a wide variety of possible responses/techniques for self-defense and escaping).

Recovering from an Abduction

Abduction causes suffering not only for the victim, but also for the victim's loved ones. The complete lack of control over one's own safety plagues the victim while the uncertainty on the part of the family if the victim is alive or dead is the ultimate anguish. If you survive being abducted, seek professional help immediately. Do not assume that there will be no psychological repercussions. In addition, strengthening your personal security will assist you in feeling safe during your recovery period. The vulnerability you may feel in the future about your safety will clearly be impacted as a result of what you went through during the abduction. Taking charge of as much of your personal security as possible will empower you to recover and move on with your life.

Responding During a Rape

One of our biggest motivating factors for writing this book is that we believe that women do not have adequate resources (especially in the form of affordable training) to protect themselves. We also know from experience that surveillance detection is a powerful tool that will help women to prevent these crimes, yet it has been sadly reserved for the elite. Our intention is to introduce this practice into the mainstream so that women everywhere can protect themselves. Since so many rapes begin with a surveillance stage, practicing surveillance detection on a regular basis provides you with the greatest proactive opportunity for spotting a potential rapist who may be targeting you and for helping you to prevent becoming his victim. Please remember that you can apply the information in this chapter to yourself or to a child you may be trying to protect.

Some women are raped by people they know and some by strangers. It can be more difficult for a woman to detect signs of surveillance from a person she knows, in that her habits may be known to this person already so he has a jump-start on the information collection process, (again this is why we promote protecting your identity and personal information, including your schedule). What you can detect is behavior on his part that feels suspicious or out of the ordinary and nudges your intuition towards fear. If a man you know (a neighbor, a work associate, a friend) starts making you feel uneasy or surrounds you with an uncomfortable tension, pay attention to these signals. If you sense he is watching you or monitoring you somehow, trust your instincts. Perhaps he is recording your voice on the phone or is name-dropping or bragging about his association with you. Perhaps he is asking others about you and is trying to elicit information or trying to pinpoint your location. If you feel tension in his presence, heighten your situational awareness and surveillance detection practice. Break any patterns you have with him, inform your SUPNET, and report him to the police if anything threatening happens. You can also conduct a misinformation campaign by instructing those to whom he is talking about you to give him false information. Or you can give him false information directly. You can also hire a private investigator to collect information and evidence against him if you feel he is a viable threat.

If a predator is unknown to a woman, the surveillance can be more difficult to detect because she is not looking for a specific person, but rather for indicators that someone is watching her. On the other hand, this predator is at a disadvantage because he does not know her schedule and habits and must come out in plain sight in order to collect this information. A woman who practices surveillance detection on a regular basis will very quickly notice if a rapist has her under surveillance. Since some rapists will act rashly and quickly, it is important for you to take any surveillance you detect seriously. Report the man to the police. Tell them you fear you are under surveillance by this man and you do not know why. Take serious measures to avoid placing yourself in ambush or attack locations. Take the threat seriously and change your patterns.

If you did not receive any early warning signals or failed to take them seriously and you find yourself in a high threat situation where you are certain to be raped, you can still take action to either prevent the rape or to mitigate the consequences and avoid being injured or killed. Every rape is different, thus there is no formula that will work under all circumstances. However, we can address some common defenses you can develop and implement. First, remember to maintain your situational awareness. It should be at its highest level at this point, meaning you are not in denial and your intuition, senses, and awareness are heightened to match the threat level. Having situational awareness means noticing the reality of what is happening and embracing the situation while remaining cool. No need to panic or let fear overpower your rational mind. Do not buy into his story or threats. Do not let him control your focus while he is engaging in his behavior. Without being obvious, scan the area and identify any other threats, as well as any exits or weapons you can use to create an opportunity to escape. Stay in the present and look for any openings. This may mean that you use your feminine wiles to negotiate yourself out of the dangerous situation. Many women have talked their way out of being raped by telling their rapists that they are infected with some life threatening or sexually transmitted disease. Some women have pulled on the sympathy strings and have convinced their rapists to leave them alone and not harm them by telling them they are pregnant, have a sick child, or have some illness. Other women create a ruse to delay the rape so they can escape it.

One young woman in Kentucky was attacked by two men when her car broke down on the side of the highway in a rural area. She was about to be raped and used her quick thinking to convince these men to change location so they could relax. She gave them the idea to go buy some alcohol and get a motel room so they could party and have sex all night. They bought into her ploy, went to the motel, and got so drunk they passed out and she called the police. Obviously, there was some risk involved in her choice. It could have all gone wrong for her if they had not been drunk. However, having them go to the motel created witnesses and a paper trail that would help the authorities lead to them post incident. It also put her in a more populated area, thereby increasing her chances of finding help. On the other hand, she could have been killed at the motel. The point is, it is impossible to armchair quarterback this situation. She sized up the situation and made an assessment about her attackers' personalities. She then used her situational awareness, cunning, and her gut instinct about these men and created a successful escape scenario. This is all any woman can do if a man is about to rape her and she has no other means of defending herself.

Even if you are totally overpowered and are raped, remember you still have power. You have the power to collect and preserve evidence so that you can prosecute your rapist. This is why it is important to report a rape immediately and to go straight to a hospital before changing clothes and bathing, thereby unintentionally destroying any DNA evidence. You may have collected evidence under your fingernails, in the form of bodily fluids, or in the form of fingerprints (especially if the rapist used any type of weapon he left behind or any materials for gagging or binding you). Many rape victims are so traumatized that they want to literally "wash away" the incident and forget it ever happened. This is certainly understandable, but given that many rapists are recidivists, deciding to prosecute them may protect you and other women from their violent acts in the future. Support groups can assist you in minimizing your level of involvement post attack by advocating for you so that you can focus more on your recovery.

Recovering from a Rape

We do not wish to try to pass ourselves off as experts on the subject of rape. Nor do we intentionally want to skirt over or appear insensitive about aspects of the dynamics involved in reporting a rape. In addition, we want you to understand that we are in no way trying to add to your suffering by coaching you on "what you could have done to prevent it." Although we do preach the motto that foresight is twenty-twenty, we never want a woman to feel she is to blame because she did not do more to prevent a crime. However, we ask you to consider the actions you take carefully if you are ever in the position where you must decide whether or not to prosecute your rapist.

If you are victimized by a rapist and do not take action against your aggressor, it may stunt your recovery from the trauma. If you take a pacifist type of approach and allow your attacker to victimize you without consequences, you are nudging your attacker along and you become a willing participant in his attack success rate. Remember that rapists will generally do whatever they can get away with quickly and easily. They will opt for what is safest for them, meaning how they can rape without getting caught. When women fail to prosecute rapists, rapists learn what works, what is safest, easiest and most effective. And then they rape again.

Deciding to avoid prosecuting your rapist can negatively impact your ability to move on because you are never vindicated. On the other hand, if you take back the power and pursue your attacker legally, your actions may influence your recovery and boost your sense of self-esteem and empowerment. If you take action by prosecuting your rapist, you set an example for women in the future and embolden them to come forward as well. This collective effort on the part of women has power. In the end, you must decide what is right for you, but we do strongly recommend that you preserve evidence so that you at least retain the option to prosecute your rapist in the future. We also recommend you seek professional support during your recovery (see Appendix E).

We heard one story about women on a college campus who took cans of spray paint and painted "rape zones" around areas of the campus where rapes had occurred. This is an example of a creative and powerful way to bring attention to the problem. Any collective efforts that bring attention to the crime of rape are worthy ventures and empower women to uphold their right to be protected against violence.

Responding to an Attempted Murder

Because the crimes of abduction, rape, and murder are so often intertwined, your response to any of these crimes must be immediate and unencumbered by denial. If you make plans for responding to these threats and rehearse them in your mind you will be much better able to survive if you are ever confronted by a potential killer. You will have fear, but fear is an asset you can use to overcome freezing so that you can get moving. You can redirect your fear into resolve to survive and reverse the element of surprise and steal his power. Stun and run or go compliant and then explode with sudden action.

Immediately heightening your situational awareness is critical to your survival. Your strongest early warning signal will likely come from your intuition and may be in the form of fear or an unsettled feeling. Pay attention to, trust in, and act upon your intuitive nudges. Your survival instinct is talking to you! You are now a character in someone else's story. You have to read your attacker's story, pay attention to where it is headed and how he sees your role in it. You then have to maneuver to either notice or create an opening for your escape. You cannot do this if you are in shock or denial about the gravity of your present situation at the hands of this potential monster. Having a plan will help reduce the shock and remove the denial.

If all of your defenses fail and you are at the mercy of another, you must fight for your life. Even if you truly are at his mercy, decide not to be at his mercy. Let that be your motivator to take charge. It is totally naïve on your part to trust him to be merciful or hope that he will let you go. There is a strong chance that he is a recidivist. He has already crossed the line by attacking you. He may be part of the three strike rule and he is going to prison for life anyway so he has nothing to lose. He is completely unpredictable. He is likely a liar, dysfunctional, irrational, unbalanced, anti-social, and a fatalist. He is operating under a twisted moral precept, in that he puts no value on human life. He has what they call in prisons "shark eyes," meaning he is already dead to the world in terms of emotions such as human compassion. His heart is cold and ruthless. His self-esteem was likely long ago destroyed. His depraved indifference to human life is your immediate and impenetrable enemy. You have no choice but to fight for your life.

You must do whatever is necessary to take back some control, either by reversing the surprise, using self-defense techniques, weapons, negotiation, or a complete uploading of whatever force you can muster against this attacker. Use your mind. Perhaps you can feign unconsciousness if he hits you to buy yourself time to plan a way to reverse the surprise on him. Perhaps you will employ your feminine wiles and attempt to seduce him. You might feign some attachment to him or eagerness to go along with his plan. Survival is instinctive; your body will respond if you can prevent it from going into shock (see Chapter Thirteen). If you must explode with force, you must commit one hundred percent to doing what your intuition tells you to do and act upon it immediately, without holding back anything. You must completely focus your force so as to deliver it successfully. And you must never give up, even if the fight lasts a long time. Your ultimate act of self-esteem in life is to value yourself enough to survive any attempt to end your life. You are worth it.

Recovering from an Attempted Murder

We strongly suggest seeking immediate medical and professional support in order to begin the recovery process from an attempted murder. Depending on the severity of the experience, your body and emotions may be seriously traumatized. In addition, your whole world will likely have been turned upside-down in terms of how you view your personal security. It will be absolutely normal for you to go through a period of time where you experience paranoid fears about being attacked again. Do not hesitate to seek professional support as soon as possible.

In addition, if you are involved in any kind of criminal prosecution of your attacker, you will be dealing with the event on an ongoing basis for a time and will be questioned about, reminded of, and forced to revisit the event. This will take enormous strength on your part and having the support of your SUPNET and professional support will be instrumental in expediting your recovery.

One Woman's Survival Story

The following is a story about an abduction and rape that has important lessons about what happens when that fear of being attacked by a stranger turns into a reality. Beatrice's story is by far one of the most disturbing in this book. When interviewing her, we were at once fascinated by her will to survive and confounded by the choices she made once she was freed from her aggressors.

Beatrice sits on her couch eager to begin. We go through our usual disclaimer and tell her that we will allow her to read the interview before we publish the book, just in case she changes her mind about sharing her story. She assures us she will not. We let her begin, unaware of how difficult it will be for us, not her, to process the information.

"I was seventeen, traveling on my own in the south of France. It was 1974 and in those days it was pretty safe and common for women in Europe to hitchhike. I was heading to Nice and got a ride with a man with whom I ended up becoming intimate. I immediately regretted it and went through a traumatic few days staying at his home. He and his brother wanted more than I was willing to give. I denied them, they became angry, I left. End of story. I continued on to Cannes alone. When I arrived I was not feeling very well. I was in a public area trying to get some help from these gypsies. I had very little money and was trying to figure out how to use the phone so I could call my mom in the States. During this whole interaction with the gypsies, who turned out to be no help at all, I had the distinct feeling I was being watched."

Our first reaction was that Beatrice obviously had made similar bad choices that many young women make and then end up regretting (hitchhiking, sexual intimacy with a total stranger). At seventeen it is understandable. As she continued her story, we began to realize that the dynamics of becoming the victim of a total stranger cause an impact that is elusive and complex.

"As I was struggling with the gypsies, a young, attractive man approached me and asked if I needed help. He was also American, so that made me feel comforted. I explained my situation and he said he would help me but only on the condition that I promised to go to Switzerland with him. I was flattered. He was nice. I was a young, free spirit. I went to Switzerland. He insisted we cross the border at night, well…three in the morning actually. I felt fear, dread, and knew I was in trouble. My recent experience with my last ride seemed to be an omen for what was to come."

We were a bit baffled that Beatrice would have made such a choice, but then again she was alone, vulnerable, almost out of money, only seventeen, and was admittedly lured in by the comfort factor of a fellow countryman offering to help her.

"He took me to a residential neighborhood near Baden-Baden. When we entered the apartment I realized that my nightmare was just beginning. Another man, also American, was sitting on the couch, naked. He was overweight and repulsive looking. He immediately grabbed me and took me into a pitch black

room. He gave me a piece of advice that ended up being the thing that saved my life in the long run. He said: 'You can be really smart, or you can get really hurt.' He then brutally raped and sodomized me."

We thought it might be time to take a break, but Beatrice wanted to continue. She was eager for us to know how she prevailed. She needed us to know because we were her ticket to other girls and women reading her story. Beatrice is all about helping anyone she can to survive a similar ordeal.

"They took me up into the mountains to a house. I was a prisoner. They literally watched my every move. I had to leave the door open when I went to the bathroom. Once, they let me outside near the cow pasture to breathe some fresh air, but I was on a short leash and could not seek help. I slept in the same large bed with them and they passed me back and forth for sex. I survived it by thinking during the sex, which at this point was not violent. I would think my way through it, like a means to an end. It was apparent to me that the older man was in charge. I decided to befriend him. On one occasion he wanted to take a bath with me. I started to let myself have a good time with him. We talked about all sorts of things. He was Jewish, nouveau riche, into art, spirituality, being a vegetarian, and cocaine. I partied with them to win rapport, though I never allowed myself to get too out of it. It is amazing how little drugs and alcohol affect you when you are making a conscious effort to stay alive. When we took that bath together I knew I had him. I realized he underestimated me and thought I was some uneducated, country girl. When he realized I came from a cultured, upper-class life, his attitude towards me changed."

At this point we began to realize how this seventeen year old girl turned the tables on her attackers. Even though they had overcome her physically, she took back the mental control by deciding to avoid becoming emotionally devastated and therefore destroyed by the danger she faced. She did not panic, but rather slowed down and listened. She did not allow any internal monologue of self-doubt inhibit her ability to survive.

"After a couple of weeks they came up with a plan for me. They told me they wanted to fly me to Canada with a cast on my leg filled with cocaine. This terrified me because they warned me that, if I tried to turn myself in, I would surely go to jail. I was obsessed with figuring this out. I knew in my gut that if I *went to Canada, my fate would be unknown. Who would meet me there? Would I be sold into white slavery? I was the perfect candidate: young, blond, beautiful. I was trapped and needed to figure out an escape. Fortunately for me, the younger man left to go research this Canada trip and to pick up the cocaine.*

For several days I was alone with the boss and knew I had to make it count. I intensified the intimacy that was developing between us. We would talk, laugh, have sex, and take baths together. It became like a love affair that most people dream of having in some chateau in the Swiss Alps. I played the role and my opportunity finally arrived; his wife was coming to visit. I talked him into taking me to a hotel since it was obviously completely inappropriate for me to stay at the house while she was in town. When we got to the hotel the concierge immediately registered something very wrong was going on. I slipped him my mother's phone number and asked him to take my plane ticket and book me a flight out the next day. I then took my captor out to dinner, saying that I really appreciated him trusting me enough to take me to the hotel. This gesture basically sealed the deal for me to get a ride to the airport from him the next day."

At this point we were baffled. Why did she not tell the concierge to call the police? Why did she not seek immediate rescue from someone...anyone?

"I know it sounds strange, but I just knew from the relationship I developed with him that he would let me go. But I also knew I had to play it out right. And don't forget, I had been conditioned to obey them in order to survive so, on some level I think I was scared to do anything too rash or yell for help. He did take me to the airport the next day. When I returned to the States I ended up sending him a book on the 'I Ching' and thanking him for letting me go."

We had read about Stockholm Syndrome but had never interviewed anyone who had experienced it. Basically a victim who is suffering from Stockholm Syndrome becomes emotionally attached to her/his captor. The victim will develop a sense of loyalty and will even defend her/his captor after being freed. Patty Hearst is the most well known example. Beatrice had never heard of Stockholm Syndrome but told us that she became obsessed with watching the Patty Hearst trial on the news, which occurred not long after Beatrice's release.

"I never sent the authorities after him, even though I knew his name and had an address on him. I guess I thought I had won because I managed to outsmart

him and get away. We did develop a kind of relationship. It was weird, to be sure, but in the end I felt it was best just to move on and leave it in the past."

It is certainly a woman's choice to put past traumas behind her and move forward. It is also understandable that some women who are abducted and raped do not want to extend their suffering by going through a trial. On the contrary, many women want to put a stop to predators so that they do not strike again. This is an admirable and positive contribution to society. As adult women, if we report our attackers we are taking our social responsibility seriously. Given that so many predators are recidivists, the likelihood that they will harm other women in the future is high. We do not feel it is our place to judge any woman for the choices she makes after surviving an ordeal in which she was victimized both physically and psychologically, but we do applaud those who are able to find the strength and courage to bring their attackers to justice.

Beatrice's story has several insights worth discussing. First, she basically ignored her intuition and situational awareness before she was taken captive. She knew someone was watching her when she was interacting with the gypsies, yet she was desperate enough that she ignored this hunch and went to Switzerland with the American man. She also relayed that she knew she was in trouble when crossing the border, yet she did not get out of the car and ask for help from the border guards. Because she willingly allowed herself to be taken to a second location, she raised her risk level of being raped and murdered.

Once attacked and held captive, her survival instinct and situational awareness kicked in again and this time she listened. She was able, even while being raped on multiple occassions, to think clearly and figure out a solution. Part of what allowed Beatrice to survive is that she knew herself and was able to capitalize on parts of her personality. She is an attractive and naturally flirtatious woman who says she has always been at ease with men and, as a result, has always received a lot of attention from them. This part of her personality may have worked against her and partially caused her to draw the attention of her predator in the first place, but it also worked for her in that she used it to survive. The salient point here is that Beatrice's forgotten instinct (her situational awareness) was always present. She simply made bad choices and ignored her situational awareness, thus she ended up in a high threat situation.

When we refer to SA as a forgotten instinct, we mean that women are forgetting to use what is already present inside of them. If we could all simply remember to listen to this innate voice and ability, we would advance leaps and bounds ahead of our predators. Why do we not listen? We are too busy, too young, too distracted, too worried about offending someone, but most importantly too *disconnected from ourselves.* Oddly enough, the more westernized women become, the less connected they seem to be to their basic instincts and to their physical bodies. It is time to reclaim ourselves and redefine empowerment. We can do this easily by making a simple choice to listen to our survival instinct and reconnect with our ability to live our lives using situational awareness on a regular basis. When we combine situational awareness with surveillance detection, we fortify our ability to protect ourselves.

The next step is obviously for mothers to become role models for their daughters by openly practicing and discussing situational awareness and surveillance detection. Do not be afraid to share this practice and live as an example for all of the women in your life, including your daughters, sisters, friends, students, neighbors, and work associates. Any mother reading Beatrice's story will absolutely shudder at the decisions this seventeen year old girl made. The truth is that teenage girls or young college women are making these kinds of bad choices all the time. They do so for a variety of reasons, but the common reason is that they have untrained, immature instincts. They may have also gotten away with making some wild, dangerous, risky choices and this may reinforce their confidence level that nothing bad will ever happen to them. Even if they have been told to be careful a thousand times by their parents, teenage girls and young college women must be *trained.* They must be *shown* how it works, by examples of real situations. You can show them by rehearsing 'what if' plans from stories in the news. You can show them by pointing out how being SASD works when you are out on the streets. But the best way to train them is to be their role model; be a woman who practices situational awareness and surveillance detection in their presence. One of the most important things you can give to your daughter is a course in basic street smarts.

Conclusion

The crimes of abduction, rape, and murder are the most serious threats women face. Remember, many abductors, rapists, and murderers will study their targets before attacking. Getting SASD is your best preventative measure for avoiding being victimized by these predators. What you must also consider is that in a split second your life can change and you could be confronted by one of the worst predators in existence. We never really know whose path we might cross from day to day. If that split second change impacts your life, you will be required in a brief moment to make choices. Reading this book alone is an act of readying yourself to make the right choices to defend your life. Your mind right now is considering these attacks as possible realities and educating you as to possible early warning signals and defenses. Any training you can give yourself (mental and physical) will be stored in your memory and in your body. Your attitude, in addition, is critical. This book is our way of challenging women to empower themselves to refuse to accept the violence against them at the hands of the worst predators by educating themselves about prevention and increasing their awareness and knowledge of how these heinous acts of violence occur. Think of it this way: If everyone started paying attention to what everyone else was doing, all would be visible. Predators are successful at attacking us because we are not paying enough attention.

It is an uphill battle introducing situational awareness and surveillance detection into the mainstream. But imagine if every woman in our country received affordable training in just these two preventative measures. Our belief is that the many tragic stories of abductions, rapes, and murders would appear in the news much less frequently. Women have the ability to become empowered to prevent the violence against them; they just need information, training, and guidance. Sadly our judicial system is endangering us by releasing these predators and allowing them to roam unsupervised. Women must realize that, until the judicial system is reformed so that women (and children) are protected from these sick predators, it truly is our duty to do more to protect ourselves and our children. Yes, the Constitution affords us the right to live under the protection of the law, but unfortunately it no longer provides us with the privilege to be safe. Our best hope is to work to reform the system so that the laws protect us rather than endanger us and to take charge of our own personal security until the law catches up and functions as it was intended.

Situational awareness and surveillance detection skills will help give back some of the control to you. When you can use your analytical, objective mind to assess the threats against you, those threats lose some of their emotional pull on your 'fear strings' and you are able to empower yourself with survival *skills* rather than a basic emotional desire to survive that is not reinforced by action. Imagine a mother whose child fears a monster is living under her bed. The mother knows to look under the bed to confirm or deny if anything or anyone is under there, even if only to ease her child's fears. She does not ignore her child and allow the child to go on suffering in quiet apprehension and anxiety. In the same way, if you approach your own underlying fear of being abducted, raped, or murdered and address it rather than denying it, you can confront it proactively by getting SASD rather than living with a subtle but constant, silent apprehension. By remembering that the worst crimes against us do not "come out of nowhere," we protect ourselves and our families from the devastation of their impact.

CHAPTER TWELVE

DEFENSIVE TACTICS
AND TOOLS

*"It is necessary to develop a strategy
that utilizes all the physical conditions
and elements that are directly at hand.
The best strategy relies upon
an unlimited set of responses."*

--Morihei Ueshiba

Brace yourself; our approach to this topic is somewhat unconventional. Our diverse backgrounds in physical training and mental conditioning shape our perspective on this topic. We have fused our experiences in order to offer you a unique perspective and a host of useful principles and techniques that will apply to your physical safety. We want every reader, no matter how short, tall, thin, over-weight, young, old, able-bodied or disabled you are, to know that everything in this chapter is for you. Even if you cannot physically manage the technique, some principle will apply to your ability level and will bolster your physical security.

We both come from backgrounds in a variety of types of movement training and mental conditioning practices. My training in meditation and in the internal martial arts (a decade in Taiji and two years in Aikido), my seven years as an improvisational dancer, and my current practice of yoga shapes my perspective. Bill comes from a background of twenty-five years of soldiering. He was a U.S. Army Special Forces operator and is a highly skilled warrior. He has trained in and tested techniques from the martial arts and self-defense schools. He has the unique perspective of being both the hunted and the hunter in urban and rural environments. He has clocked years of implementing hard, decisive tactics in realistic training environments and real world scenarios, including patrolling in woods and implementing rapid assessment, decision making, and survival skills. Bill also participated in the Trojan Warrior Project, in which he and a group of Special Forces operators spent six months conducting intensive meditation and martial arts training as a means of enhancing the warrior spirit and abilities.

When discussing this chapter, we decided that women can benefit from the warrior perspective and apply it to their own self-defense practice in creative ways that are more suitable to their feminine disposition. In other words, by tapping into the elite operator mindset women can access proven techniques and hidden mechanisms that apply to any type of confrontational situation or attack. You do not have to train like a male warrior in order to learn to protect yourself and glean the value of the warrior mentality. At the same time, we decided that an internal, meditative approach was also particularly valuable for women, especially when it comes to things like improving balance, stability on one's feet, and centeredness in one's body, mind, and emotions.

In this chapter we will guide you to open your mind to the topic of self-defense. You do not need to be totally in shape and agile in order to defend yourself. We encourage you to take a bit of time to explore, both internally and externally, the principles and techniques we think are most valuable to you. You will be able to use this chapter as a resource that you can revisit from time to time so that you can establish a defensive tactics plan and then refresh your skills whenever needed. What is important is for you to begin developing a defensive plan in the event you are ever attacked so that you reduce your odds of becoming a victim. That plan may include use of self-defense techniques and defensive tools. In this chapter our objective is to provide you with some basic ground truths about self-defense training and use of defensive tools. We will also encourage you to know yourself and be realistic about your capabilities when deciding which techniques and tools might work for you and what type of self-defense training you might like to pursue.

The truth is that with any physical defensive art, it takes years of dedication and practice to become proficient enough to handle yourself in any attack situation. Unless you are an expert in an art, it may just over-amplify your confidence and give you a false sense of security. The same can be true for use of a weapon; it often takes extensive training under a professional instructor to become proficient with traditional weapons, such as firearms. Yet any confrontation can still become a hit or miss venture. Even police officers and soldiers with years of training lose sometimes. However, any training in either defensive tactics or in the use of weapons will help increase your situational awareness (even if the only action you take comes in the form of reading this book and discussing it with others). In a perfect world you would not need any training in the use of tactics or weapons, but since that perfect world is not happening, we would like to explore these topics using what we consider to be a realistic approach.

Defensive Tactics

Our Philosophy

We are providing this chapter and readying you to handle yourself when under physical attack because we are not naïve about the dangers women face. Even if you practice everything we have taught you in this book, we cannot guarantee that you will never be at the hands of a man who is bigger than you, stronger than you, and who intends to beat you, rape you, or kill you. If you ever find yourself in these dire circumstances, having a plan will empower you to be able to channel your fears into energy and focus so that you can perform and survive. Thus we encourage you to make the choice now to learn as much as you can about defending yourself during an attack so that, if you ever are attacked, you will respond in the best way possible. By empowering yourself with and rehearsing defensive principles and techniques you will begin to carry yourself physically in a stronger, more self-reliant way because you know you have a back-up plan. You will also develop an apparent discerning awareness and self-confidence which will enable you to spot predators early on and deter them from targeting you in the first place.

Although your goal is to avoid confrontation by getting SASD so that you can see and sense trouble and steer clear of it *before* it escalates into an immediate threat, you must also prepare yourself to handle an attack. Detecting early warning signals is critical to being able to maintain your mental focus and strategize during an attack. By reading this chapter and having a plan to survive an attack you will increase your chances of being able to process the early warning signals, respond appropriately, and escape the danger. Every attack includes many random variables and chances to make a mistake and be injured or killed. The reality is that most women are just not as physically strong as most men. If we throw into the equation a man who is under the influence of drugs, has mental problems, or is a career criminal we realize that even a woman who is a trained martial arts expert could be physically overpowered. Physical prowess is only a small part of physical self-defense. The larger part is tactical ability or the ability to strategize.

We strongly advocate receiving self-defense training if you have the time, the inclination, and the capability. All self-defense training will assist you in expanding your knowledge base and adding more tools to your personal security toolbox. Perhaps one simple technique you learn in self-defense training will save your life one day. For that reason alone, we strongly encourage all women to receive some scenario based self-defense training at least once and the sooner the better. In any self-defense class you can always work to your ability and accommodate whatever physical limitations you have. Once again it is important to know yourself. Signing up for an aggressive martial arts self-defense class at a crowded dojo when you are already time taxed, perhaps out of shape, and over-tired may only make you feel more stressed. Do not set yourself up for failure or make yourself feel disempowered.

Instead, consider obtaining training in self-defense as a group with other women (friends from work; neighbors; friends from church; at your health club; through the YWCA or Junior League, etc.). Make it affordable and use each other as a support system so that you can make it fun and inspiring. Be bold and use collective bargaining to have your employer pay for self-defense training or organize an event to raise money for the tuition. College and high school students should request and try to organize classes as part of the school curriculum, through the physical education training program.

We recommend classes that are specifically oriented towards women and are based on practical training with mock attackers wearing full protective equipment. Make sure the training is not a single person operation; you want training that incorporates multiple instructors, both male and female, and uses common attack scenarios. Ideally you should be learning progressively to handle everything from verbal harassment to full-on surprise attacks. The idea is to gradually expose you to the fear and shock you feel when harassed, threatened, or assaulted, and teach you how you can best respond. The training goal is to manage the fear and shock of an attack so you minimize and prevent "freezing" (the most common reaction by women who are attacked). Your responses should also cover the full range from verbal warnings and boundary establishment to immediate and explosive defensive measures when they are warranted. Training should also include scenarios where an attacker has you pinned to the ground and grabbed from behind. Organizing high quality, collective self-defense training with other women is the ideal. In our vision of a responsible world all girls would be offered self-defense training before they reach adolescence.

Although we present some simple self-defense techniques in this chapter, we do not consider them to be a replacement for training. We would like to first introduce you to programs in existence that we find beneficial. One program that we think is excellent is called *IMPACT Personal Safety* (see Appendix E). Through *IMPACT* you can receive full-force self-defense training and you will have the opportunity to practice the techniques on men who are wearing full protective gear. *IMPACT* also gives women the opportunity to practice defending themselves against multiple assailants. *IMPACT* training is centered on the belief that "Good communication skills are the foundation of personal safety and well-being." They offer on-site personal safety and assertiveness training for corporations, community organizations, and schools. They also have several locations throughout the country where they offer classes for women, teens, children, and men. Their certified instructors are "dedicated to ending the cycle of violence." What we like about the *IMPACT* program is that it focuses on realistic scenario training and on helping women and children improve their awareness, self-esteem, and confidence.

Another excellent self-defense training program is conducted by Melissa Soalt (a.k.a. Dr. Ruthless). Melissa, a Black Belt Hall of Fame recipient, has DVD and video programs of her techniques and conducts training for women's organizations all over the country and internationally. What we like about Melissa is her feisty attitude. Her underlying philosophy is in alignment with ours in that she encourages women who are under attack to "shed their conditioning and summon their animal selves." She advocates "shifting from shock to fierceness" when under attack. In her seminars and DVD's she instructs her students to practice releasing their most basic animal instinct to survive, and teaches them how to channel this power into focused, full-force methods that facilitate escape. Melissa has dedicated her career to helping women evolve to a place of physical and emotional empowerment so that, if the worst prevails, they are ready and able to perform and survive. She teaches women to "bring to bear their physical strength and will to survive by learning gross motor skills they can use against their attackers' vulnerabilities." We commend her for her work. What we like about Melissa's techniques is that they do not require a lot of strength or agility. Women of all shapes, sizes, and ages can perform the majority of her techniques. We recommend you look at her website (especially if you are in a high threat situation) where she provides women with useful self-defense tips and insights (see Appendix E).

Regardless if you have already taken self-defense classes or are unable to do so, the following self-defense strategy will help you get started on your way to reconnecting with your physical instinct and ability to survive an attack.

Introduction to GAME ON!

GAME ON! means the attack is happening and you must immediately go on the offensive and implement the following:

1. Rapid Decision Making: Because the threat has escalated, you have limited time to make decisions. Use your intuition, decide, and immediately commit to executing that decision. You must commit 100% to each decision you make. If one does not work, try another.

2. Surprise: In order to surprise your attacker you will immediately and with a 100% commitment deliver decisive and explosive defensive techniques and/or mental strategies. Because your attacker will never be expecting you to "fight dirty" like a street fighter or behave in an unexpected way, you may be able to surprise him and create an opening to escape. He is expecting to control you, so a radical shift of any kind on your part will surprise him. You may talk with him in a manner that creates this radical shift (for example by pretending to be attracted to him or complying with his wishes).

3. Movement: Your response to the attack will involve some type of movement, even if it is as simple as turning sideways to allow your attacker to pass as he is approaching you. Whether you are implementing one of the techniques we describe below or are simply moving around your attacker, your emphasis should remain on surprising him and escaping. You might use side-stepping, reversing direction, entering, blending, speed variations, and stillness as part of your movement strategy. The point is to understand that you must employ your body and surprise your attacker through your movements.

10 Steps to Preparing for GAME ON!

Before we describe specific defensive moves, we want to introduce some basic principles that apply to preparing yourself for GAME ON! These are principles you can use to strategize your way out of the attack successfully. The very act of reading these principles will help you shift your mental template towards this subject and assist you in formulating a plan. Perhaps you have some vague notion in your mind as to what you would do if attacked (for example, many women carry their keys between their fingers because they have been told that this readies them to defend themselves against an attacker). Our objective is to teach you to plan proactively rather than taking last minute measures that may or may not work. The weight of fear that many women feel about being attacked is partially the result of their lack of understanding that they do possess many instinctive skills upon which they can rely during an attack.

1. Develop Your Resolve: Know yourself and know in advance what you feel is worth defending. In other words, could you take a life if it meant defending your own? Would you take a firm stance and resist your attacker by defending yourself during a violent encounter? Would you be willing to fight for what you believe in and who you are? Where do you draw the line in the sand? Some women are determined never to be raped and would fight their way out of it or die trying. Other women would surrender their bodies in order to preserve their lives. You must develop your resolve in your mind so that you mentally prepare yourself to respond with whatever level of engagement you are willing to accept. When you begin to ready yourself mentally for the prospect of a physical attack you will be more likely to respond as you intend to respond, thereby retaining some level of control during the attack.

2. Be a Moving Target: If you remain in motion, it will be more difficult for your attacker to control you. It is dangerous for you to stand still and be even-weighted in your stance because you make it easier for your attacker to knock you off balance. When a tennis player is waiting to receive an opponent's serve, he/she will shift his/her weight back and forth between his/her legs and create a slight jumping motion in order to remain ready to move in any direction when the serve lands in the court. If under attack, you too should shift your weight back and forth and have a spring in your step so that you are ready to move in any direction and escape.

Make it a habit to avoid passing through or spending time in any dangerous areas. If you must pass through a dangerous area, identify this ahead of time and move through the area quickly and unpredictably. Develop 360 degree awareness. If you feel uncomfortable, get moving and scan the entire area. Remember that you can always turn, spin, reverse direction, or join up with a group of people in the area as a means of moving away from or avoiding an attacker. Often an unpredictable move on the victim's part will foil a predator's plan. That last second, unexpected change will alert the predator that the victim knows she is about to be attacked and may cause the attacker to decide against pursuing this unpredictable victim.

3. Look for Pre-Attack Indicators: Pay attention to the posturing and gestures of someone approaching you. What is his demeanor like? Are your instincts telling you he is trouble? Is he being verbally hostile or aggressive with you? Is he talking down to you, dominating the conversation, or trying to shame you or attack your self-esteem? Is he ignoring your "No"? Is he trying to close the distance between you or herd you into an isolated area? Is he blocking your access to an exit? These are the last second early warning signals, so pay close attention.

Keep your distance (end the conversation, cross the street, pick up the pace), maintain your balance (physical and emotional), and do anything to put an obstacle between you and him (walk next to another pedestrian, enter a public location). Radiate an attitude of confidence, alertness, and determination to defend yourself. Let him know through your body language that you see him and are unwilling to play his game. Or, if you sense your best option and the least dangerous path is to become friendly or placate him then take this approach for the moment. Follow your intuition and notice the early warning signals he is presenting. Assess the situation and location for possible escape options. Does he seem like an attacker who will respond to a negotiation? Use your best judgment and if one tactic fails, try another. Rely on your situational awareness, intuition, cunning, and even your feminine wiles to estimate the situation and find a safe way out of the danger. If you make a choice not to defend yourself, let it be because you have realistically assessed the situation and have determined it is far too dangerous, at least in the moment, to use self-defense tactics or tools.

4. Accept the Attack as Real: Many women who have survived violent attacks have reported that they experienced disorientation, confusion, or a surreal, dream-like numbness. Many say they went into shock and were paralyzed by fear. If under attack, you must embrace your situation. Denial of either the fact that you are on the verge of being attacked or that you actually have fallen under attack is your number one worst enemy! Denial is neither a tactic nor a tool; it is a solid concrete roadblock obstructing your path to survival. *You must accept your reality as it is in order to be able to function within it.* Do not allow your internal monologue to make such statements as: "This can't be happening." If you are lying to yourself about being attacked or are pretending it is not really happening you are handing your attacker your life on a silver platter. Immediate acceptance of the sudden or unexpected escalation in the level of violence will free your mind so that you can focus on your escape strategy. You can obtain acceptance automatically by virtue of deciding in advance to recognize danger and follow your training. In other words, you do not have to coach yourself when under attack by saying: "This is really happening." Rather, by reading about this concept right now, accepting it as authoritative, and filing it in your mind's database you are already on the way to being able to respond automatically with acceptance of the reality of any dangerous situation.

The most common reactions to an attack are shock and the inability to move and respond. If you are SASD, the likelihood that you will be taken totally by surprise is reduced significantly. Even if you are surprised, just saying the word "attack" to yourself will help you deflate the effect of the shock. If you practice rehearsing in your mind being attacked, saying the word "attack" to yourself, and visualizing yourself responding by escaping or fighting back in a way where you prevail, you can pre-instruct your mental template towards surviving. If you move out of being frozen, you can then move in to becoming as fierce as you need to be given the specifics of the attack. You must give yourself permission, psychologically at first, to be that fierce animal using her instincts and cunning to prevail. It is okay to see yourself this way; it does not mean you are any less feminine. On the contrary, conceptually speaking you are like a wild cave woman protecting herself against primitive man. Take ownership of your evolutionary role and flip on that switch in your mind first so that your body will be able to follow the commands of your brain.

If you are surprised by an attacker, momentarily sink your center and ground yourself internally, while retaining that spring in your step so that you are ready to move in any direction. Keep your balance and focus your body and mind. You can practice this by having a partner approach you and grab onto to your shoulders or upper body. As he/she grabs you, sink your weight slightly, exhale slowly, and steady your body and mind. Do not ground yourself to the point where you freeze and become stuck. The idea is to momentarily center your body and mind, while maintaining the intention to get moving out of the attack as soon as you regain your composure from the initial jolt.

5. Break Contact: Your immediate and ultimate goal in any attack situation is escape. Do not worry about revenge or counterattacking. Get away from the danger to the nearest safe location. Breaking contact when you sense an attack is imminent is the quickest, surest way of escaping. During an attack keep looking for any possible way to break contact and escape. Drop and abandon anything that inhibits your ability to move quickly, such as any bags you are carrying. Things are replaceable; you are not.

6. Reverse the Surprise: Take the lead in the attack. No matter how stunned or surprised by the attack you are, turn it around and take the lead in the attack by stunning your attacker and breaking contact. Look for any way you can surprise him either mentally or physically, whether it be by shouting and screaming at the top of your lungs, catching him off balance, or using a strike when he least expects it. If you detect he wants to see fear in you, surprise him by going neutral. Perhaps you will carry an air horn or personal alarm for surprising him. Perhaps you will stun him with something you say or do that is out of the ordinary. For example, if you are about to be raped and see no way out, you might surprise him by pretending to be interested in having sex with him and even by offering to make him more comfortable. Or you might shock him by saying you have a sexually transmitted disease or by telling him you are on your period. No matter how you accomplish it, the idea is to reverse the surprise and then stun and run.

In every attack there are openings that the victim can exploit. Your attacker will have vulnerabilities. Look for them as the attack is happening. His body shape, size, and position in relation to your body could present you with some type of opening. Perhaps he is leaning forward and you can pull him to the ground. Perhaps your hand is conveniently located in close proximity to his groin or eyes. As the attack moves, move with it and look for openings so that you can participate and regain some control.

Sometimes an opening relates to the psychology of your attacker. For example, if he keeps making threats this usually means that he is not confident that he has you under his total control. If he can see by your reaction to his approach that you are not convinced he is the one in control, then he will continue making threats in order to build his confidence and to get you to capitulate. You can use this opening as ammunition to maintain some of the control and then reverse the surprise. You can manipulate him into *believing* he has total control so that he develops a false sense of confidence and may relax, thereby providing you with an opening for escape.

7. Stun and Run: If the opportunity presents itself, deliver an explosive and decisive counter-attack (usually a strike or blow) to stun your attacker so that you can run away. An unexpected and immediate blow to your attacker should give you an opening to run to a safe location. Be ready to run immediately and do not wait to observe your attacker's response to your strike.

We recommend you make up your own personal stun and run mantra that you can use to coach yourself during an attack, such as:

- Stun and run!
- Not this time!
- Take that!
- I knew it!
- Like hell you will!

Rehearse it under your breath as you practice the various strikes (discussed below) in slow motion. Coordinate saying your mantra to the delivery of your strike. This will help you to deliver smooth and unexpected strikes and to focus the power of your body.

8. Proximity and Closing the Distance: An attacker wants to close the distance between you and him. Do your best to prevent him from doing so, but remember that many men are faster in a short footrace and are physically stronger than most women. If he succeeds in closing the distance between you, turn this to your advantage and draw him in even closer so that you can use the proximity as a context for self-defense techniques that will work at close range (some of which we will give you later in this chapter). By moving into his attack instead of struggling to get away from him, you can trick his mind into believing he has accomplished his objective of grabbing and controlling you. Once he thinks he is in charge, he will relax his guard. You are now within reach to deliver a decisive counterattack. Once he senses that you are no longer struggling or fighting to escape, you can then surprise him by using close range defensive techniques.

9. Multiple Strategies: The best defense in any attack is what works in that particular situation. There are endless variables to every attack. You must assess the situation, on the spot, with acceptance and a will to survive by escaping. An attack is an evolving progression of movements and other elements. Consider yourself to be dancing with an enemy and move in an out of sync with him with the objective of breaking contact from this dance partner. Look for every opportunity to interfere with his ability to dominate the dance and control your body. This may involve creating a diversion or temporarily becoming compliant until an opening appears for you to take control. Yell, bite, plead, flea, reason or negotiate with him--do *whatever will work* for your specific situation. Embrace an empowered attitude and never give up on strategizing your way out of the attack. Realize that you may be required to fight for a long time before you are able to escape. Commit now, even as you read this, by imagining yourself surviving an attack that lasts for thirty minutes. Activate your will to survive and strengthen it so that it becomes far superior to your attacker's intention to hurt or kill you.

10. Avoid Being Taken to a Second Location: Never allow your attacker to take you to a second location. This may be unavoidable but do your best to prevent it from happening. If you end up at a second location, it is not necessarily a death sentence. It will, however, require you to go through much more in order to extricate yourself from the control of this person because you are now being introduced to the unknown. If you are under attack and he tries to take you somewhere else, do everything you can to talk him out of it, fight your way out of it, or elicit help to avoid it. If that means intentionally steering the vehicle you are in into a parked car or jumping out of a moving car in a location where help is right there, your odds of surviving the crash/jump may be better than the unknown that lies ahead with your attacker.

If your attacker succeeds in taking you to a second location, he now has the advantage of having you isolated and time is on his side. Even if he drags you off a jogging path and into the bushes, he gains the upper hand. Whenever an attacker attempts to take you to a second location, your response should be to fight or surprise him and make it as difficult for him as possible to move you anywhere. If he succeeds in taking you to a second location, do not give up! Keep looking for a way to escape.

Self-Defense Moves for GAME ON!

All defensive techniques revolve around one thing: movement. No matter what your physical abilities and limitations are, any type of movement training is beneficial in that it will promote greater awareness of your body and will build your confidence. Since your primary objective is to move out of an attack situation, any previous movement training will contribute to increasing your odds of escaping. If "knowledge is power" then self-awareness through movement training is empowerment. In other words, the more you know how to move, the more empowered you become.

Any type of exercise or movement you do helps you become more confident in your body. Studying any style of dance is excellent movement training; it helps maintain balance, equilibrium, and the ability to redirect an attacker and get out of his way to be able to escape. It is also a lot of fun! Yoga is great for focus, balance, strength and relaxation, all of which are key elements to surviving any kind of physical attack. Any martial art will help you train your concentration, alertness, and self confidence in your physical being. Kickboxing and self-defense classes are valuable in that they teach you about the vulnerable parts of your attacker's body, but since attacks involve so many dynamics you cannot guarantee that the opportunity will arise for you to effectively apply the techniques you have learned. Likewise, the size of the attacker is unknown, so, for example, a joint manipulation to the wrist might not be an option if your attacker's wrist is so thick that you cannot grip it appropriately to execute that particular technique.

There are some general techniques you should learn and integrate into your mind and body. First, if under attack, do not focus on the person. Rather, relax your vision and expand your peripheral vision, looking for weapons, escape routes, and help. Your primary goal is always to avoid or stun the attacker so that you can get away. Use your voice and create as much of a clamor as you can. Move as quickly as you can away from the attacker and towards help. If this fails and you are under his physical control, use your instinct. Every attack is different and there are no rules of engagement that are absolute. For example, if your attacker has you pinned on the ground, you may need to become compliant. Or, your instincts may tell you to scream and kick and fight. Retaining situational awareness is your best chance of survival because it will allow you to make decisions that are based on the reality of what is happening at that moment versus relying on something you rehearsed in a class once but that may not really work in this particular situation. Your adrenaline will be pumping like crazy, but keeping your mind clear is what will save you. Any attack will require you to make multiple choices in a very short span of time. You do have an enormous ability to help shape the outcome, especially if you have a plan and do not freeze or get side-tracked worrying about what to do. Remember, your attacker is a human being with emotions, cognition, reasoning capabilities, and some degree of logic. Even a seriously mentally disturbed attacker or one who is under the influence of drugs or alcohol can be manipulated. Your body may not be your primary tool in surviving most attacks; your mind, however, is an invaluable asset.

The value of any movement you practice is that, over time, you program your body's muscle memory. Your muscles can literally remember movement. The more you train, the stronger your muscle memory will become and you will be more likely to respond physically in an appropriate way to keep yourself safe. When you train in any kind of movement, you are creating a plan for your neuro- pathways to follow. When under attack your body is likely to respond according to what you have practiced the most, what you have practiced recently, or with the response you have planned and visualized. The more you train your body and mind, the more apt you are to invoke an appropriate response if under attack.

We are limiting the techniques in this chapter to those that the majority of women can do successfully, no matter their physical condition, shape, size, or skill level. As with all forms of movement, we recommend working to your ability level and taking care of yourself. If you have any injury or condition that limits you when conducting the techniques below, then just read about the techniques or practice them in a way that works for your body (for example, in slow motion).

Your Voice: Find your rebel yell (a blood-curdling, forceful yell that you can sustain). This is easy to do and will only require a small amount of practice on your part. Once you find your rebel yell you will easily be able to retain it and use it at any time. To find your rebel yell you want to imagine an explosion of sound. Put your hand on your belly and inhale until you feel your belly rising and your hand moving. Blast out a sound as you tighten your belly and lean forward a bit. The type of sound you make is not what matters. What is important is for you to experience that sudden, powerful verbal detonation that is loaded with the intention to stun and surprise an attacker. Experiment with pitch until you find what feels the most powerful for your voice. Practice both a short blast of sound and a longer sustained yell. You are using your voice as a weapon so that you can stun your attacker and run. Learn to release your rebel yell so that you can use this instrument in a powerful and intimidating way during an attack. Finding your rebel yell will empower you and practicing it will allow you to increase your projection level so that you can deliver your yell as strongly as possible. It will boost your confidence and allow you to relax knowing that you are "armed" with your rebel yell at all times.

Your voice is a powerful tool if utilized properly. Fear and freezing during an attack may inhibit your ability to project your voice. Some women literally cannot speak due to fear when they are under serious threat of physical harm. The best way to capitalize on your voice is to practice. Your vocal chords and diaphragm are basically muscles you can train by doing simple vocal exercises. Singing loudly to the radio when driving will help you strengthen the power and projection of your voice. Rehearse what you would yell. Practice barking orders like: "No!" or "Back off!"

You must also practice what you would say if addressing strangers to get help while you are being attacked. Would you say: "Call the police" or "Help me" or "Call 911"? Practice and try to keep your phrases short and to the point. Practice delivering them as commands, not pleas. You must relay a sense of authority with your voice when commanding someone to help you. If you yell "Somebody call 911 now!" you will give an instruction that someone can follow. It would be better if you make eye contact with and point to a specific person and command: "You, call 911 now!" or "You, watch which direction he runs in." On the contrary, if you yell "Please help me" you are requesting something and relying more on someone's charity than on his/her ability to follow a simple instruction. People may be more apt to get involved if you deliver it as a command versus a request they can mull over and decline.

Finger Jab: Find a spot on a mirror that is slightly higher than your head and is within reach of your arm's length. Begin by using your index finger only. Reach up and gently poke the mirror in that spot. Repeat this several times. Now, open your hand and using all of your fingers reach up and gently touch the mirror in the area of the spot you picked. Next, back away from the mirror and reach out your arm, fingers spread, and strike the air more forcefully (do not hit the mirror and break your fingers!). Practice this with alternating hands and repeat it several times. You will look like you are a boxer jabbing the air with your fingers. If it helps, watch a boxing match so that you can see this jabbing motion in action. Also, you can practice on your car visor while you are stuck in traffic. Just pick a point and jab gently.

The finger jab is an effective technique and does not require strength. The objective of this technique is to quickly jab your attacker in the eyes with your fingertips so that you can compromise his vision, cause him pain, and surprise him. You only have to hit one of his eyes in order to cause both of them to close immediately, giving you an opening to run away. If he is wearing glasses strike him just below his glasses on his cheek in order to push his skin up into his eyes.

The finger jab is one of the most difficult strikes for a predator to avoid because it is a fast flick delivered at arm's reach, thus your attacker has little time to see it coming. This technique is most effective if delivered as your attacker is lunging towards you and before he has you under his control. You can master the finger jab very quickly, regardless of your limitations. By practicing this technique you will prevent yourself from freezing during an attack. Plus, you will bolster your self-confidence knowing that you can very easily execute this technique if you will just take the time to practice it. Do not worry about hurting yourself, breaking a fingernail, or being too aggressive. Some women misinterpret this technique and think they are required to gouge out their attacker's eyes. This is not necessary; a simple, abrupt jab to the eyes is all it takes. Put aside your squeamishness and realize that you could be defending your life using this technique one day.

Head Butt: (Note: If you have any neck problems, we advise you to practice this very slowly and work to your limit). The head butt is a useful technique if your attacker is in close to you. Your head, if used properly, can get you out of many dangerous situations. Like the finger jab, the head butt is effective because it is a quick strike, one which your attacker will not expect. The head butt is easy to learn and practice. It is a useful technique if your attacker has grabbed you and you are close to his face. His nose is the target of your head butt.

Butt your head into his nose with either the right or left corner of your forehead. The crown of the head is too soft, so do not use it for a head butt. Only butt with the center of your forehead as a last resort because doing so may impair your vision as you run to escape. The best parts of the head are located above your brow on either side of the front of your forehead. You can feel how hard the bone is on both sides of your forehead.

To practice, hold up a pillow close to you and pretend it is your attacker's head. Pull the pillow towards you and very slowly toss your head into a center spot (perhaps indicated by something in the pattern on the pillowcase). Practice using both sides of your forehead for several repetitions. Try not to telegraph the movement by leaning the head back to wind up and create momentum. This will give your attacker an early warning signal that you are about to head butt him.

Elbow Strikes: Like the head butt, elbow strikes are effective when you are trapped in close proximity to your attacker. Elbows are hard and pointed, thus are best used when you are next to an attacker who is trying to grab and embrace you. If he has grabbed you and you know he has the upper hand, relax momentarily. In this way you will steal his mind because you will make him believe he is in total control of your body. Tricking his mind like this will also enable you to get within range of your target (ideally, his nose or under his chin). When you are in range you can reverse the surprise by striking him with your elbows.

With minimal practice you can deliver powerful, stunning blows. Stand where you have some space around you. You can begin this exercise slowly and then work up to stronger, more forceful strikes. Work to your ability level. First practice using your elbow to strike an imaginary person in front of you. Keep your hands in a fist during each strike. Alternate elbow strikes from the right and left arms for several repetitions. Now do the same but out to the sides of your body (as though your attacker were standing next to you rather than in front of you). Alternate right to left elbows for several repetitions. Next pretend as though your attacker were standing behind you. Alternate right to left elbows for several repetitions.

Your elbows can also be used to form a shield. If you lock your fingers together and arc your elbows out to form an isosceles triangle, you can create a shield with your arms and use it to protect yourself as you move out of an attack. Practice with a half opened door. Form your shield and use it to push the door open and run away. The idea is that the half opened door is your attacker and you would be using your shield to push him aside as you move forward to escape.

Heel of Hand Strike: You can also strike using the heel of your hand (the bottom area of your palm). Delivering a sudden and explosive strike to the nose or temple of your attacker may buy you time to escape. You can strike hard using the heel of your hand without hurting yourself but still inflicting pain to your attacker. Striking with the heel of your hand is more stable than punching with your fist. You can practice these strikes the same way you practice the elbow strikes above (to the front and sides only). The idea is to snap the heel of the hand onto the targeted area (your attacker's nose or temple).

High--Low--High: This technique is a way of combining all of the techniques you have just learned. You can resort to this technique if the stun and run technique has failed and your attacker has not released you. Therefore, you must continue your counterattack until you have an opportunity to escape. High—low—high will allow you to capitalize again on the element of surprise because he will not be expecting you to fight. If you are predictable in delivering your strikes, he will see your pattern and will cut around you or turn away and get behind you. By alternating techniques and targeted areas of his body, you can continue to reverse the surprise and keep him guessing.

The idea is to start high and deliver a finger jab to his eyes or a head butt to his nose. Next, immediately move low and deliver a strike or kick to the groin area, the knee caps, or a stomp to his foot. Then, as soon as he bends over from the low strike, you move high again towards his upper body, face, or head and deliver a third strike, such as an elbow strike to his nose or throat. You can also try to pull him down to the ground. As soon as you have the opportunity, run away. Do not stay in the fight because you are taking the risk that he will regain the upper hand.

You can practice by using a pillow wedged into a door jam or with a partner. When you practice this combination of techniques, move very slowly and carefully. Your objective is to train your muscles and your nervous system so that your body integrates this drill. Save the high speed, heavy training for the punching bag at the gym or for your self-defense class. Slow, smooth practice will prepare you to be able to deliver quick, controlled strikes.

Improvisation: Improvisation is the ultimate manifestation of situational awareness because it requires you to be totally present and respond appropriately in the moment. One of the most useful skills you have at your disposal is improvisation. Anytime you are inventing or executing something in the moment or on the spot, you are improvising. We all improvise in our daily lives whether in conversations with strangers, in situations that require our attention, or when trying to provide solutions to problems at work.

Musicians, dancers, actors, and artists use improvisation in their work. This means they develop techniques and skills that they can then apply freely to their mediums with creativity and spontaneity. You too have skills and abilities you can call forth to improvise your way out of dangerous situations. The beauty of improvisation is that it is so easy to practice: all you have to do is stay present and creatively approach situations. For example, even if you are home cleaning the house, you can practice improvisation while moving the vacuum cleaner around by amplifying your awareness of the spaces around which you are maneuvering the device. You can make quick 90 degree turns, controlled spins around and in between the furniture (even by holding the cord as though it were your child's hand). This might sound silly to you, but translated to self-defense it means that you will be training yourself to move quickly and fluidly around obstacles, a very useful technique during any attack.

Always remember that your primary objective during any attack is to escape as quickly and safely as possible. If you choose to take a self-defense class, you could help yourself immensely in terms of your physical safety. However, if you are unable, for whatever reason, to study self-defense you can still read about it and at least train your mind to think through attack scenarios. None of us enjoys the idea that we might come under attack one day. Being an empowered woman means allowing yourself to embrace this possibility proactively, even in the midst of the fear that may arise when you think about the subject.

Defensive Tools

Defined, defensive tools are any traditional weapons or other objects that can be used to aid in self-defense. Traditional weapons include such things as guns, knives, and pepper spray. Objects that can be used as weapons include baseball bats, ashtrays, and keys. Ideally you should only need to use defensive tools if you are in a situation where the threat is escalating or if you suddenly come under a surprise attack. All defensive tools supplement your physical self-defense skills. You would greatly limit yourself if you relied solely on defensive tools. If you are SASD, you should not need them at all, because you will detect danger early on and avoid it altogether. However, if you are in a high threat situation or fall under attack you might want to consider using defensive tools.

Our Philosophy

Defensive tools and weapons are not a panacea or a guarantee of your safety. However, they can and may save your life one day. If you intend to utilize them, be realistic and do not allow yourself to have a false sense of security. Weapons tend to offer a false sense of security in that they allow you to relax a bit mentally because you are relying on the weapon to save you, versus relying on your situational awareness and mental prowess. A weapon is best viewed as a possible accessory to your defense, not a solution. Even though carrying some kind of weapon or defensive tool can mitigate your fears about being attacked, you must also consider that any weapon or tool can be used against you if your attacker is successful in taking it away from you. Each attack is a unique story and a weapon that is appropriate in one situation, may end up hurting you in another. You must use your instincts and situational awareness to decide if utilizing a weapon is a good choice.

10 Rules for Using Tools in GAME ON!

1. Weapons only Support Your Security: A weapon or defensive tool is like having a reserve parachute or spare tire and jack in the trunk of your car; you use them in emergencies and only as an added means of support. You should not rely solely on any weapon because too many things can go wrong. For example, the weapon might malfunction or your attacker might take it away from you and use it against you.

2. Choosing a Weapon: Know yourself. Does the thought of owning a gun make you feel pressured or fearful? Does the mention of pepper spray make you nervous? What tools would you be comfortable using and having in your home and vehicle? What would help you feel safer because it would bolster your confidence? Does sleeping with a baseball bat under your bed appeal to you?

Would you be willing to spend time receiving training in how to use any particular tools or weapons? Stay inside your comfort factor when choosing defensive tools. Realize that responsibilities arise when you purchase and possess a weapon. You must receive professional instruction in order to handle and use weapons responsibly.

3. Accessibility/Carrying Defensive Tools: Whatever tools you decide to use, be sure you carry them appropriately. It will not do you any good to have your pepper spray or TASER device buried in the bottom of your purse while walking to your car in a secluded parking garage. If you are going to carry any tools then you must literally carry them in your hands, even if your hands are in your pockets. Know when to carry your tools. Normally you will carry them during transition times (such as right before you exit your workplace to walk to your car or when you are passing through dangerous areas). At home, make sure your tools are within reach and are pre-positioned and ready to go.

For example, keep your pepper spray on the floor near the bed, within reach of where you sleep.

4. Equipment Checks: Be sure to keep your defensive tools in good working order and conduct equipment checks on them periodically. You will not actually use your tools very often, but when you need them, you will need them 100%. Make sure the batteries are charged and test to be sure everything works properly. Perhaps you have a can of mace that your brother gave you for Christmas ten years ago and when you tried to spray a dog that was charging you, it did not work. Do not "live and learn" the hard way. If you are in a high threat situation, you should be performing regular checks of your equipment. Doing so will help you become empowered and build your confidence.

5. Practice: Whatever tool you decide to carry or keep in your home, practice using it. Make sure you are comfortable with its controls, buttons, noises, and effects. For example, if you carry pepper spray, practice using it outside so that you know how the mechanism works and you have experience in spraying it. Even a simple tool like a flashlight or personal alarm requires some practice. You must know exactly where to turn on each device and you must be familiar with the brightness of the light and the sound of the alarm so that you do not end up frightening yourself. You can use mock weapons for training, if necessary (for example, pepper spray kits sometimes provide a training device). At a minimum you should practice making the transition between carrying the tool in the ready position to presenting the tool when an attack is imminent. Repeat this several times to integrate the drill into your muscle memory.

6. Presentation: The way you present a defensive tool during an attack is a critical element of its effectiveness. Since your objective is to escape, you must utilize your tools in such a way as to capitalize on their role in helping you reverse the surprise. Remember: Stun and run. This means that you want to carry the tool discreetly and present it in a way that takes your attacker by surprise. If you telegraph your movements or actions, you give your attacker greater ability to defeat you because you have taken away the element of surprise: he sees what is coming.

Another possibility for presentation is an open approach where you tell your potential attacker you have some type of weapon. This would be right before the attack and would be a strategy for deterrence. In some cases this could work. For example, if you called out: "I have a knife" or "I have mace" your attacker might decide to leave you alone. The potential problem with this approach is that you are giving him information and ruining your ability to surprise him. He now knows what he is up against and can quickly calculate a defense or counterattack. If you are carrying a handgun or a weapon that can inflict lethal force, you are wise to present the weapon and warn him to stay away from you (see section on Reasonable Force later in this chapter).

7. Prioritize: If you are confronted by more than one attacker and cannot escape, eliminate the greatest threat first. When deciding your priority target, realize that it will be situation dependent. For example, you may need to go after the nearest attacker, the most dangerous, the weakest, the one who has a weapon, or the one who is in the way of the exit. You must use your best judgment given the circumstances. Remember that you can reverse the surprise because the attackers are expecting you to be intimidated because you are outnumbered.

If you have multiple attackers, do not become overwhelmed. Move and do your best to surprise one of them with a decisive counterattack. If you are successful, the others may cut loose and run away because they see you are a difficult target who has just caused them trouble. If they continue to come after you, keep moving and look for opportunities to escape. If you cannot escape, continue to prioritize so that you can remain on the offense. You will likely be required to use weapons at hand (improvised tools) to reinforce your efforts against multiple attackers.

8. Stun and Run: Your ultimate goal is to break contact and escape the attack. Defensive tools are accessories that will aid your successful escape. If you are able to surprise your attacker and can steal his mind for even a brief moment, you may be able to create an opening for your escape. No matter which tools you opt to use (if any), you are not using them to stay in the fight and prevail over him. You are trying to escape. If you use a tool and are able to successfully stun him, run away immediately. If you are forced to stay in the fight because you cannot escape, then the circumstances will change and you will likely be required to fight to defend your life.

9. Shock Rebound Shock: If you are momentarily shocked by your attacker and you cannot move, embrace this moment of shock so that you can shift to your plan to rebound by delivering some type of decisive counterattack which will, in turn, shock your attacker. In addition, learn to capitalize on his shock. For example, if you sound an alarm and he is taken by surprise, do not wait for him to regain his composure. Keep moving your defense forward and give him another shock. Do not waste that critical moment when he is shocked by your decisive use of a defensive tool or technique.

10. You are Surrounded by Weapons: Anything can become a weapon. Open your mind and define the word weapon creatively. If you look around any room in your home, you will see lots of things that can be converted into weapons, such as lamps, chairs, small end tables, clocks, pictures on the walls, books, doors, and any stick-like object such as a cane. Anything is a weapon if you are creative enough to come up with a way to utilize it as one. Look for weapons at hand. You can practice this right now by looking around the room or area you are in and creatively assessing what could be used as a weapon in a moment's notice if you had to defend yourself. Bear in mind that your goal is the same: to escape or stun and run. This principle should help you relax because it gives you confidence that, in a pinch, you will be able to find a weapon. However, if you are in any high threat situation, do not rely on weapons at hand. Instead, choose and carry a weapon with which you feel comfortable and have practiced using.

Defensive Tools/Weapons for GAME ON!

Cell Phone:

What is it?
At this point in history you would have to be from another planet to need an answer to this question, but if that is the case... it is a small, portable, wireless telephone.

How does it work?
When you turn on the phone it sends signals to a tower allowing you to receive service and make and receive phone calls.

How is it used?
As a defensive tool, a cell phone can be used in a number of ways. First, it can be your lifeline for calling the police or 911 in the event of an emergency. If you have a cell phone camera you can use it to take a photograph of someone who is putting you under surveillance or who is threatening you. If you have a cell phone with a GPS device, your phone may be the authorities' best chance of finding you should you go missing. You can also use it in less threatening situations to call someone in your SUPNET to inform them about a potential threat or ask for help.

Where can I get one?
Many cell phone providers exist and offer a variety of calling plans. It is best to use a provider that offers the most roaming service in your area. It is also important when you travel out of your area to update your roaming capabilities so that your phone will work as well as possible when you are far from home.

   If you are in a high threat situation and cannot afford a cell phone you can try contacting women's advocacy groups in your area for assistance and support in obtaining one.

How can I get training?
Your phone will come equipped with an owner's manual. If you have problems learning how to use any feature on the phone, call your provider or go into one of their stores and ask for training. We strongly recommend you practice using the features of your phone so that if you need to access them in an emergency, you are capable of using them.

Why we like a cell phone:
We like cell phones because they offer you a way of getting help in an emergency. We also like the GPS feature that can be used to track your whereabouts. Cell phone cameras are excellent for your surveillance detection practice so that you can document images of suspicious people or vehicles. Cell phones can also be used to deter a predator (because he sees you have a way of calling for help). You can also use them to create a ruse to avoid a predator. For example, if a man is bothering you at a party, you can say: "Excuse me; I have to call my boyfriend to tell him to come meet me."

Special remarks:
Most cell phones will not allow you to program 911 on your speed dial. If you are in a dangerous area or situation, dial 911 and carry your phone so that all you have to press is the "send/enter/call" button to connect the call.

Take the time to know your phone well. Do not fall into the mindset of "This stuff is too technical for me." Cell phones are designed for normal people, not rocket scientists. You can operate your phone and all of its features if you are willing to take the time to learn and practice.

Whistle:

What is it?
A small device which produces a shrill, whistling sound.

How does it work?

Air is forced into the cavity of the device causing a small ball to turn and produce the high-pitched sound.

How is it used?
You can carry a whistle and easily blow into it when you wish to attract attention, make noise, and deter a predator.

Where can I get one?
Whistles are available in toy stores, at Army/Navy surplus stores, and online. We recommend the Fox 40 Classic whistle, as it has up to 115 decibels with an omni-directional sound and is therefore one of the loudest, most piercing sounds available in a whistle. It also has no moving parts inside of it (no ball) so it will not malfunction (www.fox40.com).

How can I get training?
Just put your lips on the mouthpiece and blow.

Why we like a whistle:
A whistle is inexpensive, easy to carry and use, and a simple tool for signaling for help and for attracting attention. You can have multiple whistles pre-positioned strategically in your vehicle, your home, your office, and on your person. Whistles are great defensive tools because they are easy to use, especially for children or people who are handicapped. They can also function as a back-up signaling device. For example, you can have whistles positioned in your home so that children or disabled family members can use them to signal for help in the night.

Special remarks:
A whistle is best used in combination with your voice. Alternate blowing the whistle with cries for help, so that bystanders do not ignore the whistle sound thinking it is a child playing.

Do not tie the whistle around your neck on a chain or string unless it has a break-away cord. Make sure you have your whistle out and ready for use when walking to your vehicle or making transitions from one location to another.

Personal Alarm:

What is it?
A small device that you can carry and trigger to sound an alarm to attract attention. The alarm will be louder and different from that of a car alarm.

How does it work?
Personal alarms usually come in a keychain or pager style. They are relatively inexpensive and are battery operated. When you press the alarm button you trigger a very loud, piercing sound. Some newer models are designed so that if you release your grip on them or remove a pin the alarm will sound.

How is it used?
A personal alarm is used to shock or dissuade an attacker by attracting attention. When you present a personal alarm during an attack, get it as close to your attacker's ears as possible. Literally jam it into his ear if he is in close range of you. He should react by trying to move away from the sound and this will give you your opportunity to escape or rebound with another defensive technique if necessary.

Where can I get one?
Personal alarms are widely available in technical equipment stores, in retail discount stores, in large hardware stores, and online.

How can I get training?
Read the instructions of the alarm you purchase and practice using it at home so that you familiarize yourself with the sound and decibel level. You do not want to shock yourself with the alarm, so become acquainted with its features and noise level. Practice using the buttons, carrying the alarm, and triggering it.

Why we like a personal alarm:
They are loud and are great for attracting attention and surprising your attacker. They are easy to use and carry and are affordable.

Special remarks:
Choose a personal alarm that does not sound anything like a car alarm. The sound should be so loud that it literally hurts your ears and forces you to cover them. Since personal alarms are battery operated, test them periodically to make sure the batteries are still good.

Air Horn

What is it?
An air horn is a small device that includes a rubber ball which you squeeze to make noise from the end of the horn.

How does it work?
You either squeeze the rubber ball or press a button to sound the horn.

How is it used?
It can be used to signal for help, as the sound is loud and unusual enough to attract attention.

Where can I get one?
At a party store, toy store, discount chain, or online.

How can I get training?
Read the instructions on the particular horn you purchase and practice using it.

Why we like an air horn:

They are easy to operate and make an unusual sound that is not so familiar that people will ignore it.

Special remarks:
Small air horns are good for carrying in your vehicle. However, they are generally too big to carry discreetly in your hand.

Flashlight:

What is it?
A hand held device that produces light.

How does it work?
Normally there is a button or switch you use to turn it on and off. Sometimes you turn a ring to operate the flashlight. Flashlights are battery operated.

How is it used?
We are strong advocates of carrying a small flashlight at all times. Flashlights are psychologically empowering because you can surprise an attacker and stop him in his tracks if the light is powerful enough. Light is a key element to survival if you are stranded someplace at night or are taken somewhere and put in a darkened room. It is important to be able to see to survive. In addition, a flashlight can be used as a striking instrument for self-defense.

You can use a flashlight to illuminate darkened areas you are approaching or areas where you hear noises before you commit to entering them. Shining light on an attacker will deter him because you will have taken away his element of surprise. If he is close to you, you can seriously impair his vision by temporarily blinding him so that you can get away. You can also use a light to signal for help if you are trapped somewhere. You can flash the light using Morse code for the internationally recognized distress signal SOS (three short flashes, three long flashes, three short flashes).

Where can I get one?

There are many inexpensive plastic flashlights that are widely available. The best, however, are the new generation of lights that were designed for use by police and the military. Our favorite is the SureFire E2D Executive Defender (www.surefire.com). You can buy a cheaper flashlight at any hardware store, Army/Navy surplus store, discount chain, or online.

How can I get training?

Flashlights are easy to operate. Depending on the type you purchase, practice turning it on and off.

Why we like a flashlight:

We like any flashlight because it provides you with a crucial component to your survival: light. We like the SureFire E2D Executive Defender for several reasons. First, it fits comfortably in your hand and has a clip attached to it so you can hook it on your purse strap. Second, it is easy to switch on and off using your thumb to click once on a button on the end of the flashlight. This is a very bright flashlight (60 lumens output for seventy-five minutes). It is impossible to stare into it without wincing or closing your eyes. It can temporarily blind your attacker if you shine it right into his eyes.

Special remarks:

The SureFire light can also be used as a striking weapon because it has a hard body that is constructed from aero-space grade aluminum. The best feature, however, is the Crenellated Strike Bezel (both ends have a wavy, sharp edge) allowing it to be used to strike someone or stun him. You could begin by shining the light into your attacker's eyes and, if you could not escape, you could rebound by striking him in the temple with the sharp edge of the light.

Since all flashlights are battery operated, inspect them often to be sure the batteries are working. Also, carry the light in your hands when transitioning in and out of your vehicle or walking alone at night into your home.

Kubotan:

What is it?
A kubaton is an ancient Japanese martial arts weapon used for striking. It is a short rod that fits comfortably inside your hand and extends out from either side about one inch. Traditionally it is made of wood and is about the diameter of a broom handle. Both ends should be rounded or tapered and blunt. You can strike from either end of a kubaton.

How does it work?
You simply hold the kubaton in your hand and, using a jabbing motion, strike your attacker, either from the front, to the side, or from behind. A kubaton channels the force of your strike into the blunt end of the device when it makes contact with your attacker. Since the force impacts the end of the kubaton, you do not have to be concerned about hurting your hand or wrist when delivering an explosive strike.

How is it used?
You can use a kubaton to strike your target in the nose, face, or head. Any hard, boney area is a good focus for your strike. Look for vulnerable or exposed areas on your attacker that you can strike to stun him and impair his ability to move or come after you. You can also strike his hand or arm if he has grabbed you. It is easy to carry discreetly and its power can be devastating, even though it is a simple design and is easy to use. Because your attacker normally will not see it in your hand, you can reverse the element of surprise and stun him and run. He will not see the strike coming if you carry the kubaton low or off to the side of your body before you raise your arm to deliver the strike.

Where can I get one?
Traditional kubatons are available online, in sporting goods stores, or martial arts supplies stores. You can also make a kubaton out of a piece of a broom

handle or any hard piece of wood or metal. Imagine a shortened chopstick or knitting needle that is thicker and blunt on both ends.

How can I get training?
If you purchase a traditional kubaton it may come with an instruction book that shows you various strikes. You can practice carrying and presenting this weapon by imagining an attacker and striking the air.

Why we like a kubaton:
We like its simplicity and power. We also like that any woman can carry it discreetly and learn to use it easily. You can also improvise in a pinch and use a ball-point pen or fork as a kubaton.

Special remarks:
Some kubatons are on key chains. We do not recommend keeping your keys with your kubaton so that your keys will not be left behind if you are forced to drop your kubaton and run away.

Pepper Spray or Gel/Mace:

What is it?
These are defensive sprays that contain strong irritants that affect the skin, eyes, and respiratory system upon exposure.

How does it work?
Most bottles contain a safety device so that you must turn a lever or flip a switch before you can press the button to spray. Some include a practice device so that you can safely learn to fire the device.

How is it used?
These sprays are used when in close range of an attacker. You spray into the attacker's face, while shielding or turning away your own face to prevent exposure. Normally your attacker will immediately drop to the ground or

cover his face and move away from the spray. This is your opportunity to run away and you must take it immediately since some attackers are not affected by these sprays for very long.

Be sure to spray as close to your attacker's face as possible. Do not telegraph this weapon because he will create distance and then might figure out a way to take it from you. Hold it low to the side of your thigh and when he is right up on you raise it and spray it directly into his face, while turning your face away from the spray or shielding your face from the residual mist.

Where can I get one?
You can order these sprays online or purchase them at Army/Navy surplus stores or gun stores (including sporting goods stores that sell firearms). You can also ask a local police officer where to purchase these sprays in your area.

How can I get training?
If your device includes a practice device you can train yourself. If not, thoroughly read the instructions and examine the device so that you feel comfortable using it in an emergency. Most manufacturers suggest that you test fire the device once in the sink or outdoors and they will instruct you how to do so.

Why we like pepper spray/gel and mace:
This tool, if administered properly, will give you the ability to stun your attacker and provide you adequate time to run away from him. Of all the varieties of available sprays, we prefer the mace spray that contains pepper gel. It does not create a mist when sprayed but rather shoots out a gooey gel that adheres to the attacker's skin.

Special remarks:
Some women feel very uncomfortable with these devices due to their own sensitivity to the spray. When you test fire a spraying device you will be able to discern if you have a hyper-sensitivity to the product (if you begin choking

and gagging even from a great distance). If this is the case, we do not recommend choosing this tool.

TASER Device:

What is it?
A TASER device is a defensive weapon that looks like a plastic gun and weighs approximately seven ounces. It is considered to be an energy device and it is the most advanced stun gun available.

How does it work?
The TASER device fires probes with wires that travel as far as fifteen feet and transmit an electric shock. Once the darts make contact with the target, it shocks the target.

How is it used?
The TASER device is used just like a hand gun. You point and shoot it at your attacker. You must keep it out of reach of children and use it responsibly. Never leave a TASER device unsecured.

Where can I get one?
Go to www.taser.com. Be sure to research information on permit requirements for owning and operating a TASER device in the state in which you reside.

How can I get training?
TASER International, Inc. manufactures all TASER devices. They provide training upon purchase of a TASER device and have excellent video training support.

Why we like the TASER device:
TASER devices are non-lethal weapons. They are easy to fire and do not make a loud noise. They provide women with the ability to take down an

attacker without inflicting lethal force. Many women do not wish to take on all of the responsibilities involved with owning handguns. TASER devices are a nice compromise, as they will allow you to temporarily control your attacker so you can escape.

Special Remarks:

The newest models of TASER devices are equipped with a cartridge that shoots out tiny confetti which contains the serial number of the specific device fired. This will become evidence in a police report. If a TASER device is stolen it can be traced because each device will only work with a registered, numbered cartridge. Thus when the thief orders a new cartridge, the company can trace the stolen device.

Be sure to receive training. You must announce your presentation of a TASER device, thereby warning your attacker and giving him the chance to stand down before you fire the device.

Firearms:

What is it?

Any firearm, be it a handgun, rifle, pistol, or revolver is capable of delivering deadly force to an attacker.

How does it work?

All firearms shoot bullets through a barrel and can inflict lethal force.

How is it used?

Firearms can be used to deter an attacker by presenting the gun and warning your attacker to stand down. They can also be used as a last resort for defending your life, either by inflicting injury on your attacker or by inflicting lethal force if you have no alternative in order to save your life.

Where can I get one?

Contact the National Rifle Association (NRA) for a reputable dealer in your area.

How can I get training?
Contact the NRA for a trainer in your area. More than likely the store from which you purchase the firearm will provide trainers.

Why we like firearms:
If you need the stopping power of a firearm, nothing else will suffice. Yes, firearms are lethal weapons and owning them involves great responsibilities. However, if you are in a situation where you need a firearm to defend your life, you will need it 100%.

Special Remarks:
In the strongest possible terms we recommend that you consider ownership and use of a gun with the utmost care and seriousness. Guns should be reserved for life-threatening confrontations where all other attempts to avoid or de-escalate the situation have failed. If you are faced with the prospect of such a lethal attack and you are trained and prepared to use a firearm, then nothing will help you defend your life better than a firearm.

Understand that this tool is often misunderstood and misused. Owning a gun in and of itself is not enough. You must own it legally, have it registered, and receive proper training. A gun is worthless (and potentially dangerous) if you do not understand how to use it properly. In addition, you must be prepared to take on the serious responsibilities of owning a gun, especially if you have children. Many women are simply not comfortable with guns because they are powerful, deadly weapons. If you have doubts about owning and operating a handgun responsibly, then we recommend you opt for a TASER device.

Improvised Tools:

What is it?

Any object at hand that can function as a defensive weapon.

How does it work?
Usually an improvised defensive tool will be some type of striking or piercing implement, such as a stick or a ball-point pen.

How is it used?
An improvised defensive tool can be used to strike, pierce, distract, burn, or temporarily blind an attacker (such as throwing hot coffee in his face). The idea is to surprise your attacker by using some improvised tool so that you can buy time to escape the attack.

Where can I get one?
If under attack, look around you. Be creative and see what defensive tools are at hand or if there is anything you can use to improvise a tool.

How can I get training?
You can practice at home with available objects. Consider how each is best used in a defensive capacity and take time to train yourself to use it. You can also rehearse scenarios in your mind. If you are out in a public place and you imagine a man attacking you, look around and imagine what you could use to defend yourself and how you would use it against him.

Why we like an improvised defensive tool:
Mostly we like them because you must be engaged in the moment and have your situational awareness operating if you are to be able to think quickly enough to improvise a defensive tool. We also like that they do not cost money.

Special remarks:
You cannot count on the availability of an appropriate tool in every attack situation, thus if you live, work, or travel in dangerous areas you should

consider carrying a more traditional tool, such as one of those mentioned above.

Morse Code for SOS

We believe every woman should know how to send the internationally recognized distress signal SOS. In Morse code these letters are represented by the radiotelegraphic signal: ... _ _ _ ... and are used as a call for help. Morse code is a system of communication that uses short and long patterns (the dots being short and the dashes being long) to represent letters of the alphabet. You do not need a radiotelegraphic device to communicate using Morse code. You can communicate the SOS distress signal by using sounds, flashes of light, or wigwags of a cloth or flag. For example, you could use your flashlight and make three brief flashes of light, then three longer flashes, then three brief flashes. You could do the same by making three short, three long, and three short sounds on your whistle.

Vehicle Defense

In this section we focus on how to use your vehicle to protect yourself by driving and maneuvering away from danger. Your vehicle can be used more aggressively as a defensive weapon in certain attack situations which we discuss later in this chapter. However, we strongly recommend receiving evasive driving training if you are in a high threat situation and fear you may be attacked en route or while in a parked vehicle (see Appendix E).

Transitioning In and Out of Your Vehicle

Approaching Your Vehicle: Remember that smooth is fast. This means your movements during transitions should be smooth so that you develop the ability to be fast and react quickly if the threat escalates. As you approach your vehicle, scan the area and practice surveillance detection. Do you see any sudden movements or anyone correlating with your movement? Scan the area around your vehicle. As you approach and get closer to your car, look underneath it and inside it before unlocking it. Is anything out of place? Does it appear that anyone has been tampering with your vehicle? If you notice any flyers or papers have been placed on the windshield, scan the area and look for anyone in the vicinity who may be watching you. Do not worry about removing the flyer before unlocking the vehicle if you feel you might be at risk. Drive out of the area before removing it. Sometimes carjackers will place a flyer on your front or back windshield so that you will get in and start the car and then get out again to remove the flyer.

Initial Entry: Once inside, lock your vehicle, start the engine, and scan the area and practice surveillance detection again. Do you notice any vehicles within line of sight of your vehicle starting their engines too? Are any pedestrians in the area approaching your vehicle?

Departing: As you pull out, scan the area and practice surveillance detection. Did anyone pull out after you and begin following you? Did anyone pull out in front of your vehicle and impede your forward progress? Is any vehicle correlating with your movements? If you suspect you are being followed, drive to the nearest safe location.

Arriving and Parking: Slow down and scan the area and practice surveillance detection when you arrive at your destination. Remember you can also do a drive-by where you drive near your destination to assess the area before you commit yourself to entering the area. On your drive-by you can check out who is in the area and where you feel safest parking. Identify your options for exiting from your parking spot.

If it is dark, park under lights. Once you park, rescan the area, using all of your mirrors before unlocking the doors and dismounting. This will only take a few seconds but is well worth the attention, given that an attacker may be present and you will want early warning. Developing this habit of scanning quickly becomes easy to do because your instinct is to protect yourself. Allowing yourself the opportunity to reboot this instinct will help you to relax and empower you. Once you dismount your vehicle, scan the area by listening to what is happening around you. Do you hear any footsteps, engines starting, vehicles pulling out or approaching? Again, this takes only seconds to do but you will be activating your ability to detect any early warning signals of danger. This is what having situational awareness is all about so make it a habit to use every available opportunity to practice it. You should consider that any transition time in and out of your vehicle is of interest to a predator since women are very vulnerable during these transitions.

10 Steps for Preparing Yourself for Vehicle GAME ON!

1. Know Your Vehicle: Every vehicle has controls and tools that can assist you in preventing an attack, such as a horn or car alarm. We recommend you know your vehicle controls intimately. Be aware especially of how to turn on your hazard lights. Practice driving in reverse while using your mirrors whenever possible so that you are used to doing it if you are ever in an emergency situation that requires you to back up at high speed. If you have either OnStar or a GPS device, be familiar with how to operate it. Take an evasive driving course if you are in a high threat situation so that you receive adequate training in maneuvering your vehicle if under attack.

2. Maintain Bubble Space: Creating distance between your vehicle and other vehicles gives you more time and room to maneuver your way out of an attack. You will also reduce your risk of antagonizing another driver if you avoid tailgating or allowing another vehicle to follow too closely. At traffic lights, you do not need to pull up right beside the car in the next lane, especially if the driver gives you the creeps. Drop back a bit so you are aligned with the back end of his car. Allow yourself room to maneuver your own vehicle. If you can see the tires of the vehicle in front of you, then you will have room to move out of the area. If you are threatened, you can maneuver left or right to drive away from any vehicle stopped in front of you.

3. Line of Sight Awareness: Practice surveillance detection. Remain aware of who is in line of sight of your vehicle, especially when it is parked and you are making a transition by entering or exiting your vehicle. If someone is watching you with the intent of following you in your vehicle, he will have to be in line of sight so that he can determine which way you will travel. As you continue to drive, use your mirrors to detect if you are being followed. Pay attention for any indicators that someone is trying to control your vehicle. Keep your distance from other vehicles.

4. 'What If' Escape Routes: Develop the habit of mentally rehearsing 'what if' escape routes. For example, if you approached an intersection you drive through daily and another vehicle tried to control your movements, what would you do? How would you escape the danger? This mental exercise is a training method which will enable you to have a quicker response to a real attack. You can practice this mentally when you are stuck in traffic. Imagine different attack scenarios and how you would escape.

5. Drivable Terrain: If under attack, you must think very creatively about what constitutes drivable terrain. You may be required to drive on the sidewalk, over someone's perfectly landscaped lawn, or through penetrable barriers such as wooden fences in order to escape your attacker. Obviously you must avoid harming innocent bystanders when doing so.

6. Look Where You Want to Go: Always look where you are going--literally. If you must make a sudden sharp turn, your eyes should be looking in the direction of where you want to go, not at the obstacle you are trying to avoid hitting. Your hands will steer in the direction in which your eyes are focused.

7. Concentrate on Steering and Driving in Control: If any vehicle is harassing you and trying to forcefully control your vehicle, immediately concentrate on steering and driving your vehicle in control, doing everything possible to break contact and escape. You must control your vehicle and drive to safety. As soon as you have control of your vehicle call 911 for help.

8. Drive Away from the Threat: Do not exit your vehicle unless you know you are safe. If you have no safe location, keep driving until your car runs out of gas or dies. Your vehicle is your best means of escape. If any kind of road rage incident occurs, break contact from that vehicle, even if it means going out of your way and being delayed. Avoid driving in secluded risky areas when trying to break away from a threat. Practice surveillance detection en route to your safe location.

9. Identify Safe Locations: Quickly identify the nearest safe location if you sense a threat. Safe locations can include police stations, fire stations, hospitals, or any busy public location where you can find help. Focus on driving there in control and not exiting your vehicle unless you are certain you will be safe doing so. Practice surveillance detection before dismounting your vehicle and entering the safe location.

10. Maintain a Neutral Demeanor: Do not use aggressive expressions or hand gestures which might aggravate the situation. Instead, change lanes or allow the vehicle to pass you. Be courteous and avoid eye contact with other drivers. Do not engage in aggressive behavior that might start a road rage incident. Coach any passengers in your vehicle to do the same. Do not flip off the driver of another vehicle, no matter how angry you are. Just take a deep breath and let the person drive on ahead of you so that you do not aggravate the situation. It does not matter who is at fault; what matters is retaining your safety.

Moves for Vehicle GAME ON!

Drive By/Loiter: If you are entering an area and feel threatened do not park and get out of your vehicle. Drive by the area conducting visual scans and practicing surveillance detection. You can also loiter in a nearby location from which you can observe the area before entering.

Use the Phone: Your cell phone is your best defensive tool. Keep it on, accessible, and do not hesitate to call 911 if you identify a threat and are unable to get out of the area to safety without assistance. If you have no cell phone, safely get to a nearby phone or ask another driver to call the police for you.

Break Contact: Drop off if any vehicle is aggressively pursuing you or you feel you are being followed. Act on your intuition and break away to the nearest safe location. If you are unable to break contact, call the police for help.

Turn Unexpectedly: Making a last minute, unexpected turn may allow you to lose any vehicle that is aggressively following you. You will make the turn at the last second and will use your turn signal only if you have to warn another driver behind or in front of you of your sudden move. Only use this move if you can do so safely without endangering other drivers or yourself.

Reverse Out: If possible, you may reverse your vehicle in order to escape an attacker. For example, if you are at a stop sign and your attacker is approaching you head on in an effort to block your forward progress, you may reverse and turn your vehicle around to head in the opposite direction. Again, reverse only if you can do so safely.

Bumper Car Rules: One vehicle attack technique is called a "bump and rob." Here the attacker will purposefully bump into your vehicle in order to use the supposed accident as a means of stopping you and then robbing you. If someone bumps into your vehicle, call the police while you are still inside the vehicle and immediately put on your hazard lights to attract attention. If possible, drive to a safe location before stopping. Crack your window to discuss the accident with the other driver. Tell the driver you have called the police. Do not dismount your vehicle until the police arrive.

If another driver tries to control you by bumping your vehicle or forcing you out of your lane, concentrate on steering and controlling your vehicle. It may terrify you but realize that you are now basically in a bumper car ring. However, just because another car is bumping into yours that does not mean your car will suddenly break down or you will be forced to stop. Steer in control and look where you are going. Understand that your attacker has violated the normal driving rules and you may be required to do the same in order to survive. Your response will be terrain and situation driven. As in any attack, your objective is to escape without harming yourself or any innocent bystanders.

Ram: Remember that every vehicle weighs a minimum of over one ton of metal. Vehicles are difficult to stop when moving. This is why police chases go on and on because it is actually quite difficult to stop a moving vehicle if the driver does not want to be stopped. A moving vehicle has roughly two and a half times its weight in kinetic energy. This means that if a vehicle keeps moving, it can push its way through obstacles with ease. For example, if an attacker were trying to control your vehicle by pulling out onto the road perpendicular to your car, it would not take much movement or speed for you to be able to ram his vehicle out of the way with yours. You would either point your right headlight across to his front wheel or point your left headlight across to his rear wheel and then drive into the wheel to push the car off to the side so you can drive past it. This maneuver should *only* be used if you feel your life is in danger and you have no other recourse. Of course, we strongly recommend you receive proper training in this maneuver if you are in a high threat situation and are afraid of being attacked en route.

Do Not Be Distracted: If you fall under attack by another vehicle, continue to scan the area and do not become too focused on the attack. Your attacker could be attempting to distract you with one maneuver while his partner could be waiting in the wings in another vehicle ready to surprise you. Stay in the present and take in the whole picture rather than having tunnel vision.

If Your Vehicle Breaks Down: If possible, exit your vehicle and enter a safe location. Scan to be sure no one is waiting on foot to attack you. If you are in an urban environment and your vehicle breaks down, use a phone to call for roadside service and wait in your locked vehicle or inside a safe location until help arrives.

When on the freeway, you must take extreme caution if your vehicle breaks down. First, if possible, pull off at an angle onto the shoulder. This will help you attract the attention of highway patrol. Keep your hazard lights on at all times. Call for help immediately (if you have no cell phone you may need to walk to the nearest emergency phone). Use mile markers and exit signs to pinpoint your location if your vehicle has no GPS device. Even at night it is generally safer for you to dismount your vehicle and move away from it while waiting for help to arrive, in the event that another vehicle accidentally crashes into yours.

Realize that you are in a potentially precarious situation if your vehicle breaks down on the freeway. Predators use freeways because of the availability of victims, the lack of law enforcement, and the low risk of public intervention due to the high speed of other travelers. Serial killers often find their victims on freeways. Any woman alone on the side of a freeway with a broken down vehicle is an easy target. When you move away from your vehicle, do so discreetly and try to find a location in which you can be concealed yet still watch your vehicle and the shoulder of the freeway. You want early warning if anyone stops to help.   Take any defensive tools with you and be ready to use them. If possible, make yourself look like a man (put on a hat, a coat, walk like a man, etc.). Most people are driving by at high speed so you can easily trick their eyes by making yourself appear to be a man. Ditch the high heels and anything that screams femininity to onlookers passing your broken down vehicle.

Types of Attacks in Vehicle GAME ON!

Foot Attack: If you notice someone approaching your vehicle on foot and you feel threatened, drive out of the area. If you followed the instruction on parking above you should have already identified the nearest exit and all other exit options. Keep your cool and drive in control. Remember that your vehicle is equipped with all sorts of defensive tools. You can honk your horn, press your OnStar button, or sound your car alarm. Use your mirrors to keep a watch on him. Even if he starts pounding on your windows, drive away in control. If you see him brandishing any kind of gun, duck as you drive away quickly and in control of your vehicle. Your chances of surviving are greater if you drive away quickly and in control than if you surrender to his control. Even if he has a gun the odds are in your favor that he will miss hitting a moving target. And if you are wounded it does not mean you will die. Drive to a safe location and seek medical attention.

Remember, you are under no obligation to roll down your window if someone approaches your vehicle, ostensibly to ask for directions. If you do decide to speak with the person, just crack your window.

Obvious or Aggressive Vehicle Follow: If any vehicle is obviously following yours or is aggressively following yours, drive immediately to a safe location. Collect any identifiable information on the vehicle and call the police to report it. If the vehicle disappears before the police come, report any information. Then vary your routines and practice surveillance detection so that, if the driver of the vehicle comes after you again, you will notice him early on and can continue to evade him.

Reckless Endangerment/Forced Control: If a highly aggressive attacker is after you realize he will stop at nothing to control your vehicle or cause you to have an accident. Your response will be terrain driven and may or may not include unexpected turns, reversing out, bumping, or ramming. Your primary objectives are to escape the attack, call for help, and find a safe location. Stay focused on steering in control, looking where you are going, and utilizing all drivable terrain. Be prepared for surprises or multiple attackers. The game is on and your job is to survive.

Impersonation: An attacker may attempt to use impersonation as a ruse for gaining proximity to your vehicle. For example, an attacker may pose as an undercover police officer using an unmarked vehicle with a siren and flashing light. He may instruct you to pull over and he will then impersonate an officer who is threatening to arrest you for speeding. Request to see his badge and do not exit your vehicle or roll down the window more than a crack. Tell him you would like his name and the number of the station or local dispatch so that you can call to check that he is a legitimate officer. Any real police officer will understand and appreciate your need to confirm his legitimacy. If he refuses to cooperate, tell him to call for back up before you will consent to exiting your vehicle. Obviously if he presents a firearm, you will be required to do whatever the situation dictates to keep yourself safe.

Blocking: An attacker may initiate his attack by blocking your vehicle from the front or behind. If he is working with a partner they will use two vehicles and trap your vehicle between them. Remember you can ram either while moving forward or in reverse. Again we recommend evasive driving training if you are in a high threat situation so that you can safely practice these maneuvers under the guidance of professionals.

Broken Down Vehicle: Another ploy is the broken down car on the side of the road. Here the attacker is hoping that some kind person will stop to help so that he can rob her/him or worse. You can be that kind person by calling for roadside assistance but never stop to offer assistance; unfortunately the risk of danger to you (especially if you are alone) is just too high.

The Good Samaritan: An attacker may pose as a Good Samaritan, offering to assist you in some way. If you are having car trouble or have been in a minor accident, he may use this as a means of gaining proximity to you and your vehicle. He may also use the role of the Good Samaritan as his method of approaching your vehicle so that he can car jack you. Pay attention to early warning signals and act on your intuition. Do not unlock your doors if you are inside the vehicle and be ready to call for help.

The Force Continuum: Using Reasonable Force with Defensive Tactics and Tools

The use of defensive tactics and tools does not come without responsibilities. One of those responsibilities involves using what is known as "reasonable force." The "force continuum" is a guide you can follow to understand how to respond to your attacker with a reasonable amount of force given the situation. The force continuum provides you with a scale you can follow to discern what level of force is appropriate. Basically, you are bound by law to use the least amount of force necessary to protect yourself. That means if you can move or talk your way out of the attack before it escalates or somehow control your attacker, such as by using a joint lock (such as a wrist or elbow manipulation that causes pain), you must. However, if you are faced with a more aggressive situation, you might need to move up the force continuum and respond by using some type of non-lethal weapon, such as pepper spray or a kubaton. Next on the scale would be to use some type of defensive technique that may harm your attacker but will not seriously disable or kill him. For example, you might use an elbow strike or a head butt. Finally, if you are in imminent danger of being killed by your attacker, you can move to the top of the continuum and use lethal weapons, such as guns, knives, or improvised lethal weapons (make sure to register your gun and have a permit to use it). Still, you can only use lethal force if that is your only option for staying alive. Put simply: You do not have carte blanche to kill a man just because you are angry that he attacked you. You are only allowed to use enough force to reasonably defend yourself.

Following the force continuum will allow you to save your own life, to stay within your legal right to defend yourself, and to respect the life of your attacker (as odd as that may sound, since he may not be respecting yours). Think of it this way: If your attacker were drunk and unarmed, you should be able to either escape the attack or somehow prevent or stop the attack by using reasonable force. Even though he is in the wrong for attacking you, you cannot cross the line and use excessive force to defend yourself.

The same is true if you are the victim of abuse; you do not have the right to use excessive force against your abuser, unless doing so is your only option in that moment for saving your own life. In other words, you cannot accumulate the incidents of abuse as a means of justifying using excessive force during an attack where less than lethal options were available to you and you could have survived that specific attack without killing your abuser. Although these laws may seem unfair or in favor of the attacker, the reality is that numerous women have gone to jail for using excessive force against their attackers. This is why, if you are attacked and you do use any kind of force against your attacker (with or without any weapons), we recommend you call a lawyer immediately.

Part of having a plan regarding use of defensive tactics and tools is to understand the force continuum and prepare yourself mentally to respond with appropriate force. As an attack unfolds, the force continuum levels may shift. For example, an attack may start out on the low end of the scale, meaning you have the option to negotiate your way out of it somehow. This may fail and you may then have to climb up the scale and respond by using a higher level of force. For example, you may need to strike your attacker or spray him with mace. Stay in the present, use situational awareness, and be flexible enough to understand what level of force is reasonable for the immediate circumstances.

If you are in a high threat situation, we strongly recommend that you research the force continuum further so that you have a clear understanding of your rights and limitations. You can do so by conducting a keyword search on the internet or by consulting a lawyer who specializes in criminal defense (as you might be the one who is viewed as the criminal if you are charged with using excessive force).

Conclusion

Very few women wake up in the morning thinking, "Hmmm…I will probably be attacked today." Yet, every day women are brutally attacked. All women will become more empowered if they make attack prevention part of their daily lives. We realize this may sound like an extreme burden. Actually, it is the opposite. It is simply instinctive. Most women would do absolutely anything to protect a child; it is instinctive. Each woman is someone's child. It should be as instinctive to protect ourselves and each other as it is to protect children. Just as children are at a disadvantage because they are weaker than adults, women too are at a disadvantage because we are physically weaker than most men. Rebooting our instincts to survive will help us in reclaiming our right to be safe and to live without constant fear. If you combine being SASD with use of defensive tactics and/or tools, you will greatly increase your ability to avoid being attacked (or to survive being attacked if you are unable to prevent it). Equally important, you will feel less vulnerable and more empowered because you are informed and prepared. You will have customized a security plan for your life with which you will be comfortable and which you can expand if your threat level increases. In the next chapter we take you deeper into the attack process and instruct you on ways you can respond to and survive an attack, in the event that you have no other alternative.

CHAPTER THIRTEEN

WHEN ALL ELSE FAILS... RESPONDING TO AND SURVIVING AN ATTACK

Why is he staring at me? Maybe if I'm nice he'll go away. He'll go away.
No, thanks... Uh, I'm going now. No... I really... I have to go.
Stop... please. Oh my God; this isn't happening!
Okay, okay, I'm doing what he asks. Oh, please don't! You're hurting me...

Shock is a woman's worst adversary in any attack. A predator will use the element of surprise as a means of getting his target to go into a state of shock so that he can attack her successfully. If we fail in preventing attacks, then our last chance is to manipulate this element of surprise upon which the attacker so relies. We do this by training our bodies and our minds to handle shock, reduce the effects of it, and speed our recovery from it. Once we are in a state of shock, we literally cannot function. If you are attacked by a predator, even though your adrenaline will surely be rushing throughout your body, you will still be able to respond if you are not surprised and you do not go into shock.

We have all experienced what it is like to be surprised or startled by someone, even if only momentarily. We gasp, our body immediately tenses, and we breathe a heavy sigh of relief when we realize we were simply startled and are not really in danger. We have also all experienced, on some level, an adrenaline rush. If we use the example of a rollercoaster ride we can learn to distinguish the difference between being surprised and having an adrenaline rush. On the rollercoaster we know that a thrill is coming. It could be around the next turn or it could be over the crest of the next hill. We do not know for sure exactly when, where, or how much the ride will thrill us, so our adrenaline gets pumped up as we anticipate the next little or big thrill. However, we are not surprised or startled by the thrill because we know we are on a rollercoaster and the thrill is to be expected. The thrill is what we paid for and why we are there, thus we can function and (theoretically) not pass out from the ride. Perhaps you know someone who is an 'adrenaline junkie.' We can learn a lot about the difference between the effects of surprise on the body and an adrenaline rush from people who intentionally put themselves into dangerous situations in order to obtain a thrill. These thrill seekers have prepared themselves in such a way as to minimize their risk of surprise but maximize their risk of thrill, so that their adrenaline starts pumping vigorously but their bodies can continue to function.

All of the preventative measures you have learned so far should help you avoid being surprised by an attacker. However, if you are unable to avoid being surprised then you increase your risk of going into shock. If you are taken by surprise when under attack you may experience an "adrenal dump" that induces a biochemical reaction involving changes in levels of sodium and potassium that cause the body and brain to experience some degree of the following symptoms:

- Tunnel vision (your eyes cannot focus and your peripheral vision is compromised or your vision may even blur).
- Auditory exclusion (your hearing may become impaired or you may hear a loud ringing in your ears).

- Memory distortion (your ability to move and negotiate the space and objects around you may be altered and time may seem to slow down dramatically).
- Severe muscle tension and the overall inability to allow the body to follow the commands of the brain. Your muscles may seize and no matter how hard you try to move it may seem as though you are paralyzed. At a minimum, your fine motor skills will be compromised.

Obviously you can see how hard it would be to survive an attack if your body experiences this "adrenal dump" and you cannot see, hear, or move well. When we are startled by something and our body shuts down we become an easy target and a probable victim. Attackers know this and it is why they try so hard to exploit the element of surprise.

It should be registering with you now why situational awareness is truly a survival instinct. Even if the worst happens, your situational awareness is what will help you in surviving an attack because it will prevent the attacker from being able to surprise you. If you heighten your awareness and then find yourself under attack you may be able to survive because, although your adrenaline will certainly be rushing, your body will still be able to perform. You will not be paralyzed as a result of being surprised.

We have shared some of the most powerful prevention methods available in this book and we believe in their effectiveness whole-heartedly. However, we are realists; the truth is that no prevention method is foolproof. There are so many particulars that impact any attack situation. You could be a black belt in Karate, a highly skilled intelligence operator, or an expert markswoman and still an attacker may, under the right circumstances and with extremely calculated planning, be able to overcome you. Part of the problem is that the possible attack scenarios are simply too numerous to defend against completely. Predators learn from their mistakes and the mistakes of others. They evolve and they continue to find creative solutions in order to bypass any obstacles to their success. If they are able to bypass your early warning system, you do have a last chance and a way to survive or, at a minimum, to do damage control in the event of an attack. If you come under attack, know that it is not over until it is over. Even if you have more than one opponent your potential for surviving any attack will improve if you prepare yourself to avoid being surprised and going into shock.

Your ability to survive an attack depends greatly on your readiness to do so. When you implement situational awareness and surveillance detection, you are training your mind to ready itself for the *possibility* of an attack, but not the attack itself. Still, this training is valuable in that it increases your alertness and keeps your mind focused on the idea of an attack. On some small level you are taking away the element of surprise from the attacker by virtue of the fact that you are studying his probable tactics, his attack preparation in particular. Anything that you can do to detract from the attacker's element of surprise will be helpful to you and detrimental for him.

The attacker has two tactics which help in building up the element of surprise: patience and distance from the target. An example of a patient attacker might be the one who follows his target, studies her routes, and opts to wait to attack her on a day when she is traveling on an unfamiliar route that is not part of her routine travel. This attacker may have to come out and follow the target time and time again before she goes to his ideal attack location, but because he is patient, the attacker will wait until he has the opportunity to have the circumstances and location of the attack his way.

Another option that strengthens the attacker's element of surprise is distance from the target. If the attacker is able to collect information on his target while maintaining a safe distance between himself and the target, he will be able to capitalize on this element of surprise. A good example of this is cyber stalking. Someone who has even basic information on you, such as your name and address, can use the internet as a tool for harassment. This is why we are so concerned with blogs and the amount of personal information an attacker can collect from a distance. If a young girl releases information such as her 'favorite hangout' on her blog profile in conjunction with her photo and the name of her school, the attacker now has an edge and can easily surprise her in either of these locations because he knows what she looks like. We have to be smarter than our potential adversaries. We must take away this element of surprise. However, if for some reason we fail in doing so, we must be ready to respond and survive an attack.

In the following story, the potential victim was able to walk away unscathed because she was prepared to handle being surprised by an attacker.

Arlene, a sixty-four year old widow, lives in a quiet, somewhat rural neighborhood outside of Santa Fe, New Mexico. Arlene is a painter, so she works out of the studio behind her modest home. Since her husband's death five years ago, Arlene has become concerned that, because she now lives alone, she might be targeted by a predator. Her old Labrador, Jesse, is her alarm system, although he is pretty easy to manage with a dog biscuit or anything that smells like food.

Arlene lives a quiet life. She paints in the mornings when the light is good and tends to her flower garden in the afternoons. Most evenings she is at home reading or watching television. Her social life is moderately busy with art openings and gatherings with friends. Late at night she often feels the dread of living alone after so many happy years with her husband. Sometimes that dread is compounded by the fear of being attacked in her home, causing her to lose sleep and wrestle with anxiety.

Arlene takes many precautions where her home security is concerned. She is an avid fan of keeping doors and windows locked, even while inside her home. Her house is equipped with exterior motion lights and she always keeps her curtains drawn after dark. After her husband died, she had a carpenter reinforce her bedroom door and install a deadbolt. Since she lives in a one story home, she was not concerned with getting out in case of a fire. Arlene locks her bedroom door when sleeping. Jesse sleeps on the floor at the end of her bed.

One morning Arlene awoke at four a.m. to a strange sound coming from her kitchen. Jesse stirred and began barking loudly. Arlene put the phone in her hand and walked over to her locked bedroom door to listen. Since Jesse was obviously more agitated than usual, she became frightened. Arlene remained locked in the bedroom, unsure if she should call the police yet too afraid to investigate the source of the noise. Suddenly she heard a loud bang in the hallway. A voice cried out, "Shut that dog up or I'll shoot him!" Arlene dialed 911 but the phone lines had been cut. She quickly turned on her cell phone that was charging next to her bed and dialed 911. She was terrified but was determined to survive.

She was able to quiet Jesse and shouted out with a stern, commanding voice: "I just called the police on my cell phone. They will be here any minute so I suggest you get out while you can." Suddenly her bedroom door almost burst out of its hinges. He was trying to get in and she realized she had very little time to respond. Arlene grabbed her panic alarm, ran to the window, opened it, and sounded the alarm. Her nearest neighbors were close by so she knew they could hear the alarm. She had spoken with them about her intention of sounding the alarm if she was ever in trouble.

Moments later, although it seemed like an eternity to her, the police arrived. They caught the intruder while he was running away. Her neighbors saw him heading down a small road behind Arlene's house.

What is significant about Arlene's story is that she obviously spent the time and energy to assess her security risks. She knew that she was vulnerable so she made a 'what if' plan and thought ahead. Because she invested the time and attention to consider this attack possibility, she was mentally prepared to handle it. Arlene did not panic or go into shock. Even though she was terrified, she was able to function in an emergency because she was *prepared*. Prevention is all about preparation. Remember: Foresight is twenty-twenty.

One tenet we preach in our trainings is to trust your instincts and always err on the side of caution. A funny thing happens psychologically when you are under threat: on some level you may judge yourself and think you are being too paranoid. So, for example, if a college student had already identified a blue van parked near her dorm and she was concerned that the driver of that van might be watching her, it would make sense that she would then become suspicious of any blue van. If she were walking back to her dorm one night and she saw a blue van parked with its engine running, she might become afraid, but she might also start to second guess her instincts and judge herself for being too paranoid. Her internal monologue might kick in and cause her to doubt her suspicions. This lapse in her personal security practice might cause her to walk right past the van in order to enter her dorm. Or, perhaps she is too tired to walk away from the threat because she just wants to get in her room and study. Whatever her reasons, if she ignores the potential threat, the consequences could be deadly.

Pre-Attack Indicators

It is possible that you will only receive minimal advanced warning that an attack is imminent. Some general indicators include:

- Someone fixating his attention on you.
- Someone following you, especially closely.
- Anyone who antagonizes you or threatens you verbally.
- Anyone closing the physical distance between himself and you.
- Anyone whose demeanor or bearing appears threatening.
- Physical contact that is inappropriate and could lead to violence (grabbing your arm; tripping you or bumping into you 'by accident'; cornering you; backing you into a wall; approaching you by surprise from behind; raising an arm or hand towards you).
- Presentation of a weapon of any kind.
- A ruse/lure to get you to a secluded location.
- Anyone approaching you as you are entering your vehicle.
- A moving vehicle that is aggressively manipulating your vehicle.
- Anyone attempting to isolate you in a secluded area of a building (such as stopping an elevator between floors; following you into a stairwell; waiting for you in a parking garage; following you into a restroom).
- Key dates, scheduled events, or significant anniversaries that somehow increase the threat of an attack (for example, an upcoming date for finalizing a divorce might increase the risk of some type of retribution from the estranged spouse).

Last Chance Attack Prevention

Our emphasis in this book is on prevention because we know that the sooner you detect danger, the more time you will have to respond appropriately and the less likely you will be to go into shock. However, since every attack is different, your ability to respond will be determined by what is happening in the moment. Several options exist for you to prevent and avoid an attack, including:

- Detecting and sensing the early warning signals and pre-attack indicators.
- Avoiding or evading the possible danger (for example, if you are walking and see someone suspicious, turn around and go the other way or go into a public location to avoid coming in closer contact with that person).
- Using your demeanor, eye contact, or gait to send your attacker the message "stay away."
- Creating a distraction, a public display for attention, or a ruse to redirect the attacker and foil his plan (for example, if someone was approaching your vehicle and you felt uneasy you could honk your horn or set off your car alarm).
- Delaying the attack by placing obstacles between you and your attacker to buy yourself time to get away.
- Going into an offensive mode and fighting back with all of your might. Do everything you can to stun him.
- Run away; move out of the attack; escape!
- Report the details of the attack (or attempted attack) to the authorities. This may prevent your attacker from returning to try again.

What Not To Do

Some common reactions to being attacked that will *reduce* your chance of survival include:

- Freezing with fear.
- Denial and disbelief.
- Talking yourself out of accepting the attack as real by allowing your internal monologue to convince you that the 'threat truth' is not what is happening, but rather the 'safe truth' is what you are encountering, (see Chapter One).
- Putting your head in the sand and totally ignoring the reality.
- Hoping you are wrong about the attack. Having compassion for the attacker and refusing to respond with appropriate force even when you must.

Attack Survival Options

Your attack might begin like this: you detect danger and then immediately react because he is already grabbing you and becoming physically violent. Or your attack could begin like this: you detect danger and then immediately run away to safety. Maybe your attack will begin like this: you are totally taken by surprise, without having had the chance to detect or sense it coming and then must create a ruse in order to get away. Perhaps your attack will begin like this: you are threatened by someone and you then take action to deter it by talking him out of hurting you. The list of possibilities is endless.

The most important lesson is to take *all* pre-attack indicators very seriously and act *immediately*. Take charge of the situation and disable your denial. Listen to your intuition and do what it tells you to do, immediately and with 100% commitment. Your first action should be to attempt to break contact and get as far away as possible. Do not second guess yourself. The worst that can happen if you are wrong is that you will feel a little embarrassed. So what!

If you are right and you are about to fall under attack you literally do not have even a moment to waste. Do not allow your internal monologue to dissuade you from responding immediately and taking the threat seriously. Imagine that internal voice to be a little girl whom you are in charge of protecting; you would instruct her to respond and run away from an attacker. Instruct yourself with the same advice and without hesitation.

It may be that you might need to give your attacker what he wants because your physical capabilities are inadequate for defending yourself and if you fight you may only escalate the violence level. Or, it may be that you can grab a weapon at hand and reverse the surprise by striking him so that you can escape. Perhaps you will be able to enlist the help of a stranger by shouting for help. The situation will dictate your response. Stay aware, do not give up, and remember that it is not over until it is over.

As an empowered woman, your chances of survival will increase if you expand your vocabulary of defenses through education and awareness. Give yourself some simple, easy commands, such as chants or words. Rehearse and use them in the event of an attack. We emphasize rehearsing these so that they remain accessible in the recesses of your mind. Coach yourself. Remember that when under attack you will likely revert to either your most recent experience or what you have trained in the most. If you have trained yourself with survival commands, your mind will stand a better chance of remembering and releasing those commands during the attack.

The following are examples of short commands you can rehearse and integrate into your subconscious. Choose one (or more) so that if you need a directive in a pre-attack situation, you will have one at your disposal to say to yourself to prompt you to act. If you do not like any of our commands, make up one for yourself that you believe will work better for you. Just keep it short and simple; your time is severely limited.

Bolt!
Move now!
Run away!
Escape!

Stun and run!
Prevail!
Fight back!
Survive!
Take charge!

You can also enlist the help of others either during or immediately after an attack by using the three D system: Direction, Distance, and Description. This is a way of giving clear instructions to a bystander you have enlisted for help. Attacks are time sensitive, meaning you cannot waste time with lengthy explanations of your dire situation. You need help and you need it now, thus you must effectively communicate the specific help you need. Remember that if you have just been attacked, you may look frightening to a bystander who may wonder if you are sane or sober. Even professional rescuers such as law enforcement or firefighters may have doubts if you appear to be so out of it that you are not speaking clearly. Seize control of the situation by giving clear, direct instructions for help.

Here is how the three D system works:

Direction: Point to the attacker and say: "This guy is hurting me" or "He's there" or "He ran that way."

Distance: Use nearby visible landmarks to pinpoint the distance between you and the escaping attacker. For example, you might point in his direction and say "He's there, near the dumpster on the corner."

Description: Give some minimal description of the escaping attacker so that when you point in his direction and give a distance marker, the description will allow the person helping you to distinguish the attacker from other people who may be in the area. For example, you might point in his direction and say: "He's there, near the dumpster on the corner, the white guy with the red baseball cap."

Planning Ahead:
Creating Emergency Evacuation Plans for Attacks

Let us assume you have done everything right. You have used our book and taken all precautionary measures available to prevent an attack. You have followed the progression of recommended techniques:

- Using *Situational Awareness*: Intuition, Sensory Awareness, Early Warning Signals, 'What If' Plans.
- Protecting your *Privacy and Identity*.
- Conducting a *Risk/Threat Assessment*.
- Creating a *SUPNET*.
- Developing a *Surveillance Detection Plan*.
- Conducting *Route Reviews* and *Building Reviews*.
- Training in use of *Defensive Tactics and Tools*.
- Developing an *Attack Response*, including attack commands you can rehearse and use when under attack and emergency evacuation plans to follow (see below).

Still, that horrible day comes when you are attacked. How do you cope? What do you do? You must plan ahead for it and rehearse how you will handle being attacked at home, at work, in your car, out in public, and while traveling. You can achieve this by making an emergency evacuation (evac) plan for potential attack locations and scenarios, thereby rehearsing your escapes.

An emergency evac plan is similar to a 'what if' plan in that you are projecting the future possibilities. The difference is in the immediacy of an emergency evac plan. You can use a 'what if' plan for both detecting danger and for avoiding it. An emergency evac plan, on the other hand, is used solely for escaping danger. Rehearse your emergency evac plans to whatever extent possible. This is akin to rehearsing a fire drill at school when you were a child. Practicing your evac plans will help you to integrate them into your mind and body. Your evac plan should include a list of the possible types of attacks you might encounter in any part of your life and your plan to escape in the event you are attacked.

Home Emergency Evacuation Plan:

Potential attacks in your home:

Intrusion (by a stranger, stalker, or known abuser)
Burglary
Arson or Vandalism
Shooting
Rape
Abduction
Murder
Other? (Consider if anything in your life or any particular circumstances may put you at risk of other attacks not listed)

For all of the above attacks in your home, design an emergency evacuation plan for you and your family. Your plan should include options for escape, as well as options for securing yourself inside the home in the event you cannot escape. Not everyone can afford a "Panic Room" but you may have a place where you can lock yourselves in and call for help. In your escape plan, consider all possible ways of exiting your home safely. Also consider where you would go for help. For example: Would you get in your car and drive away? Would you go to a neighbor's house? What if that neighbor were out of town? Rehearse your plans. This is especially important to do with children. You have probably already rehearsed a fire drill with them, thus it is not a big leap to rehearse a plan for "what to do and where to go if a bad person comes into our home."

Workplace Violence

(Note: You can train your children to apply some of the following tips in the event an act of violence breaks out in their school.)

Workplace violence is a growing concern as incidents of violence continue to occur and employers/employees are victimized. Simple steps you can take to protect yourself and help prevent violence in your workplace include:

- Maintain clear boundaries in conversations with male co-workers. Be aware of any misogynistic comments, such as "I hate working with women; they are always ordering me around and treating me like a dog."
- Guard your personal information and property. Be careful not to reveal key details about security procedures at your workplace to outsiders.
- Conduct a risk/threat assessment of your workplace, including your duty position, your location in the building, and your shifts.
- Assess any interfacing you do with the public in your job for risks to your safety.
- Assess service deliveries and public access to your workplace for risks.
- Become informed about the policies of the human resources department regarding hiring employees. Do they conduct any type of screening or background checks on employees?
- Determine if the nature of your job places you at higher risk (for example if you work in a government job or are part of the legal profession).

Workplace Emergency Evacuation Plan

Potential Attacks at Work:

Attack in parking garage, stairwell, elevator, or restroom

Duck and cover scenario (bomb threat)
Workplace violence (e.g., disgruntled employee with a gun)
Intrusion
Burglary
Arson or Vandalism
Shooting
Rape
Abduction
Murder
Other?

Part of your emergency evacuation plan at work will be provided by your employer. Your company may, for example, conduct "duck and cover" or bomb threat drills. It is also important for you to design your own evac plan for potential attacks at work.

Your plan should include the following:

- Identify escape routes out of the building.

- Identify hiding locations inside and around the building. These are places where you can conceal yourself until the attack is over and the police have arrived on the scene.

- Identify the locations of all fire alarms so that you can signal others to evacuate the building if an attack breaks out in your area.

- Create obstacles between yourself and the attacker.

- Suggest to your employer that access to areas of the building be restricted by using a code or badge system, locking doors, and using alarms.

- Ask your employer to implement an escort policy for service people or anyone entering sensitive or non-public areas. Proper identification should be required and service people should be vetted before entering.

- Pay attention to early warning signals of any anti-social behaviors, such as aggression from disgruntled employees or caustic remarks from hostile customers. Report anything suspicious to management and/or security. Be aware of any in-house conflicts and the presence of recently fired employees.

- Report any threats made by co-workers. Remain anonymous so that your report does not cause any hostility between you and the co-worker.

- Follow and act upon your intuition if violence breaks out. Do not be so curious as to move towards the outbreak. For example, if you hear faint popping sounds in another part of the building, do not run there to see what is happening. Rather, seek the nearest escape.

- Develop a system of signaling danger to other parts of the building should violence break out in any area. You may use some type of signaling device such as a whistle or personal alarm. Or you may develop a code for use only in emergencies.

The idea is to plan how you would get out of the building as quickly and safely as possible. You must consider all parts of the building in which you spend time. What if the attack happened in the employee lounge or in the building lobby? Where would you go to escape? You need to be aware of all the exit portals that are feasible. Be creative; some windows might provide you with an exit. In addition, determine hiding places at work in the event you cannot get out. Ideally you would have access to a phone in each hiding place (or you would keep your cell phone with you at all times). Rehearse both hiding and escaping. Even if you only rehearse it mentally, you will still be ahead of the game and better able to respond appropriately.

Vehicle Emergency Evacuation Plan

Possible Attacks while in Your Vehicle:

Break-in
Car jacking
"Bump and Jack"/ "Bump and Rob"
Road Rage
Harassment
Aggressive Following
Theft
Arson or Vandalism
Shooting
Rape
Abduction
Murder
Other?

The most important thing to remember if you are attacked in your vehicle is that you may need to immediately surrender your vehicle in order to be able to escape. For example, do not hesitate to give up your vehicle to a car jacker. Moreover, do not hesitate to leave your vehicle and seek refuge in a safe location if you are being aggressively followed, harassed, or if you are involved in a road rage incident. However, if you leave your vehicle, be sure to get the appropriate support before re-entering it after an incident. The other important thing to remember about being attacked while in your vehicle is that you are in a moving weapon that can be used either as a means of protection or as a weapon against you. If someone tries to run you off the road, for example, your vehicle can either be your safest means of escape, or it can become the chariot of your demise.

Developing an evac plan for attacks that may occur while you are in your vehicle is somewhat more difficult because of the numerous possible scenarios. However, it is important to train yourself (by rehearsing) to surrender your vehicle when appropriate or to use it as a means of escape. Granted, you cannot get out on the roads and practice fancy, high speed evasive driving techniques. But you can rehearse 'what if' plans for your regular routes (for example, identifying and using safe locations along your routes). You can also be sure to equip your vehicle with a phone and a list of emergency numbers. Calling 911 is usually the best option, but have a backup plan, such as the number of the police department in your city or county. (For more information see section on vehicle defense in Chapter Twelve).

Public Attacks/Crowd Violence

When out in public do not assume that you are safe just because many people are around. Realize that if some type of outbreak of violence occurs, you could become a victim simply because you were in the wrong place at the wrong time. You can develop habits to use in any public location or crowd situation, such as a concert, sporting event, busy subway station, or an outdoor festival.

- Habitually identify exits and escape routes when you arrive at any new location or change locations.
- Use situational awareness and surveillance detection techniques to identify early warning signals of danger and suspicious behaviors.
- If you sense danger, act on your intuition and exit the area before violence erupts.
- If violence erupts and the crowd panics, stay out of the flow of traffic and do not get trapped in the center of the crowd. Move to the side near a wall or column. Search for exits that are not blocked.
- Do not be too curious. If you sense danger or notice a crowd gathering, move away from the potential threat rather than towards it.
- If you are with small children, pick them up and carry them to safety.
- Use your arms to form a shield to protect your face and head as you move through a panicked crowd. If you are knocked to the ground, protect your head until you are able to stand up again.

- Remain focused on moving to safety. Do not allow your emotions to be swept away by everyone else's panic. Stay calm and coach yourself verbally to find a safe location where you can wait out the incident until the authorities arrive and order is restored.

Out in Public Emergency Evacuation Plan

Possible Attacks When Out in Public:

Terrorist Attack
Mob Scene/Crowd Panic
Assault
Robbery/Pick Pocketing/Purse Snatching
Battery
Shooting
Stalking
Rape
Abduction
Murder
Other?

The best way to develop emergency evacuation plans for the time you spend out in public is to look at your habits and schedule and determine the places you visit regularly. Then develop an evac plan and rehearse it for each place. For example, if you have a regular manicure on Tuesdays at a shopping mall, do you know where the exits are in the mall? Or, if you take a weekly yoga class at night that is located next to a busy plaza, do you park your car in a well lit spot and in the direction that allows you the quickest escape? Do you walk out with others for added security? Does your evac plan include carrying a panic button in case you are grabbed? Assess your habits and create feasible evac plans. Do rehearse as many evac plans as possible, even if only in your mind. For example, if a man pointed a gun at you and demanded your purse, you might want to throw the purse a few feet away so that he must distance himself from you in order to get it.

Travel Emergency Evacuation Plan

Possible Attacks While Traveling:

Assault
Robbery/ Pick Pocketing/Purse Snatching
Identity Theft
Battery
Rape
Abduction
Murder
Hate Crime
Terrorist Attack
Other?

Your emergency evacuation plans when traveling require more planning ahead and are more difficult to rehearse. However, your main objective is to identify all your resources for help as soon as you are on the ground in your new location. Carry phone numbers of local police and your hotel information with you at all times. Know the exits in your hotel and where they are in relation to your room. When you are out on the town, pay attention to your surroundings and identify a taxi company that is reliable. Bear in mind that, at a moment's notice, you may be required to bolt from any location, be it a tourist spot, a restaurant, a side street, a theatre, or even a church. This does not mean you need to be paranoid during your trip. It simply means that, because you are in a strange place, your situational awareness is slightly more elevated. (For more on traveling safely, especially in foreign countries, see Chapter Fourteen).

Having emergency evacuation plans helps you condition your mind and body with the prospect of escaping an attack. If your emergency evacuation plan fails and you are in a struggle, do everything you can to survive. Use every resource at your disposal: your voice, your body, any weapons, psychological manipulations, and, if it is your only option, excessive force. Coach yourself throughout the attack by saying "I will survive! I will survive! I will survive!"

After an Attack

Depending on the nature of the attack, certain steps must be taken immediately afterwards and for the duration of your recovery. These include: medical attention, evidence collection, and psychological support. Obviously, your first priority is seeking medical attention. You may have trouble focusing on the logical action to take immediately after an attack. Use your SUPNET and get help from the authorities, professionals, and people you trust. Take care of your body; it was just traumatized and needs to be cared for and healed. Even if you feel emotions that do not make sense, such as embarrassment, prioritize getting medical attention. Do not allow your inner monologue to talk you out of it. Even if you are only bruised, go see a doctor and get checked out to be sure you do not have a concussion or worse.

Seeking medical attention is also your first step towards evidence collection. By seeing a doctor you are creating a medical record of the injuries you sustained. If the police get involved, they can take photos of you and the crime scene and collect other evidence that may be crucial in helping them arrest your attacker. If you have been raped, do not take a shower or wash yourself in any way until you have gone to the hospital and professionals have used a rape kit to collect evidence. Again, do not allow your inner monologue to talk you out of reporting the attack. Many women allow their trauma to become the guiding force after an attack. This is why so many women do not report the crimes committed against them. Again, plan ahead. Decide for yourself now how you would respond after being attacked. Program your mind ahead of time, so that you have a plan and can act, even in the face of severe stress and trauma.

Finally, realize that your recovery will include seeking out psychological support of some kind. Initially you may just turn to family and friends for help. However, depending on the severity of the attack, you may need to seek professional help. Do not assume that you cannot afford help. There are countless organizations that can direct you to affordable help (see Appendix E). It is important for you to take the trauma seriously so that it does not continue to impact you in ways that feel out of your control. A professional can guide you through a process wherein you can confront and transcend your trauma and other emotions associated with it. The point is: you survived the attack so take the next step and commit to surviving the emotional fallout from the attack.

Part of becoming an empowered woman is to accept that you will be required to work through the psychological fallout from an attack. Think of it as similar to working through a bad breakup. There are and will be emotional consequences, possibly for years to come. Women who keep their attacks secret suffer in silence. Women who report their attacks suffer in silence too but they gain greater access to support. Being willing to work through your suffering, with or without support, is part of your empowerment process. As more women speak out against their attackers, more justice will be served and those attackers will be prevented from attacking other women. We are all in this together.

Conclusion

If we return to the idea that women tend to try to fix things and appease, we can glean the wisdom to see how crippling this can be to our personal security. Often we will ignore or seriously underestimate our sharpest defense mechanism: our intuition. It is our most powerful asset for staying safe, yet because we are socialized to be polite and to appease, we sometimes attract predators and draw them in too closely, allowing them access which endangers us. We do this simply because we have been coached all of our lives to 'be polite.' We need to reconnect with our instinct and take our intuition seriously. It is a critical part of our early warning system. When we combine our situational awareness with our surveillance detection practice, we are exponentially increasing our chances of avoiding an attack altogether. Even if these prevention methods fall short, we are at least consciously ready to respond in the event of an attack because our minds have already recognized the possibility of one.

On some level none of us wants to believe that we could become a victim. Security practices can seem like a nuisance and we often opt to hope for the best rather than plan for the worst. Security is all about planning for the worst so that you are prepared in case it happens. Even if the worst happens and your attacker prevails, if you survive, the fact that you did your best to defend yourself will assist you in recovering psychologically from the impact of the attack. If you do not survive, would you not rather die having done your very best to defend yourself versus being a sitting duck, totally unable to respond? Any woman who has survived an attack will tell you that her active participation in minimizing the harm she experienced left her feeling some dignity about her response. Sometimes this response means submitting to a rapist so that you will not be murdered or so that the attack will not escalate. Sometimes it means screaming at the top of your lungs and running away as fast as you can.

There is no pre-set formula we can give you because every attack is different and so is every woman. Your best chance of survival lies in your ability to know yourself, assess the situation as it unfolds, and do your best (whatever that entails) to live. You are stronger than you know and you can recover from an attack with the proper help from family and friends and support from professionals. Many people have survival stories and they go on to live fulfilling lives, even though they may carry scars and damage. Your survival is what counts; the scars and damage cannot destroy you if your free will to transcend them and live on is very much alive.

CHAPTER FOURTEEN

WOMEN ON THE MOVE: TRAVEL SECURITY

"Roam if you want to
Roam around the world"

--The B-52's

Women are on the move. More and more we are traveling for business and pleasure, both domestically and internationally. Women are easy targets when they travel because they are out of their familiar element and they are distracted by the newness of everything they are experiencing. Predators know this and their radar heightens when they see women in their countries who are obviously foreigners. They also know that women who are inexperienced travelers are sometimes more likely to engage in conversations with strangers because everything is new and exciting and their minds are open to adventure. In addition, many unseasoned travelers will engage in social behaviors that are more risky because they are exposed to social environments that are enticing and different from what they are used to back home. Even if you are traveling inside your own country, you will stick out in unfamiliar places unless you make a concerted effort not to. Predators also use to their advantage the knowledge that women traveling alone are often unprepared to identify safe locations, contact the authorities, or protect themselves from strangers (who may use the ruse that they are friendly locals looking to help a tourist in distress).

Regardless if you are traveling in your native country on a business trip or you are departing on an international vacation to a remote location, please bear in mind you are often more vulnerable while traveling than when you are at home because you are in transition between secure environments. Logic would lead you to believe that if you are just traveling in your home state you are inherently safer (and that may be true); still you can also make yourself more vulnerable if this feeling of safety allows you to become complacent and you stop noticing early warning signs of danger and indicators of surveillance and suspicious activity. It is neither our goal to discourage you from traveling nor to make you a nervous, paranoid wreck constantly running on adrenaline. Rather, we hope to help you to develop calm and discerning awareness. Like waves of water that ebb and flow with the changing pull of gravity you can instinctively raise and lower your situational awareness and security status when you travel through locations and situations based on the possible threats you perceive.

In this chapter we give you lists of travel tips that we hope you will consider carefully because they are derived from our experiences and are not based on theory alone. We have both traveled extensively all over the world and have lived in a variety of foreign cultures. When pooling our experiences, we discovered that common security risks exist and apply to just about anywhere you travel. In addition to our lists of tips, we will address the concerns of women who are working for international aid organizations or as missionaries, or are expatriates living in foreign countries, since they face other issues that the average traveler never encounters.

Remember to consider the current political climate when you travel. At present, the war on terrorism and the war in Iraq have implications that affect Americans traveling abroad. Use common sense and avoid discussions on politics and religion. No matter where you go you will find that people both love and hate Americans. In our experiences, we found that the majority of people we encountered love Americans. Our nation and way of life is still coveted by people worldwide because of the "American Dream" and the great opportunities and bountiful way of life we are privileged to enjoy. Our athletes, movie stars, and comparatively glamorous lifestyle entice many people living in impoverished countries. By comparison, Americans are vastly wealthy and many people try to take advantage of this. It also makes us highly desired targets for theft; pickpockets love American tourists.

Our list of travel tips is broken down into categories: Before the Trip; Arrival/Departure; Hotel Security; and Out & About. Some of these tips might sound obscure to you, but depending on the continent you visit, certain cultural practices may apply about which you may be unaware and could pose a problem for you. For example, in some parts of the world a woman wearing shorts and a sleeveless shirt is considered to be offensive. Or, sitting with the bottoms of your feet facing another is considered to be very rude. We posit that if you offend someone, even inadvertently, you may increase your risk level and make yourself a potential target, especially if you do so in an area dominated by anti-social men or criminal activity. Probably no one would shoot you for wearing shorts and a sleeveless shirt, but they might take special notice of you, harass you verbally, or even follow you. Why put yourself in a position to create conflict which may escalate into danger?

Before the Trip

- Recruit a travel partner. You will be able to relax and enjoy yourself more if you are traveling with a friend. Using the buddy system exponentially increases your security; this is why it is a standing rule in the armed forces. If you are traveling with young children, bringing a nanny on the trip will provide greater security (and convenience). Two sets of eyes are always better than one, especially if they are SASD. Even if you must travel alone you can always find opportunities to meet other women whom you can temporarily enlist as buddies.

- Before traveling, you should begin your trip at home by researching where you are going. One great resource, available on the internet, is the CIA World Factbook for each country. This gives you the specifics about all aspects of the country, including the types of crime, drug issues, and terrorist threats that the particular nation currently faces. You can also access the U.S. Department of State website to get an update on any threats or warnings relevant to the area. The Center for Disease Control website will update you on any health risks, such as infectious diseases. Sometimes these risks relate to the drug/crime problems in a country (for example: Hepatitis or A.I.D.S.). Lonely Planet is another good site for learning about local issues and customs. You can always research local newspapers to find current information on your destination. It is wise to research local customs, significant dates and events, traffic laws, and laws that pertain to conducting business. (See Appendix E for these websites).

- Be discreet about your travel plans; not everyone needs to know you are leaving for a trip or where you are going. Be careful not to broadcast the details of your trip in the presence of strangers.

- Debrief friends and family who have already traveled to your destination for insights, hotel suggestions, and for points of contact they established and trust.

- Make a checklist you can review and follow to help ensure you are prepared and do not leave something behind.

- Pack wisely; less means more because you will be less encumbered and more mobile.

- Do not use U.S. affiliated name tags, t-shirts, or anything that identifies you as an American.

- Exchange some money into the local currency at a bank near you so you arrive with the ability to be immediately self-sufficient. Exchange kiosks at international airports are often watched by criminals trying to spot an obvious foreigner who just exchanged a large sum of money.

- Learn local phrases or at a minimum make a small cheat sheet of important words like: Help, Emergency, or Police.
- Always pack and carry a small yet powerful flashlight.
- Photocopy your passport, medical insurance card, plane tickets, and your traveler's checks. Keep one copy of these at home and another with you.
- Keep your U.S. currency and your foreign currency separate so that no one sees you displaying dollars except when you exchange money.
- Make a list of everything in your suitcase, as well as a description of your luggage so that, if your luggage is lost or stolen, you can quickly make an accurate claim for reimbursement.
- Consider purchasing travel insurance for your trip.

Arrival/Departure/En Route

Now that you are well prepared to leave, we want to give you some ideas for how you can use situational awareness and surveillance detection techniques for every phase of your travel. There is no need to be overwhelmed; you can do this! In fact, you will be able to travel with greater confidence and ease if you are SASD. Because arrivals and departures are transition times, they are significant to criminals because they offer opportunities for beginning the surveillance phase of their targets and for taking advantage of distracted travelers.

- Be alert and on the lookout for indicators that you are under surveillance at the airport, train station, or bus station. Youths are often used as spotters, so do not ignore adolescents or even children. Notice if anyone follows you or fixates his/her attention on you.
- Be wary of distractions and unsolicited advances from strangers (they often work in teams; one may distract you as the other steals your

bags). Keep your eyes on your bags and do not entrust a stranger to watch your bags while you visit the ladies' room.

- Be alert for unattended bags or suspicious behavior.
- Wait to send your carry-on luggage through the security x-ray machines until you are ready to walk through. If the security guard delays your passage, keep a careful eye on your bags as they come out from the machine on the conveyor belt.
- For small items such as your purse or a camera bag, use straps with clips to attach these to your larger pieces of luggage, so that no one can snatch these smaller items if you are looking away or are distracted.
- Consider bringing either a waist or neck pouch (both worn under your clothing) for storing your passport and other important documents if you are planning on sleeping during your travel hours.
- Notice if any passengers boarding your plane, train, or bus seem to be communicating somehow, even though they do not appear to be traveling together.
- Talk with female flight attendants for information about your arrival location. Talk with female tourists as well. Perhaps they are revisiting your destination and will have helpful information to share.
- Upon arrival, by all means ask for directions if you need them. However, go to the information booth or find a female employee at the airport or station to ask. Do not bury your head in a map like a lost, helpless tourist. If you must consult your map, first scan the area to see if anyone is paying close attention to you.
- Pay attention to entrances and exits at the airport or at stations. Do not end up in corridors or secluded areas. If any disturbance occurs and police start swarming the area, try to exit immediately or at least get close to an exit or a supporting structure in the building.
- Upon arrival in a foreign country, contact the U.S. embassy or Consulate to inform them that you are visiting the country. Give them the dates of your trip, your hotel information, and information

about any side trips you intend to make. If you have any medical condition, such as a heart condition or diabetes, give them this information as well. Obtain their 24 hour emergency phone number in the event you need assistance in an emergency.

Hotel Security

Predators often plant themselves in hotel lobbies to troll for targets, conduct surveillance, and 'pick up' their targets in order to follow them as they leave the hotel. It is easy to collect information while sitting in a hotel lobby near the main desk where people are checking in and relaying personal information to the receptionist or the concierge. They may also position themselves nearby, for example outside a door but within line of sight and earshot to the reception desk.

- When checking into your hotel, pay attention to anyone in the lobby who is watching you. Keep your voice low, so as not to broadcast the details of your stay at the hotel (length of stay, room number, the fact that you are traveling alone, etc.). Ask the person at the reception desk to write down your room number rather than announcing it out loud to others who may be loitering and listening nearby.
- Request a map/schematic of the hotel and the area. Identify where the nearest police station and hospital are located and mark them on your map.
- Vary your routine and do not establish a pattern. Do not announce your plans in public. Hotel staff can be very nosy because they are in the courtesy business. Rehearse a few polite but vague answers to questions about your plans for your intended stay. If you are a frequent traveler to the same location this is especially important. If you are in a country where there is a significant terrorist presence and threat, be extra cautious and make a concerted effort to stay SASD.

- Try to stay in hotels that are not frequented by large numbers of U.S. tourists, have underground parking garages, or design features that make them more vulnerable to terrorist attacks (such as a building that is constructed using a large amount of glass).

- Request to be escorted to your room by the bellhop. Ask him to wait while you check that all window and door locks are in good working order and that balcony doors are secure. Normally hotel maintenance can easily and quickly repair any broken locks or you can request a new room.

- Do not stay on the ground floor of the hotel or in a room that is accessible from a nearby or attached rooftop.

- Know where the exits are on your floor. Read the fire escape map posted next to the door in your room. You can even count how many doors you are away from the fire escapes.

- Pack a bolt bag and keep it accessible. It should contain your valuables, a set of clothes and a pair of shoes, any defensive tools, and your cell phone (if you brought one). Never leave valuables visible and accessible in the room. You can either use the room safe or hotel safe deposit box at the main desk to store valuables.

- Use every lock on the door to your room whenever you are inside the room. When you leave the room, hang the "Do not disturb" sign on the knob (unless you want the room cleaned), so that it appears that someone is in the room. Bring a small, stick-on alarm to attach to your door which will sound if anyone opens your door while you are sleeping. You can also improvise some type of barricade by placing a chair or trashcan in front of the door to alert you if anyone tries to break in to your room at night.

- When exiting the hotel, again scan the lobby to be sure no one is conducting surveillance or initiates following you. If anyone gets in a taxi behind yours, see if that taxi follows yours. If you leave the hotel on foot, be sure no one follows you. If you notice someone following you, go back to the hotel and depart again later, possibly from another exit.

Out and About

Tourist destinations are ripe for crime. If the purpose of your travel is vacation, know that criminals are out there targeting women for a variety of reasons, including robbery and rape. Realize that the newness of the location and the many activities and interesting sights are distractions. Stay SASD so that you can relax and have a better time knowing you are being proactive about your security. If the purpose of your travel is business, realize that you are likely setting patterns everyday (eating breakfast at the same time each morning, using predictable transportation, etc.). You are also distracted not only by this new location, but also by your work. Stay SASD so that you do not make yourself an attractive target.

Bear in mind that the level of assertiveness of men in foreign countries will be different than that to which you are accustomed in the United States. Often men in foreign countries will be very pushy when they try to elicit information from you. They may not take no for an answer or will try another tack if you attempt to steer them away from a certain subject. If you tell them you are traveling with your boyfriend or husband, they may ask where he is and why he left you alone. Hold your ground and politely break contact as soon as possible if any man is crossing the line of your perception of appropriate social etiquette. He may be totally harmless, but you must prioritize protecting yourself and your information over taking care of his feelings.

- Do not broadcast your nationality or beliefs in issues either verbally or with what you carry or wear.
- *Do not hitchhike!* Even if hitchhiking is common for women in the country you are visiting, do not succumb to this habit. It is simply

too high risk since you are out of your element and cannot count on extracting yourself safely if some maniac gives you a ride.

- Vary your routine. Avoid being predictable in your schedule and in your whereabouts.

- In crowded places keep your voice down. Remember that your accent is easily detectable and foreign to others.

- If you need directions, ask your hotel concierge, an official, or a shop owner before you ask a stranger. If you must ask a stranger, choose a woman.

- Find out from your hotel concierge which cab companies are safe to use. Whenever taking a taxi, write down the number of the taxi and the driver's name (usually this is displayed on a badge or card attached to the dashboard). It is also wise to look at the driver's picture on his badge and make sure he is the one who is actually driving you. In many foreign countries the taxis have no seatbelts in the back seat. Also, the windows are often locked closed. Lock your door if possible.

- Always carry a business card from the hotel so you have the address and phone number to show taxi drivers or in the event of an emergency. It is also a good idea to obtain a pre-paid phone card that will work in phone booths. Ask the concierge where you can obtain a card (usually at a convenience or grocery store).

- Do not carry all your money in one place or display it in public. Carry what you think you will need for the purchases you have planned in a separate pocket or pouch. If you must access your cache, do so in a restroom stall so you are discreet.

- Do not broadcast the fact that you are traveling alone. Say you are with your husband, boyfriend, or a tour group.

- For daily activities, do not wear clothing or jewelry that attracts the attention of criminals. If you are going out for a fancy meal or to the theatre, be extra SASD so that you can dress up and have fun without trouble.

- Be especially careful of pickpockets (and gypsies) if you travel on buses, subways, or trains. In many countries small children are well trained pickpockets and will create diversions in order to rob you blind.
- Always have small change available for traveling on public transportation.
- If you are renting a car, be sure you study the traffic laws and road signs of the countries in which you will be driving. Always have good maps and never allow your gas tank to go below the half way mark. Also, be very careful at rest stops along the highways. If you pull off and the rest stop is too isolated, find another one.
- When out at night, do not drink too much. Criminals target female tourists who are impaired due to alcohol consumption. Again, using the buddy system will help you retain control over social situations that might put you at risk.
- Never change money on the black market. Although you will get a better rate, you are risking getting into trouble and interacting with a criminal.
- If you are using an ATM machine, find one that is inside a bank or store. Guard the screen while you type in your pin number. Scan the area before approaching and using the machine and while walking away with the cash to be sure no one follows you.

Interacting with Law Enforcement

You cannot assume that law enforcement in other countries will behave the same way they do at home. Research your destinations so that you know what to expect from law enforcement. Keep a low profile and do not instigate any unnecessary interactions if you are traveling in a country where corruption among the authorities is a known problem. Some countries have epidemic corruption amongst law enforcement and tourists often become targets of their scams to procure more income. In some places, they will use extortion by threatening to take you to jail for some petty offense unless you pay them, in cash, right on the spot. In some countries they may try to demand sexual favors before they will drop the bogus charges against you. One tactic you can try, if ever in either of these situations, is to tell the officer you are going to call your embassy or consulate to report the incident (having the emergency contact number of the embassy or consulate with you at all times is advised). This may scare him off and he may let you go. Make sure you get his name or car/license plate number if at all possible and report the incident to the embassy or consulate immediately.

Women Living and Working in Foreign Lands

Regardless if you are a missionary, an international aid worker or an ex-pat living in a foreign country, you must prepare yourself for the many threats you may face. We cannot stress enough how important the techniques in the first seven chapters of this book are for you, given that you are elevating your risk level just by virtue of the fact that you are living in a foreign country.

Many missionaries and aid workers are assigned to impoverished, isolated communities. Living in these remote locations puts you at greater risk of danger. Extreme poverty and harsh conditions can lead to social crises and crime can run rampant. If you are planning to work as a missionary or aid worker, find out the statistics of crimes against foreign women in the area to which you have been assigned. Your organization owes it to you to both inform you and protect you while you are stationed in another country (and most do). Still, ask what policies are in place to help keep you safe before accepting the assignment. In addition, know yourself. If you are assigned to an area where many women have been raped on the job, are you willing to go this far for whatever cause you are supporting? Know what you are willing to accept in terms of risk and get the facts *before you leave home*. If possible, contact another female worker who was assigned a position in the same place. Get the truth; you deserve to be protected.

If you are an ex-pat, be sure you have strong connections to the nearest U.S. Embassy or Consulate. Keep close ties to the ex-pat community as part of your SUPNET. You can even create an alert roster to update each other by telephone with information about any threats. Know the local laws and research the criminal and terrorist threats in the area. Use surveillance detection regularly, especially when traveling along your routine routes to work or any locations you frequent habitually. Practice SD when in any buildings you spend time in regularly, such as your residence and workplace. Stay SASD in your daily life so that you can experience living in a foreign land safely. Be sure to read the section on abduction in Chapter Ten, as ex-pats are often targeted for abductions by both criminals and terrorists.

Conclusion

Traveling should be an enjoyable experience. However, if you are unprepared to handle potential dangers, your trip can easily be ruined. Think ahead, before you depart, and do as much as you can to ensure that you travel safely. Traveling, whether for business or pleasure, has become a common part of our lives. Our global economy has strong momentum and many women in business are being given opportunities to travel to foreign countries. Likewise, many women are opting to travel abroad for vacations or even relocate to foreign countries. Have a plan if you intend to make a trip or to reside overseas. Your personal security practice is mobile; you can take it anywhere. If you conduct even a simple risk assessment for your trip, one that is based on your research about your destination, you will likely see that the threat level is higher than what you face at home. Make the proper adjustments and travel safely so that you can enjoy the experience and return from your trip unharmed.

CHAPTER FIFTEEN

DEFENDING OURSELVES: CAREERS IN SECURITY

*The history we shape
shapes those who follow us
and propels our gender forward*

While the majority of violence against women is inflicted by men, the majority of protection from this violence is provided by men. Chew on that one for awhile and you will begin to wonder why more women do not seek careers in security related fields. This is the great irony. We believe that there is a strong relationship between the lack of women working in security fields and the high statistics in violence against women. Look at it this way: Before women began integrating themselves into politics, many women's issues were overlooked or blatantly ignored. If women were the movers and shakers in local police departments, for example, perhaps more community programs would exist for helping women learn to protect themselves against violent crime. This is not to criticize the male heads of police departments; rather, we are simply making the point that women's issues normally receive better attention if women are pushing them forward. Look at "MADD" (Mothers Against Drunk Driving) as an example of an organization that has taken on a type of crime that has impacted their lives and the lives of their families. As more women work as activists and legislators, more laws are passed that impact the lives of all women.

We believe that the female perspective in any security related field serves as an asset. In our experience with training women all over the world in surveillance detection, we witnessed a common proficiency level in certain areas that far exceeded that of our male trainees (though they possessed other attributes that the females sometimes lacked). Across the board the women were far more patient, methodical, specific in their observation skills, detailed in their reporting skills, and able to blend into the environment more easily without arousing suspicion. Women are hard-wired differently than men and their unique perspective enhances many security practices.

Because the security industry is flooded with men, and because it is a growth industry due to the war on terrorism, this is a great time for more women to enter the field. In addition, more colleges and universities are offering degrees in security management and security related professions, such as criminal justice and forensic science. The time is ripe for women to enter this dynamic and growing field. You might be wondering why a woman would have interest in this field. Certainly, it is not for everyone. Women with careers in security sometimes feel the annoyance of being a minority in a man's world. On the job, our co-workers are predominantly male because there are so few women in the field that we are dispersed and rarely get to work together. Women working in security are often subjected to having their credibility scrutinized. However, now that you are equipped with a refined, SASD mental template regarding your own security, if you were to enter the profession you could excel quickly in this rapidly growing industry. In addition, many men working in the field have great respect and admiration for their female co-workers.

If the security world interests you, you are a hot commodity, especially if you are properly educated, trained, and are willing to travel. It is an exciting profession with a variety of career possibilities. Careers in security allow women plentiful opportunities to nurture others by protecting them, rescuing them, and ensuring their safety. Careers in security also provide perks, namely your confidence will be boosted and you will have a much better handle on keeping yourself and your family safe. The opportunities are expanding in security related fields. In addition, other fields apply to the security industry. For example, if you are fluent in a foreign language you might work for the United Nations as an interpreter on sensitive political and security related issues. With the proper education and training you can pursue a career in any of the following:

- Law Enforcement (police officer/state trooper/highway patrol)
- Forensics
- Intelligence (FBI/CIA/NSA)
- Sales (of security related products and systems)
- IT Security (Information Technology)
- Technical Security Specialist (surveillance cameras, listening devices, etc.)
- Security Trainer
- Security Consultant
- Corporate Security
- Security Management
- Education (security in schools, especially colleges and universities)
- Public Relations
- Private Investigation
- Transportation Security (TSA)
- Executive Protection (bodyguard, for executives or celebrities)
- Diplomatic Security
- Homeland Security
- Civilian Contractor (multiple private security companies exist that need more women working for them, both in this country and overseas)
- Law (criminal lawyer or paralegal)
- Politics (including lobbyist or spokesperson)
- Military

- Translator/Interpreter
- Research and Development/Manufacturing (of security related products and systems)
- Self-Defense Instructor
- Counselor/Therapist (focusing on women who are victims of domestic violence or rape)
- Hotline Operator
- United Nations Peacekeepers
- Author
- Professor

You can also work within your community as a volunteer and become involved in shaping policy and legislation that impacts women's security issues. You can participate in the evolution of empowerment, not only through your own personal security practice, but also through becoming a member of the profession. To get started, we advise researching fields that interest you (by going to the library, searching on the internet, or networking with people in the field). Once you select an area of interest, look into any available educational programs or internships in that field. If you already have a degree, continuing education is an option. Having a degree is an asset but is not a necessity in some areas of the security industry. In fact, many people in the industry have military backgrounds rather than college degrees and many employers consider this experience to be of equal or greater value.

With more women working in the field, we can strengthen and contribute the female perspective, thereby influencing the future of our own security. Think of how the sexual harassment policies have been changed in most companies due to women's efforts towards this issue. Imagine how building design features could be impacted if more female security guards were able to give their input about the layout of parking garages. Whole communities can be transformed if more women become involved in tackling the security issues and problems created by crime.

By embracing our evolutionary path to learn to protect ourselves rather than relying solely on men for our protection, we can grow into more empowered women, both as individuals and as communities working together. Just as we formed a sisterhood around the issue of having the right to vote, we must also form an alliance regarding the security of our species. We must stop complaining about our weakened position and burying our heads in the sand hoping we will never be victimized. We must also begin transforming ourselves into stronger, more capable women. Together we can be very powerful, but only if we become truly involved in shaping the laws, policies, and procedures that impact our security.

CHAPTER SIXTEEN

EMPOWERMENT: THE OTHER SIDE OF EXHAUSTION

"Life's hard you know (oh whey oh)
So strike a pose on a Cadillac."

--The Bangles

The weaker sex; we have heard it all our lives. Is it not exhausting trying to prove this is a fallacy, fearing all the while it may be true? If you are not busy enough buffing up at the gym and expending the energy to defeat the myth that you are weaker, you are frantically turning your car keys into a weapon, sleeping with a baseball bat under your bed, and working like a dog to exist safely in the reality that indeed you are weaker. Sometimes you just have to put down the laundry basket, grab that early coffee break at the office, or drift off while he is making love to you and sigh with wonder at why your strength is so often unseen, unheard, unappreciated. 'Hang on girl,' you tell yourself, and 'buck up.' If your strengths were as physical as a man's, all would stop to notice. Just because you raise the kids, cook and clean, have a career, are a dynamo in bed, and still have time to paint your nails does not mean you too cannot be afforded the privilege of walking to your car without risk of being attacked. Well…actually that is exactly what it means because you do not have that privilege. Thankfully the love, friendship, and warmth of the good men in our lives make our physically weaker position tolerable and allow us to experience how wonderful it is to relate positively to the physically stronger sex. We can and must retain our humor and feminine nature while strengthening our personal security. Like the Bangles advise us in the quotation above, we must take the hardships in stride and continue being women.

When hate, violence, and perversion arise our real strength is tested. Unfortunately we do have to face that, generally speaking, we are at a physical disadvantage and are therefore victimized by predators. We can take kickboxing classes, buy TASER devices, carry mace in our purses, and cover our drinks with napkins to fend off date rape drugs. We can trade in our feminine, passive ways and buff up our bodies and attitudes to transform ourselves into worthy adversaries. Do we lose ourselves in the process? Is not losing ourselves worth the risk of remaining a target? Do we ever really feel safe or are we living with a low level of quiet desperation that steadily runs through our nervous systems and dampens our spirits with low grade but constant stress? These are the questions that plague women living in western civilizations while many women on other continents continue to work like slaves, are forced into arranged marriages, or have their genitalia brutally removed. Even worse, in some nations women and young girls are forced to work in the sex industry as a result of economic hardship and political corruption. The road has been long and difficult for us all, yet our strength thrives and we continue to protect and defend ourselves as best we know how. As exhausting as it all seems, we can emerge out of our tumultuous history to the other side of exhaustion. The evolution of empowerment means we are entitled to and capable of existing as a notable presence in society, one which no longer tolerates the notion that our victimization is acceptable.

We have designed a very simple formula for you to memorize and, eventually begin living. It is your recipe for empowerment:

COGNATE INTEGRATE MOTIVATE ACTIVATE

The premise is that our empowerment begins when we *cognate*, or bring into our intellectual minds, the idea that we are rising above our role as victims. Once our cognitive process is underway, the next step, which will happen naturally when you begin to cultivate your situational awareness and surveillance detection practice, is to allow your empowerment to *integrate* into your being. Once you have pointed your mind in the right direction, through cognition, and your body as well, through integration, you now are ready to *motivate* change. The word "motivate" has taken on a rather syrupy, trite connotation. We see it simply as a change word, meaning it is a directive you give yourself and then just allow it to unfold in your life. You do not need a pep rally or daily affirmations or a permanent smile swiped across your face. You just need to wake up every day knowing that you are a part of a species that is evolving and your life is a contribution to that process for other women, young and old, to see. You are an empowerment teacher just by virtue of the fact that you have altered your presence and are now radiating as an emboldened spirit, rather than a cowering victim. Lastly, you will *activate*. You will have a plan for your personal security as it relates to all aspects of your life. When you *activate* it means that you will find your own path and apply all you have learned so that you can embody a new level of confidence inside yourself and emit it to the world. This confidence is inside you already; it is in all of us, but we need to awaken it and live it.

Once you follow this empowerment recipe, you will see that all of the struggles and challenges that you have been hassling with all your life will suddenly not feel so draining. Your ability to positively influence the men in your life will happen naturally, by example, without the need for a long lecture or nagging session. The thick-headed ones will no longer bother you because you will just move along and seek out the momentum of your own emboldened path rather than clogging up your time and energy with those who drain your reserves. You will quit depleting your own reserves through denial or exhaustion because you will accept that, as Ghandi said: "You must be the change you want to see in the world."

The best part is you will have discovered a new energy inside yourself, one that replenishes you regularly. This energy will begin to permeate every facet of your life. You will stand tall because you have rebooted your mind, senses, body, and emotions on a cellular level. It sounds abstract, but it is true. You are allowed input into your own evolutionary process. In a way it is the same as if you were a professional athlete. Your regular, focused training changes your body and mental template. Just as you can literally program your muscle memory through repeated movement training of any kind, you can reprogram your cellular memory and become a more alive woman through the practice of situational awareness and surveillance detection. Getting SASD is that powerful.

The more mindful you become in your life, the more responsibility you take for your own experiences. Part of what you will discover is that most men want to protect you. For example, there is no need for you to feel ashamed or embarrassed for asking a man at your office to walk you to your car if your intuition tells you something feels off and you are afraid to go alone. It does not mean you are incapable, weak, or silly. It means the opposite: You are so in touch and aware that you recognize when you need help and you ask for it. The majority of men out there love being in the role of rescuer and that, ladies, is the good news.

Men elicit help from women all the time. We sew the button back on the shirt, make the coffee at work, and provide an ear when they want to talk about their day. We nurture naturally, happily, and regularly. It is our nature and instinct. We are hard-wired to do it and that is okay! So why do we have such a hard time letting them live their instinct to protect us? We can find a balancing point in our relationships with the good men (meaning safe) in our lives wherein we do not have to carry our torch and fight at every turn to be seen, heard, and appreciated. Why exhaust ourselves this way? When we allow our feminist struggles to get the best of us, we actually make ourselves more susceptible to becoming the victims of the bad men in our lives. Why? For starters, our attention is scattered, our energy is compromised, and we are too emotionally entangled to notice the early warning signals of danger. In addition, we present ourselves as targets because we are too aggressive and confrontational or we become self-righteous and indignant.

We realize this is a lot to digest and, although it sounds great in theory, applying it is another story. Our goal with this book is to literally impact the evolution of women's empowerment by helping 'woman as victim' transform into 'woman as activated.' We realize that reading helps begin the cognition process, but that the rest of this recipe requires hands-on practice. That is why suggest you receive training to help jump-start your empowerment process and give you guidance on practicing situational awareness and surveillance detection (see Appendix A).

We also realize that the activated, evolved woman will still face the prospect of violence. What will change is her ability to now successfully avoid it and transcend it on a daily basis with greater ease and confidence. Women can now support each other and future generations by becoming activated and aware.

The evolutionary question lingers: will deer, over the ages, evolve to a point where they are instinctively programmed to recognize the headlights of an oncoming vehicle. Will they, as a species, continue to freeze and stare into the headlights or will they adapt and avoid the vehicle? If a species in the animal kingdom can adapt its instincts to keep itself safe, think of how fortunate and blessed we are because we have human consciousness as our unique asset. We have our human minds to assist and expedite the development of our instincts. You can adapt and evolve by discovering the potential of your greater being; so switch on and get SASD!

EPILOGUE

OUR EVOLUTIONARY TRUTH

The strength of women
so unseen, so unheard, so abused
lies in wait, evolving
its rewards are our lingering treasure

This book ends with a simple but powerful, exciting truth: *You are in charge of the evolution of your personal security practice.* Imagine if massive amounts of women worldwide take on this empowered approach to their personal security. Over time the lack of tolerance for violence against women will impact the world. It is a slow process, one that takes generations. We each give the ever turning cogwheel a small nudge just by virtue of being alive. We can choose to have our small nudge move the wheel in a positive, forward direction. As we nudge the wheel forward collectively, we impact change. Look at how other evolutionary processes have already occurred in our lifetime. Our senior readers remember that their mothers were not allowed to vote. Our middle-aged readers remember how hard it was for women to enter certain fields and work with men and receive equal pay. Our teenage readers remember that girls used to be forbidden to play football in school. In cultures across the globe women continue to work towards making small strides in the direction of bettering their lives. Even though the pace is slow, our lives have impact on future generations of women. The more vocal and overt we become with our security practices, the less victimized we will be.

Consider yourself nudged. The act of reading this book has instigated the process of altering your mental template. You can now activate your empowered self by integrating new, simple practices into your life. It is truly that easy. You are capable and do not have to become a victim. But you do have to participate in remembering your forgotten instinct (situational awareness) and you must apply it and other preventative measures (especially surveillance detection) to your daily routines. You have to be involved to be a survivor. You must develop plans for improving your personal security in all aspects of your life.

This book also ends with a reminder of a harsh truth: Bad, random acts of violence do happen. If they happen (or have happened) to you, give yourself a break and continue with your recovery so that the rest of your life belongs to you, not your attacker. It was not your fault, even if you realize in retrospect that there were preventative actions you could have taken to avoid the consequences of someone else's violent predisposition. Even if you have already been victimized, your evolution is still in your hands. Consider yourself to have a PHD in survival. You can decide how to process the trauma and move on with your life. You get to be the one to transform yourself into a woman who is empowered enough to take charge of her personal security from this moment on and for the rest of your days.

Cindy's story is a telling example of the value of cultivating our forgotten instinct.

Two days before the attacks of September eleventh Cindy was walking her dog in a suburb in the Boston area when she came upon two Middle Eastern men flanking a parked car, leaning on its roof while deeply immersed in excited conversation. She did not recognize their foreign tongue but noticed that they were totally out of place in the neighborhood. She walked her dog around this development every day and had never seen the men before. Her dog, Mitzy, an Australian shepherd, suddenly became skittish and uneasy. Cindy too felt the stir of danger inside, but walked on. The next day while she was again walking Mitzy she came upon the same two men near the car. This time a third man came out of the basement door of the split-level house calling to the others to come inside, again in a happy, excited manner. She got a good look at this man.

The next day, September eleventh, Cindy and every American watched in horror as the Twin Towers toppled and the Pentagon burned. Soon after, while she was at home vacuuming with the T.V. on, Mohammed Atta's photograph popped up on the screen.

"My stomach literally dropped and I immediately felt ill and disgusted. I was certain he was the third man I had seen at the door of the split-level house."

It took Cindy a couple of days and her husband's encouragement to contact the F.B.I., who interviewed her four weeks later (clearly the delay was due to the vast amount of tips they received). At the interview she identified Atta and the two other men from photographs they showed her. Later investigations revealed that the hijackers had stayed in a motel approximately five minutes away from where Cindy had seen them days prior to the attack.

Cindy was never able to find out if her report had any merit. She knows the F.B.I. staked out the home where she saw the men. She also knows that the family living there continued to occupy the home, though she said for two weeks after the attacks the screen door to the lower level of that house was left open and the house appeared to be vacant. She surmises that they may have been renting the lower level of the home to the men she identified.

"The fact that the family still lives there makes me think I might have been wrong. But then again, perhaps they just rented out their place and that is not a crime."

She also reported a description of their vehicle and it turned out to be a similar vehicle to the one the authorities found at the Portland, Maine airport. We asked Cindy what it was that made her feel so sure that the men she had seen were Atta and the other hijackers.

"My dog's reaction was really significant because she is always a friendly dog to people and other dogs alike but this time she clearly had an uneasy reaction. Also, I had never seen these men in the neighborhood before and, after 9/11, I never saw them again. But the most powerful sign to me was when I first saw Atta's face

on T.V. and I had such a strong intuitive and physical reaction. I immediately felt guilty that I had not reported him the day I saw him because, intuitively even then, I felt something was off about all three of these men. Of course I realize now that, even if I had reported them, no one would have taken me seriously because 9/11 hadn't happened yet. But still, I struggled for a long time with the idea that maybe I could have prevented part of that horrible day if I had only trusted my instincts and valued them enough to inform someone about what I saw. It's funny how we talk ourselves in and out of things. On the one hand, I feel bad that I sort of betrayed my intuition by not listening to it immediately. On the other hand, I was probably also afraid of being scoffed at for calling the police and saying my dog and I both felt suspicious about these men. Women's intuition ends up being the butt of a lot of jokes and on some level I think that impacted me too."

Cindy's story has collective value. Homeland Security keeps telling us all to be vigilant, but they do not give us clear instruction as to how we can be vigilant. Getting SASD will give you the added perk of noticing both people who are out of place and people who are engaging in suspicious activities. As more of us start paying closer attention to indicators of surveillance and the early warning signals of attacks, whether we are near a sensitive facility such as a nuclear power plant or in a busy public location such as a crowded subway, more crimes and acts of terrorism can be thwarted.

The other issue that looms in Cindy's story, and about which we are often asked, is racial profiling. Some people immediately assume that conducting surveillance detection is equivalent to profiling. Nothing could be further from the truth. In fact, we believe that profiling is actually quite detrimental to both personal and national security. When you profile, you narrow your focus and run the risk of missing indicators of surveillance, attack preparation, and the attacks themselves. If you just go on what someone looks like, you may miss seeing the potentially dangerous actions and behaviors of others simply because you ignored them because you thought they looked innocent.

Although Cindy did mention a valid indicator when she noticed that the men she saw "looked out of place" in the neighborhood, her main indicator was her intuitive feeling that something was off about them. Granted, if she saw the same thing and reported it today, it is likely the authorities would respond and profiling would be a part of the reason for their response. The logical reason for the profiling is that so many terrorist organizations are comprised of young, male Muslim extremists. However, Timothy McVeigh, the bomber of the Federal Building in Oklahoma City, was not Middle Eastern or Muslim. *The beauty of surveillance detection is that it is an equal opportunity preventative measure.* What makes surveillance detection so incredibly effective is that it removes the spotlight from what people look like and focuses it instead on their location, behaviors, and actions. You are actually being profoundly politically correct when you conduct surveillance detection appropriately because you consider everyone you are watching (regardless of what they look like or their ethnicity) with the same level of discerning awareness, until they *do* something to warrant further scrutiny.

Criminals who target women come in all shapes and sizes. If all you do is look for the stereotypical sleazy, creepy guy, you will likely overlook the well-dressed white collar predator at the office, or the athletic, down to earth stalker, or the Ted Bundy-esque charming but brutal rapist and murderer. Women have to be smart enough to use the techniques that we teach in this book intuitively and objectively, without allowing themselves to be influenced by any tendency towards profiling or stereotyping. By now it should be obvious how detrimental to your own safety profiling can be. "Do not judge a book by its cover." *Anyone can be a predator.*

Some believe thoughts are matter. We believe: *What you think about yourself matters!* If you think you are a victim, you will likely become one. If you think you are empowered, you will become empowered. Your actions will follow your thoughts, so shape your thoughts carefully, with integrity, dignity, and realized empowerment. Just as you cultivate your mind with education, deepen your spirit with religion, and shape your body with diet and exercise, you can also activate your evolutionary momentum with awareness and action. By getting SASD you can integrate a successful personal security practice into your daily life without overwhelming yourself or becoming burdened by fears about security. Rather, your fear will function as an early warning signal and you will be able to respond appropriately. Be patient with your security practice. Give yourself time and experience to implement what you have learned in this book. Find that balanced place in your approach so that you do not become overly paranoid or insufficiently observant. Your security practice is an ongoing process; every day you will add one more log for the woodpile to feed the fire you light from within.

NOTES

On the quotations at the beginning of each chapter: Passages at the beginning of each chapter that are *not* cited quotations are the original work of Laura Clark, with the exception of the passage at the beginning of Chapter Thirteen, which was written by William E. Algaier.

Chapter One

Quotation at beginning of chapter: Thich Nhat Hanh, *The Miracle of Mindfulness* (Boston, Beacon Press, 1975).

Chapter Four

Quotation at beginning of chapter: Sheryl Crow, *"Lifetimes"; Wildflower* (A&M Records, 2005).

For more on mind mapping see: Tony and Barry Buzan, *The Mind Map Book: How to use Radiant Thinking to Maximize Your Brain's Untapped Potential* (Penguin USA, 2006).

Chapter Five

Quotation at beginning of chapter: Massive Attack, *"safe from harm"; Massive Attack Blue Lines* (Circa Records Ltd, 1991).

Chapter Six

Quotation at beginning of chapter: Marc Cohn, *"Strangers In A Car"*; *Marc Cohn* (Atlantic Recording Corporation, 1991).

Chapter Seven

Quotation at beginning of chapter: Tracy Chapman, *"Why?"*; *Tracy Chapman* (SBK Records, 1988).

Chapter Eight

Quotation at beginning of chapter: Cowboy Junkies, *"Good Friday"*; *Miles From Our Home* (Geffen Records, 1998).

On the statistic about abuse against pregnant women: Miranda Harry, *Domestic Violence, Plum Magazine* (New York, Groundbreak Publishing, Inc.; Fall/Winter, 2005, 130-131).

On indicators that your partner may become abusive:
www.womanabuseprevention.com
www.actabuse.com
www.policeone.com

On having an emergency evacuation plan for domestic violence:
www.awaic.org
www.hruth.org
www.caadv.org

Chapter Nine

On the definition of stalking: *The American Heritage Dictionary of the English Language* (Boston, Houghton Mifflin, 1969).

For more on EMDR see: *EMDR:* Francine Shapiro and Margot Silk Forrest, *The Breakthrough "Eye Movement" Therapy for Overcoming Anxiety, Stress, and Trauma* (New York, Basic Books, 1997).

Chapter Ten

On sexual seduction techniques against adult women: Interviews with men who attended sexual seduction seminars and used supplemental materials to learn techniques.

On the process of sexually seducing minors ("grooming"; "the collection") and on the signs that a child is being sexually abused:
www.vachss.com
www.aacap.org
www.stopitnow.com/warnings.html
www.dioceseofbmt.org

On paraphilias: www.medicinenet.com/paraphilia/article.htm

On pornography industry statistics:
www.familysafemedia.com/pornography_statistics.html

On Eve Ensler's quotation: Cynthia Billhartz, *V-Lady Takes on Body Politics* (St. Louis Post Dispatch, Jan. 3, 2006, F1-3).
For more about Eve Ensler see: www.vday.org

Chapter Eleven

On the proclivities of rapists, murderers, and serial killers: John Douglas and Mark Olshaker, *Journey Into Darkness* (New York, A Lisa Drew Book/Scribner, 1997).

Quotation by the authorities regarding target of opportunity in strangulation case: In an article by the Associated Press (June 6, 2006) Sheriff David Davenport was quoted regarding this aspect of the investigation of the murder.

On acronym SURVIVAL: U.S. Army Special Forces Field Manual (3-05.70) for the SERE School (Survival/Evasion/Resistance/Escape).

Chapter Twelve

Quotation at beginning of chapter: Morihei Oeshiba (translated by John Stevens), *The Art of Peace* (Boston, Shambhala, 1992).

On the force continuum:
www.martialarts.jameshom.com/library/weekly/aa021201a.htm
Escalating the Level of Force Appropriately to Subdue an Opponent

www.crimedoctor.com/security_guards_2.htm
Security Guards and Officers Use of force Continuum, by Chris E. McGoey

Chapter Thirteen

On the body's reaction to surprise and the "adrenal dump":
The Cooper Color Codes (Jeff Cooper's attack recognition and response system).
www.sfuk.tripod.com/articles/kaliphilselfd.html

www.spa.ukf.net/spaadren.htm

On workplace violence: Loren W. Christensen, *Surviving Workplace Violence* (Boulder, Paladin Press, 2005).

Chapter Fourteen

Quotation at beginning of chapter: B-52's, *"Roam"; Cosmic Thing* (A&M Records, 1989).

Chapter Sixteen

Quotation at beginning of chapter: The Bangles, *"Walk Like an Egyptian"; Different Light* (SBA Records, 1986).

PART THREE

HELP YOURSELF

SECURITY SPEAK

THE JARGON OF SELF-DEFENSE

Language is powerful. Think of how certain expressions and buzz words take hold and become part of our everyday speech. Below we provide a jargon women can use to warn each other about predatory behaviors and potential dangers. Our objective is to make it easier for women to communicate with one another about the types of threats they face. For example, if you are at a party with a friend and you see a guy who you think might be planning to drop a date rape drug into her drink, you might warn your friend by simply saying: "Watch out for him; he might be a dunker." Or, if you are out in public and you notice a man intently watching another woman or a child, you could approach the woman and say: "Excuse me; I wanted to let you know you have a gazer. He hasn't taken his eyes off of you for a minute so be careful of him."

Some of the terms below are made-up, some come from military jargon, and others you will have heard before out on the streets. Part of our objective is to insert a bit of humor into an empowered woman's security practice. Women are entitled to have a little fun with this otherwise serious and intense subject. One caveat: Do *not* use any of this jargon as a name calling device towards potential predators. It is never a good idea to insult someone who is considering harming you; you only make yourself a more attractive target!

SECURITY SPEAK

Aggro: (adjective) Used to describe a person who gets angry easily, or someone who is in an angry, negative, hostile, or aggressive mood.
Example: Ignore that guy; he's aggro.

ASAP: (Acronym) As soon as possible.
Example: Come meet me ASAP; this date is not going well.

Break Contact: (Phrase/Command) Get away *immediately*, regardless if it means ending a conversation, exiting a location, getting away from someone who is in physical proximity to you, or even ending a relationship. This is a good command to rehearse for yourself so that you can coach yourself verbally. You can also use it to advise others.
Example: You should break contact; he is showing signs of being abusive.

Catcaller: (Noun) A man who makes animal sounds or noises at women in order to harass them.
Example: Are you aware that the men working for the contractor on your construction site are catcallers and have been harassing me every day for the past week?

Check Your Six: (Phrase/Command) Look behind you or watch your back. This comes from the military clock direction method of reference when patrolling in the woods. 12 o'clock is always the direction of travel, therefore 6 o'clock is behind you.
Example: Will you check my six while I walk to my car?

Chester: (Noun) Short for Chester the molester, a pervert cartoon character from *Hustler Magazine.*
Example: Pay attention to the Chester in the red jacket approaching.

Crack On: (Phrase/Command) Continue on with what you are doing; move on and do something else; get over it and move on.
Example: This relationship has really damaged me, but I've just got to crack on and forget about this jerk.

Curb-Crawler: (Noun) A man who cruises red-light districts and other bad areas of town with the intention of harassing women or trying to interact with women.
Example: Can you believe what that curb-crawler just yelled out the window at us?

Decepto Boy: (Noun) A man who is talking in circles or is being deceptive in any way.
Example: Decepto boy called me again to ask me out; he still thinks I don't know he has a girlfriend.

Dunker: (Noun) A man who drops date rape drugs into women's drinks.
Example: Did you notice that dunker trying to get his hands on that woman's martini?

DX: (Verb/Acronym) Direct exchange. Get rid of it. This comes from military jargon (for example, if your issued equipment breaks you can go to the supply room and DX it for new equipment).
Example: DX that guy; he's a total loser!

Eyes On: (Phrase/Verb) To read or assess a person, location, situation, incident, or event. To see or watch carefully.
Example: Why don't you stay here while I go get eyes on the situation.
Go ahead; I'll keep eyes on your jacket.

Emergency Evac: (Noun/Command) Emergency Evacuation. Use this when you need urgent, immediate help to get out of a dangerous location or situation. This should be a code word you share with people in your

SUPNET. For example you could send a text message to a friend saying "EE" and designate your location. Now your friend knows to help you get out of there.
Example: Let's go. We need to do an emergency evac for Susie. She's at the corner pub and is in trouble.

Gazer: (Noun) A man who tends to stare, leer, or look at women in a sexual manner.
Example: No, let's not go to that bar; it's full of gazers.

Ground Truth: (Noun) What is actually going on; the real situation. It includes the visual or eyes on truth as well as the overall truth about any person or situation.
Example: I need to get ground truth so I can figure out if my daughter's boyfriend is abusing her.

High Risk: (Adjective) Describes a man who is of questionable character or reputation and is potentially dangerous.
Example: Sure he's kind of cute but definitely high risk. Did you see how he pinched that waitress as she walked by?

Hinky: (Adjective) Suspicious; odd; creepy; uncomfortable; uneasy; freaked out.
Example: This place is hinky; let's get out of here.
      That guy is acting hinky and is scaring me.

Hosty: (Adjective) Short for hostile.
Example: He may be a hottie, but he's also a hosty!

ID: (Verb) To identify.
Example: Did you ID if someone was following you?

Interval: (Noun) A safe distance from a potential threat.

Example: Keep your interval from the car in front of you so you have room to maneuver.

Later Loser: (Phrase) To be used as a signal to your friends to get rid of a man you think might be trouble. Abbreviate it to LL to use it as a code, whisper it, or say it in private; do not say it directly to the man (he may get aggro!).
Example: It's time to say LL and get away from this guy.

Lech: (Noun) A man who is displaying lecherous behaviors; a pervert.
Example: That lech is trying to look down my blouse.

No Duff: (Phrase) For real or no kidding. To be used to communicate an emergency situation. You should never joke with this phrase; it should be reserved for use only in true emergencies.
Example: Hey, let's get out of here. I'm feeling really hinky about that guy, no duff!

No Me Molesta: (Phrase) Spanish for "Don't bother me." You can say this to yourself (inaudibly) if you are in the company of a man who is pestering you. That way you will give yourself a prompt to break contact with him.
Example: (to yourself) Ugh—why is this guy hitting on me? No me molesta, creep. Time to go.

Pull Security: (Verb/Command) To watch over the situation or people and focus on security. (Note: Women can support each other by pulling security but they should also take responsibility for their own security).
Example: It's your turn to pull security tonight while we are out at the rave.

Punch It: (Command) Move fast *now* (can be used while driving to indicate acceleration or when on foot to prompt yourself or someone to speed up and move away from the danger).
Example: Let's punch it and get in the car; I'm afraid that guy is following us.

Radar Ready: (Phrase/Command) Be alert; pay close attention; stop being distracted and focus on potential danger.
Example: Okay, girls, radar ready because we have to park in this dark lot.

Rendezvous (RV): (Verb) To meet at a designated location in the event you get separated, either at a set time or if something happens like a disturbance or an emergency. Choose a safe and easily recognizable location.
Example: OK, let's RV at 9 p.m. at the drugstore on the corner.

Scope: (Verb) To watch intently (not necessarily with optical devices such as binoculars).
Example: He's scoping us big time; let's get out of here.

Secure: (Verb) To guard or keep in a safe place.
Example: Go ahead and dance; I'll secure your drink.

SITREP: (Noun) Situation report. Update. The most recent information and/or an assessment of the situation.
Example: Give me a SITREP please; I can't find Karen and Amanda and this party is getting too crazy.

Snapper: (Noun) A man who is sneaking photos with a cell phone or hand-held camera or video camera.
Example: Check out the snapper over there behind the bushes photographing those kids.

Spacie: (Noun) A woman who has no situational awareness, is not security conscious, or unwittingly takes foolish risks.
Example: Don't be such a Spacie when you walk home to your dorm at night.

Stand To: (Command) Everyone should immediately stop what they are doing and be 100% alert!

Example: Whoa, stand to! I think that guy has a gun in his jacket pocket.

Stare Boy: (Noun) A man who stares blatantly at a woman.
Example: Did you notice stare boy over there by the exit?

Sweep: (Verb) To observe carefully; to investigate or check out.
Example: Let's sweep the room before we decide what guys look normal enough to talk to.

Switch On: (Phrase/Command) Get with it; understand; become aware of.
Example: She needs to switch on that the guy is a lech!

Trick Meister: (Noun) A man who uses deception or trickery against a woman.
Example: That trick meister told me he worked at my bank. I found out he totally lied.

Uncle Pervie: (Noun) Term for a man who displays perverse behaviors or makes perverted comments.
Example: Watch out for uncle pervie over there in the three piece suit.

Wing Girl: (Noun) A woman who functions in a supporting role regarding security issues.
Example: Can you be my wing girl and call me while I am out on this blind date?

Wingman: (Noun) A man who is working to support another man in any endeavor against a woman (including endeavors that threaten the woman's security).
Example: He's got his wingman over there. I'm sure they are working as a team to pick us up.

Wolf-Whistler: (Noun) A man who whistles aggressively at women as they pass by.
Example: I am so sick of these wolf-whistlers who think they are God's gift to women. Are they just clueless about how unattractive that behavior makes them?

360: (Noun) An all around defense, as in the 360 degrees of a full circle.
Example: I spotted that gazer when I was doing my 360 when I got out of my car.

APPENDIX A

TRAINING OPPORTUNITIES AND CONTACT INFORMATION

For Consulting or Training (Individuals or Groups)
Contact:

Laura Clark:
www.securityforwomen.com
sec4women@yahoo.com

William E. Algaier:
www.gatorwerks.com
gatorwerksllc@yahoo.com

Other Titles Available by the Authors:

SURVEILLANCE DETECTION, The Art of Prevention

Available through www.cradlepress.com (or can be ordered at your local bookstore or online).

APPENDIX B

PERSONAL SECURITY PROFILE

The purpose of filling out this questionnaire is to augment your risk assessment by identifying both your current security measures and the gaps in your personal security. This profile will also help you when you are creating your route and building reviews by reminding you to focus your attention on your routine behaviors and activities. Obviously once you complete this questionnaire you will want to use discretion when handling this document, as the information herein should be protected.

Personal Security Profile

Fill in the blanks and answer questions as honestly and specifically as possible.

1. TRAVEL FROM HOME TO WORK

Departure time:
Arrival time:
Method of transportation:
How many routes?
Do you vary your routes randomly?
Any routine stops? (for coffee or newspaper, etc.)

Do you drive yourself? (if not then do you carpool or have a driver?)
Do you have any security detail traveling with you?
Where do you park at work?
Is there security protecting your vehicle when it is parked?

2. TRAVEL FROM WORK TO HOME

Departure time:
Arrival time:
Method of transportation:
How many routes?
Do you vary routes randomly?
Any routine stops? (the health club, shopping, child care, etc.)
Do you drive yourself?
Do you have a security detail traveling with you?
Is your neighborhood gated or otherwise secured?
Where do you park your car at home?
If your car is not secured in a garage, is it parked within line of sight of your home or a surveillance camera?
Do you hide a key anywhere on your vehicle?
Does your gas cap lock?

3. ROUTINE APPOINTMENTS AND SOCIAL ACTIVITIES

Routine appointments and social activities include things like: regular doctor's appointments, hair care, manicures, sports, church, child care, bridge club, book club meetings, volunteer work, etc. Follow the format below for *each* routine appointment or social activity.

Appointment / Activity:
Day of the week:
Departure time:
Arrival time:

Routes traveled to location:
Method of transportation:
Security presence at location (guards, cameras, etc.):
Is your vehicle parked in a secured location?

4. SECURITY AT YOUR HOME

Does your home have an alarm system?
Is there a locked or guarded entrance gate to your home?
Are there any surveillance cameras around your home?
Do you have a dog?
Are any neighbors' homes within line of sight of your home?
Do you have motion lights?
Is your street part of a Neighborhood Watch program?
Do the police drive on your street frequently?
Did you change the locks when you moved into your home?
Do you have any firearms or weapons in your home?

5. SECURITY AT YOUR WORKPLACE

Is there a uniformed security presence?
Is there an under cover security presence?
Are there surveillance cameras?
Are the entrances and exits secured by gates or any kinds of barriers?
Is employee parking secured?
Is public parking mixed with employee parking?
Does the public have unrestricted access to the building/s?
Are employees required to wear any type of badge, uniform, name tag, etc.?

6. SITUATIONAL AWARENESS

Rate your level of situational awareness for each item that applies to you. Be honest and write in any specific comments that will clarify your answer.

1=poor   2=average   3=good   4=excellent

While driving I pay attention to see if anyone is following me or watching me along my routes:

When riding in a vehicle I pay attention to my surroundings (rather than talking on the phone or reading the newspaper, etc.):

When at home, I pay attention to foot and vehicle traffic on my street, especially near my home:

When at home I look to see if anyone is watching me, my family or my home:

I keep all doors locked while I am home:

I lock all doors when I am away from home:

I pay attention to my surroundings when parking my vehicle and when re-entering it after time away:

I keep my vehicle doors locked while I am driving and whenever my vehicle is parked:

When I am attending social activities, my situational awareness is compromised (e.g. by distraction, consumption of alcohol, relaxed mental state, etc.):

APPENDIX C

SAMPLE REPORT FORM

DATE / TIME SUBMITTED:
REPORTED BY:
DATE OF SIGHTING:
TIME OF SIGHTING:
ACTIVITY DESCRIPTION:

PERSON: MALE   FEMALE   UNKNOWN
BUILD: PETITE   AVERAGE   SLENDER   SKINNY   WIREY
STOCKY   MUSCULAR   CHUBBY   MODERATELY FAT   OBESE
OTHER _____
SHAPE OF HEAD: OVAL   ROUND   SQUARE   TRIANGLE   EGG
HEART
OTHER_____
FACIAL FEATURES:
  BROW: SHORT   MEDIUM   HIGH   OTHER_____
  EYES: ROUND   ALMOND   CLOSE TOGETHER   FAR APART
BLUE   BROWN   GREEN   HAZEL   LIGHT   DARK
OTHER_____

EARS: SMALL MEDIUM LARGE OTHER_____

NOSE: LONG   SHORT   PUG   SKI SLOPE   BULBOUS
OTHER_____

CHIN: POINTED   SQUARE   DIMPLED   ROUND
OTHER_____

HAIR TYPE: BALD MILITARY SHORT MEDIUM SHOULDER
LENGTH LONG DREADLOCKS AFRO WAVY CURLY BUSHY
KINKY STRAIGHT OTHER_____

HAIR COLOR: NATURAL   COLOR TREATED

SHADE: LIGHT MEDIUM DARK

COLOR: ORANGE   RED   BLOND   BROWN   BLACK   BLUE
PURPLE GREEN GREY OTHER_____

FACIAL HAIR: MOUSTACHE: THIN   THICK   LONG   HANDLE-
BAR OTHER_____

BEARD: STUBBLE   5 O'CLOCK SHADOW   MEDIUM   FULL
BUSHY LONG GOATEE PATCH OTHER_____

COMPLEXION AND SKIN: LIGHT   MEDIUM   DARK   SMOOTH
RUDDY FAIR SUN TANNED   POCK MARKED   SCARS_____
TATOOS_____   PIERCINGS_____   OTHER_____

GEOGRAPHIC ORIGIN: CAUCASIAN   ASIAN   BLACK
MULATTO LATINO
MIDDLE EASTERN   UNKNOWN OTHER_____

CLOTHING: CASUAL FORMAL SPORTY BUSINESS UNIFORM
OTHER_____

COAT: JACKET   RAINCOAT   OVERCOAT   SUIT
(SINGLE/DOUBLE BREASTED)   SUEDE   LEATHER   WOOL
OTHER_____

TOP: T-SHIRT   V-NECK   POLO SHIRT   COLLARED SHIRT
SHORT SLEEVES   LONG SLEEVES   BLOUSE   TANK TOP
SPORTS BRA   TUBE TOP   HALTER TOP   SWEATER
SWEATSHIRT VEST OTHER_____

BOTTOM: BELT SASH TROUSERS JEANS SHORTS CARGO
PANTS COURDEROYS SWEAT PANTS SUIT PANTS DRESS

PANTS SLACKS CAPRI PANTS SKIRT (MINI MEDIUM LONG) DRESS (MINI MEDIUM LONG) SKORT SARONG SARI JUMPSUIT OTHER_____

CLOTHING ORIGIN: AMERICAN EUROPEAN ASIAN MIDDLE EASTERN AFRICAN INDIAN LATIN OTHER_____

SHOES: DRESS CASUAL SPORTS SANDALS BOOTS HIGH HEELS LEATHER MILITARY UNIFORM FLATS OTHER_____

ACCESSORIES: CELL PHONE CAMERA VIDEO CAMERA VOICE RECORDER PDA LAPTOP BINOCULARS BRIEFCASE PURSE SATCHEL BACKPACK FANNY PACK PLASTIC BAG PAPER BAG SHOPPING BAG UMBRELLA CANE CRUTCHES BABY CARRIAGE SUITCASE DUFFLE BAG GYM BAG BASKET OTHER_____

HEAD COVERINGS: BASEBALL CAP UNIFORMED CAP TURBAN SKULL CAP STOCKING CAP SHEMAGH (ARAB HEAD SCARF) FEDORA HARD HAT BERET FEZ VISOR BANDANA SCARF PAGE BOY HAT COWBOY HAT STRAW HAT HEADBAND SWEATBAND DOO-RAG LEATHER HAT OTHER_____

JEWELRY: WATCH BRACELET NECKLACE RINGS WEDDING RING EARRINGS ANKLE BRACELET NOSE RING LIP RING TONGUE RING EYEBROW RING EAR CUFF CUFFLINKS CHAINS TIE CLIP WORRY BEADS ROSARY RELIGIOUS MEDALS/SYMBOLS OTHER_____

DISTINGUISHING ATTRIBUTES: POSTURE GAIT LIMP DEFORMITY TATTOOS BODY PIERCINGS SCARS BIRTHMARKS HAIR LIP WIDOW'S PEAK CLEFT PALATE IRREGULAR PIGMENTATION (ALBINO BURNS FRECKLES AGE SPOTS) OTHER_____

IMAGE RECORDED: YES NO

VEHICLE: SEDAN   CONVERTIBLE   SUV   MINI VAN   PICK UP TRUCK   DELIVERY   COMMERCIAL   MOPED   MOTORCYCLE BICYCLE   BOAT   OTHER_____

STYLE: 2 DOOR   4 DOOR   OTHER_____

MAKE:

MODEL:

YEAR: USED   NEW   OLD

APPEARANCE: CLEAN   DIRTY   TINTED WINDOWS   DECALS BUMPER STICKERS   REAR VIEW MIRROR DÉCOR   DENTS SCRATCHES   PAINT JOB   OTHER_____

COLOR:

LICENSE PLATE NUMBER:

LOCATION:

DIRECTION OF TRAVEL:

IMAGE RECORDED: YES   NO

APPENDIX D

STALKER INCIDENT LOG

Date:

Time:

Location:

Incident Description:

Stalker Description:

Stalker Vehicle Description:

Stalker Direction of Travel & Location Last Seen:

Specific Threats:

Implied Threats:

Witnesses to the Incident:

Contact Information:

Evidence Collected:

Action Taken:

Reported to:

Law Enforcement/Case Number:

Advocacy Representatives:

APPENDIX E

RESORCES

The following is a list of resources we have compiled. Some of these include people we know and with whom we have worked. Others are resources we used when conducting research for this book. We do not endorse any of these groups. We are simply providing you with contacts and information. Please realize that, although we are providing you with the most current information possible, we cannot guarantee that the addresses, phone numbers, and websites will not change.

Abduction/Kidnapping

Clayton Consultants, Inc
5927 Balfour Court, Suite 109
Carlsbad, CA 92008
(760) 431-0304
www.claytonconsultants.com

Background Checks

www.backgroundchecks.com
(866) 300-8524

Domestic Violence and Abuse

National Domestic Violence Hotline
(800) 799-7233

National Coalition Against Domestic Violence (NCADV)
1120 Lincoln Street, Suite 1603
Denver, CO 80203
(303) 839-1852
www.ncadv.org

National Clearinghouse for Defense of Battered Women
125 South Ninth Street, Suite 302
Philadelphia, PA 19107
(215) 351-0010
(800)903-0111

Evasive Driving Training

Anthony Scotti Schools
16 Hillside Avenue
Medford, MA 02155
(781) 395-3097
www.SecurityDriver.com

Reichel Driving Concepts
Bruce Reichel
(304) 229-5322
dbreichel@msn.com

Identity Theft

Identity Theft Clearinghouse
Federal Trade Commission
600 Pennsylvania Avenue, NW
Washington, D.C. 20580
(877) 488-4338
www.ftc.gov

Privacy Rights Clearinghouse
3100 5th Avenue, Suite B
San Diego, CA 92103
(619) 298-3396
www.privacyrights.org

Social Security Administration
SSA Fraud Hotline
P.O. Box 17768
Baltimore, MD 21235
(877) 438-4338
www.ssa.gov

Internet Crime

U. S. Department of Justice
Computer Crime and Intellectual Properties Section (CCIPS)
(202) 514-1026
www.cybercrime.gov

Legal Assistance

Legal Help USA
www.legal-help-usa.org

www.victimbar.org

National Criminal Justice Reference Service
P.O. Box 6000
Rockville, MD 20849-6000
(800) 851-3420
www.ncjrs.org

Movement

Chinese Internal Arts Center
www.stltaiji.com

Zhang Xue-Xin, President
Feng Zhiqiang Taijiquan Academy, USA
www.silkreeler.com

www.yogafinder.com

Rape

Rape & Incest National Network (RAINN)
(800) 656-HOPE (4673)
www.rainn.org

National Clearinghouse on Marital and Date Rape
www.ncmdr.org

Self-Defense

IMPACT Personal Safety, Inc.
5450 Slauson Avenue, #230
Culver City, CA 90230
(800) 345-5425
www.impactpersonalsafety.com

MELISSA SOALT AKA DR. RUTHLESS ®
"Practical No-Nonsense Self Defense for Women"
FAX: 413. 256. 5422
www.dr-ruthless.com

Self-Help

American Self-Help Clearinghouse
(973) 625-3037

National Self-Help Clearinghouse
(212) 817-1822
www.selfhelpweb.org

Post-Traumatic Stress Disorder Alliance (PTSDA)
www.ptsdalliance.org

Sexual Abuse

National Child Abuse Hotline
Childhelp USA
(800) 422-4453
www.childhelpusa.org

STOP IT NOW!
(888) 773-8368
www.stopitnow.org

Children of the Night
Rescuing America's Children from Prostitution
(800) 551-1300
www.childrenofthenight.org

Stalking

www.antistalking.com

National Center for Victims of Crime (NCVC)
Stalking Resource Center (SRC)
(800) 394-2255
www.ncvc.org

Victim-Assistance Online
www.vaonline.org

Wired Patrol
www.wiredpatrol.org

www.stalkingbehavior.com

Terrorism

U.S. Department of Homeland Security
www.dhs.gov

Federal Bureau of Investigation
www.fbi.gov

Central Intelligence Agency
www.cia.gov

Travel

U.S. Department of State
Bureau of Consular Affairs
Office of Public Affairs
2201 C Street NW
Washington, D.C. 20520
(202) 647-5225
www.travel.state.gov

Center for Disease Control and Prevention
(877) 394-8747
www.cdc.gov/travel

Type in the words: "CIA The World Factbook" plus the name of any country in a search engine and you will pull up the CIA Factbook for that country.

www.lonelyplanet.com

Victim Assistance

Communities Against Violence Network (CAVNET)
www.cavnet.org

Office for Victim of Crime Resource Center
National Criminal Justice Reference Service
P.O. Box 6000
Rockville, MD 20849

www.ncjrs.org

National Organization for Victim Assistance (NOVA)
510 King Street, Suite 424
Alexandria, VA 22314
(800) 879-6682
www.trynova.org

National Center for Victims of Crime
2000 M Street, NW Suite 480
Washington, DC 20036.
(202) 467-8700
www.ncvc.org

Workplace Violence

The National Institute for Occupational Safety and Health (NIOSHA)
(800) 356-4674
www.cdc.gov/niosh/homepage.html

The Occupational Safety and Health Administration (OSHA)
U.S. Department of Labor
200 Constitution Avenue
Washington, D.C. 20210
(866) 487-2365 www.osha.gov

ACKNOWLEDGMENTS

We are so grateful to the brave women who contributed their stories; they did so with the intention of helping you.

We extend a special thank you to Wendy, Lloyd, Gordon, Biddy, Marie, and all those who lent their kind and generous support, encouragement, and advice during the writing of this book. We could not have made it through this journey without your support.

Thank you, Deep, for sharing your creative energy.

We also express our gratitude to Scott Eagle and Jim Mosley at Outflow Media for their patience, hard work, and creative input into this book.

ABOUT THE AUTHORS

Laura Clark has trained surveillance detection teams all over the world. She has worked on a variety of government anti-terrorism contracts and in the private sector as a surveillance detection trainer and operator. She is a longtime educator and has assisted in training women in self-defense using techniques from the martial arts.

Laura is the managing director of *Surveillance Detection Consultants LLC*, a security company specializing in women's security and surveillance detection consulting, training, and operational services in the private sector.

William E. Algaier is a veteran U.S. Army Special Forces operator who has worked as a surveillance detection trainer on government contracts. A veteran of the first Gulf War, he recently returned from Iraq where he assisted in training the bodyguards protecting the top five Iraqi government officials. Now he shares his warrior mentality and skills in order to teach women to protect themselves.

Bill is the managing director of *Gatorwerks LLC*, a security company specializing in surveillance detection training, consulting, and operational services for the military and in the private sector.

A Prayer for Evolution

Grant me my upgrowth
Allow me shift
Into remembrance of my hidden higher self
The woman whose power is so graciously endowed
The woman who continues to flower with redeeming might
Grant me my morphology
So that I may better reflect the dignity of my species
And safely guard my precious being

-- Laura Clark

Printed in the United States
68452LVS00008B/38